The Unconscious Body Image

The Unconscious Body Image espouses a completely original view of the links between physical and psychic development, providing fresh insight into our understanding of psychosomatic symptoms and child development.

Françoise Dolto describes how unconsciously held mental images of the body and its functioning impact upon the subject's feelings and ideas of themself, and conversely how emotions and ideas impact upon the body's functioning by way of these unconscious images. *The Unconscious Body Image* also presents Dolto's view of the development of mind in relation to unconscious body images generated at each stage of development (oral, anal, genital, latency and puberty), and ideas about psychic castration at each developmental stage and children's socialisation, filling a significant gap in psychoanalytic understanding of the mental integration of social law.

This book will be a key text for psychoanalysts in practice and in training, particularly those working with children, psychoanalytic psychotherapists and psychodynamic practitioners in the social sciences, childcare and education.

Françoise Dolto (1908–1988) was an acclaimed French psychoanalyst and paediatrician. In her early career, she was mentored by Sophie Morgenstern, and she later became a close friend of Jacques Lacan. She had a regular radio programme on the French national broadcast station France Inter and made many appearances on television and in print.

Sharmini Bailly is a psychoanalytic psychotherapist based in the UK. Her previous books include *The Lacan Tradition* (Routledge, 2018).

The Unconscious Body Image

Françoise Dolto
Translated by Sharmini Bailly

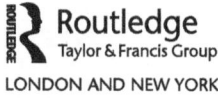

Routledge
Taylor & Francis Group
LONDON AND NEW YORK

Designed cover image: © Alécio de Andrade, ADAGP Paris, 2022

First published 2023
by Routledge
4 Park Square, Milton Park, Abingdon, Oxon OX14 4RN

and by Routledge
605 Third Avenue, New York, NY 10158

Routledge is an imprint of the Taylor & Francis Group, an informa business

© 2023 Éditions du Seuil

© Éditions du Seuil, 1984

© Catherine Dolto and Editions du Seuil, 2022 for her preface

© Anne Marie Canu and Editions du Seuil, 2022 for her preface

© Sham Bailly and Editions du Seuil, 2022 for the General Introduction

British Library Cataloguing-in-Publication Data
A catalogue record for this book is available from the British Library

ISBN: 978-1-032-32040-3 (hbk)
ISBN: 978-1-032-32038-0 (pbk)
ISBN: 978-1-003-31249-9 (ebk)

DOI: 10.4324/9781003312499

Typeset in Times New Roman
by Apex CoVantage, LLC

Contents

Preface

As Françoise Dolto's daughter, I inherited both the immense honour and considerable responsibility of holding the copyright to my mother's works, and in this role my greatest challenge and duty has been to commission the English translation of *L'image Inconsciente du Corps*. This is why the publication of this translation brings me immense joy. I am profoundly grateful to all involved in this project: Sham Bailly, who took on the daunting task of translating the book; Anne Marie Canu, who persuaded Sham to accept this task; and Lionel Bailly, who supported them. Anne Marie has been by my side since my mother's death. As a psychoanalyst who worked with my mother, was close to her and is bilingual in English and French, she had an important role this project. After completing the translation, Sham Bailly reworked the text with the help of Lionel Bailly and Anne Marie Canu. Without it being planned from the beginning, three people therefore contributed to this translation, and it happens that in the Dolto Archives Association, it has been our practice for three or more people to work together to produce definitive versions of the texts. This is because Françoise Dolto had a very particular use of language, in which when she failed to find a word, which perhaps did not exist, she would invent it; and she also used expressions and stylistic formulations that were completely original, which makes it easy for a translator, even with the best intentions, to misunderstand and misrepresent her thinking.

Françoise Dolto was among those analysts, like D.W. Winnicott, who worked to embed psychoanalysis in society. Very early on, she published many articles in the mainstream press, and later, she presented a show on national radio: 'While a Child Appears' was a huge success. She held public conferences to packed halls and published several books, some – like this one – more theoretical, and others that were easier reads. Very much ahead of her time, she became an important personality beyond psychoanalysis, having enormous influence upon how children are viewed in society. She began in paediatrics and was one of the first to consider the child, however tiny, as an intelligent being always in a quest for meaning. Before her, children in France were thought of as vaguely more sophisticated digestive tubes; after her, they are thought of as sensitive beings in the process of becoming, to be respected and understood.

The impact in the media of her death was enormous, and such were the crowds that surged forward at her funeral that police had to close the road. Now, numerous roads, schools, libraries, nurseries and hospital departments bear her name. This notoriety undoubtedly attracted some jealousy, and she found herself marginalised by academic colleagues – not for the first time. In 1939, when she published her thesis, *Psychoanalysis and Paediatrics*, many of her psychoanalytic colleagues sneered at her way of considering the baby to be capable of understanding and interaction. This was revolutionary at the time.

In the tumultuous history of psychoanalysis, she held a unique, somewhat solitary place, even if she remained close to Jacques Lacan in friendship and in institutional matters to do with the transmission of psychoanalysis. While her seminars were well attended, she said she had no students and did not want to create a school, and would often say: 'Listen to what I say, listen to what others say to you and then do as you like.' However, at Armand Trousseau Hospital she revived the principle of the public consultation, at which she would see children in the presence of trainee psychoanalysts who functioned like a Greek chorus, with whom the children would sometimes interact. Until the end of her life, she tenaciously maintained this unique tool of transmission, doing her final consultations with the help of a portable oxygen tank. It was of great importance to her to help very small children and their parents to prevent the appearance of psychological disturbances. This is why she invented the Maisons Vertes – psychoanalytic spaces for parents and children – that have proliferated the world over.

This book, *The Unconscious Body Image*, is the culmination of her life's work, having been published only four years before her death. It is a confusing book for some, shifting as it does between theory and clinical work and written in an academic style. Françoise Dolto neither refers to nor quotes anyone, even if evidence suggests that she read everything published at the time. When asked who were her teachers, she replied: 'Babies are my teachers.' In this book, Françoise Dolto follows the thread of the of desiring subject and of identity in the process of construction, while giving an essential importance to the perceptive apparatus as the receptor and filter for the small human who is always in search of meaning. Her 'person in becoming' is structured within the quest for linkage, which is inseparable from his dependence while he is in the charge of his tutelary adults. She places in the foreground the role played by the senses in the elaboration of meaning, in other words the Symbolic, essential for the humanisation, of which symboligenic castrations would then be indispensable stages. In this, her theory as well as her clinical practice are profoundly original and innovative, perhaps too much so for them to find a place in academia, which she anyway never sought out. This probably explains why it is only now, more than 30 years after her death, that the English-speaking public is being presented here with the chance to discover this valedictory book, the culmination of her works, while it was all there in seminal form in her 1939 thesis, *Psychoanalysis and Paediatrics*.

Catherine Dolto

Foreword

This is not the first attempt at translating *L'image Inconsciente du Corps*. Previous attempts have been unsatisfactory, less because of the linguistic skills of the translators than because of their ability to understand Dolto's thinking.

When Sham Bailly sent me the first draft of her translation of Chapter 1 of this book, I was moved and fascinated: I felt I was hearing Dolto's own voice, but in a form I had not heard before. I wrote to Sham as follows:

> It is, to me, more than a translation, it is a transmission. it brings to my mind the words of Françoise Dolto when she said '*J'ai parlé anglais avant de parler français. Mes parents devaient me parler anglais pour que je comprenne*'. ('I spoke English before speaking French. My parents had to speak to me in English for me to understand.') It seems to me you are giving back to her her original language: reading you, it seems to me I am hearing her, in this first chapter where from the whole book will flow, talking from this very archaic place that made her so exceptionally attuned to the very young child (present in children and adults as well), this very archaic place in her that had been wounded when her Irish nanny was sent away, the open wound maybe being what allowed all through her life for this amazing communication with the archaic in her patient, so immediate and really amazing that it was sometimes deemed brutal (it happened to me at my first session with her, at the second session I told her '*vous allez trop vite!*' and she said 'Yes, I know.'). But that wound in her, that open wound that allowed free communication with the unconscious, happened when the words in her ears, when she had yet no speech but was in total communication with one person, this young Irish nanny who had such a love of life, were English words: it seems to me you are giving her back those words. Putting the reader in communication with this archaic was so hard for her in French (I think that is why writing was so difficult to her), and now it comes so naturally, so to speak, in your Chapter One. . . . To the end of her life she talked about her Irish nanny, whose name she did not even know, whenever she was asked how she had become an analyst.

Translation is first of all listening – each one of us with his or her own ears, such as our parents have made them, listening in the way an analyst listens. Listening to babies, newborns, infants before the age of words, their language unspoiled by words, which are always insufficient. I remember discussing this with FD during analysis. 'Yes,' she said, 'it is not words that have to be listened to but the spaces between words.' All analytic listening is an act of translation – the translation of meanings that come into being in the act of being heard.

Later, when discussing with Sham and Lionel the intellectual background to Dolto's ideas, I wrote to them again:

Dolto did not have ideas, I mean preconceived ideas about any of her patients, adult or child. She listened to a baby as closely as she possibly could. And when she wanted to talk about it and no words were sufficient, she grabbed at whatever word came along to her on the spot, and the ambient words, considering Lacan's predominance at the time, were often Lacan-words. Of course. But she trusted her audience to not take them in the Lacan-sense but to try to listen, with her, to the baby she was talking about. A famous example is the mirror stage. When she attended his seminar, she told Lacan: 'I don't understand a word of what you say,' and he responded 'No matter. What I talk about is what you practice'. And he would send to her patients he found himself unable to deal with.

Late in her life, she would say, 'Lacan never had any influence on me. I was a fully fledged analyst when I met him.' But she would add, 'However, I have to say, when Lacan sent to me young analysts who had been in analysis with him, they understood what I told them.' And to these young analysts who had been attending Lacan's seminars and listening religiously to his discourse, the advice she gave them was 'Go to the park, sit on a bench close to the sandpit and stay there at least two hours, listening to the babies and the toddlers. They will teach you.'

If I were asked to describe Françoise Dolto, what I would say is that 'I have never, never, never, seen anyone listen to a child the way she listened to a child.' When questioned as to how she did it, she would answer, 'I don't know. Maybe I have always remained a baby.'

I am sure you know, having worked with babies, how they talk to each other, how they understand each other. How, in a family where one child poses difficulties and cannot make himself understood (because of an undiagnosed hearing difficulty, for instance, causing his language to be totally incomprehensible), it is the brother or sister closest in age who can become his interpreter.

Maybe FD had never left that place, where babies talk to each other, where body and mind are still one, where the whole body speaks, where words of course are always insufficient. It is a language we have all of us known at some point, and maybe some of us have remained closer to it than others. Language before words.

But then, when you try to put that into words, it can well seem obscure, unless the reader can put himself back into that stage as well. Not all analysts are there.

FD put it, in the end, like this: '*L'analyste, c'est l'enfant. Mais l'enfant tout petit, avant les mots*' – 'the analyst is the child, but a very small child, before words.'

Words are always so insufficient, yet we have to use them – they are all we have. French words? English words? Or any other language, but 'true words,' those that follow the mother's life-giving milk – 'the mother tongue,' so rightly named.

Anne Marie Canu

Introduction

Sharmini Bailly

This book is a singular attempt to form a theory of how interpersonal dynamics structure the human mind and, in turn, how that governs the functioning of the body, within the mid-century French psychoanalytic tradition. It is perhaps Françoise Dolto's most ambitious book, in which she tries to set out her own unified theory of the psychic development of human beings in relation to the development of their bodies. Her writing reflects her conceptual processes, which are brilliantly intuitive interpretations of clinical material but not always closely and logically argued. She offers a boldly abstract concept – the unconscious body image – together with the clinical cases from which she has derived her ideas about it, or vice versa, but often leaves it to the reader to build the logical, theoretical bridge between her metapsychological construct and the clinical example.

Dolto is far from being alone in this way of writing: her contemporaries Lacan, Winnicott and Bion all did the same, which is what makes reading them difficult and slow but ultimately, if you put in the work of figuring out the links, very rewarding. It could be that with all these great theorists, the lack of explanation or logical argument of their insights is due to their historical period. In the mid-twentieth century, psychoanalysis was developing with the full untutored vigour of a latency period child, and despite the quite extraordinary achievements of Freud and others of the founding generation, the mid-century analysts were still working with a quite rough-hewn set of psychoanalytic theories, all of which needed further refining; moreover, they copied the methods of their predecessors in hacking out their ideas from clinical rock – stating what they thought without always explaining how the thought was derived. In my view this is not for want of trying, as I think Lacan and Bion in particular tried very hard in their different ways to explain themselves, though without full success; but it is to their daring to venture their insights without stringent justification that we owe most psychoanalytic theory.

When Françoise Dolto was training in psychoanalysis and beginning to practice it in the 1930s and 1940s, there was little psychoanalytic theory available in translation in France. Her ideas continued to develop throughout the rest of her life, but Anne Marie Canu, who knew her very well, has told me that Dolto stated with some pride that apart from Freud, she had 'learned nothing' from any

DOI: 10.4324/9781003312499-1

living psychoanalyst with the exception of Winnicott. This I find both very hard to believe in one way, and completely credible in another.

I find it hard to believe she remained completely untouched by the thinking of others because the terminology she uses and the concepts encoded therein reflect a strong Lacanian influence; while her followers may dispute that she 'learned' this from Lacan in any formal sense, his teachings in the mid-twentieth century formed the standard framework of reference for French psychoanalysis, and she might quite simply have absorbed them by social osmosis. Whether by intention or by accident, her writing is imbued with the Lacanian concepts of the Real, Symbolic and Imaginary orders, signifiers and signification, the mirror stage, the trace of desire, fantasy, libido and a nirvana-ish death drive devoid of aggression, the phallus and castration.

If, on the other hand, I find it *easy* to believe she was little influenced by anyone else, it is because she is writing here about the interpersonal space in a way that seems completely unaware of the British object relations tradition, or of American ideas of self- and other-representations – all of which pre-date this book. And it is from this peculiar blend of Lacanian-theory-by-exposure-if-not-design and Dolto's intuitive clinical brilliance that arises the importance of this book. It is a sort of object relations theory without ever a mention of objects; instead, the interpersonal dynamic is tethered closely to the mid-century French psychoanalytic concepts listed previously. And the result she arrives at is the unconscious body image.

So, what exactly is this? In the first chapter alone, Dolto gives more than ten different definitions of the unconscious body image, and nearly as many of its counterpart, the bodily schema. And it seems that the harder she tries to explain what it is and how it is constituted, the more obscure it becomes. These are some quotations from the section 'The Body Image Is Not the Bodily Schema':

> The body image is specific to a libido in a situation, to a type of libidinal relationship.

> the bodily schema is partly unconscious but also preconscious and conscious, while the body image is eminently unconscious; it can become partly preconscious only when it is associated with conscious language, which uses metaphors and metonymy referring to the body image, as much in facial as in verbal expressions.

> The body image is the living synthesis of our emotional experiences: interhuman, repetitively experienced through elective erogenous sensations, archaic or current. It can be considered as *the unconscious symbolic embodiment of the desiring subject*.

> The body image is at every moment the unconscious memory of all the relational experience and at the same time is present, alive and in a dynamic

situation that is both narcissistic and inter-relational: it can be camouflaged or revealed in the here-and-now of a relationship, through any expression – linguistic, in drawing, modelling, musical invention, in plastic creations but also in facial expression and gesture.

it is in the body image, which underlies narcissism, that time is interwoven with space, that the unconscious past resonates in the present relationship. In the present moment, something of a past relationship always shows itself, like a watermark. The libido is mobilised in the immediate relationship but an archaic relational image can be awakened, resuscitated; the image that was repressed returns.

For the sake of non-Lacanian readers who like to be able to fit a new concept into their existing conceptual framework, I would like to suggest a definition of the unconscious body image as follows: *the unconscious body image is a self-representation created through interactive communication with the object*, the object being at first maternal and later including all other adults responsible for the child's upbringing. The communication is at first mostly through physical interactions (holding and handling in Winnicottian terms); affective value is added to these interactions through the consistency of linkage of what Dolto calls 'subtle' factors with the gross 'substantial' value of the interaction (subtle = the smell and sound of mother and the words she gives to familiar things, as opposed to substantial = the milk provided by her breast that satisfies hunger); the affective value of these 'subtle' factors creates in the child *desire as distinct from need*; then a series of 'castrations' (privations of previous modes of satisfaction of desires) channels the infant's desire into increasingly socially appropriate activities until the child is fully 'humanised.'

This book puts the complex nature of interpersonal interactions squarely in the centre of French psychoanalytic theory, where it had been missing. While Lacan may have devoted a whole seminar to 'the Object Relation' (1956–57), his 'object' is an object of desire, an abstraction derived from the imaginary phallus, rather than an ideational representation founded upon lived interactions. In my view, it is the British school's 'object' that more closely describes the mother and other 'tutelary adults' who loom so large in Dolto's work. The repeated, consistent interactions and characteristics (smell, touch, sound) unique to the mother are that which structure the baby's desire and unconscious bodily image, in the same way that the object relation structures the infant's expectations, anxieties and ultimately its self-representation. This form of object relating closely resembles Daniel Stern's Representation of an Interaction that has become Generalised (RIG), while the object itself may be the 'evoked companion' that accompanies an RIG.[1]

---

1 Stern, D. N. (1985). *The Interpersonal World of the Infant: A View from Psychoanalysis and Developmental Psychology*. Chapter four, section titled 'Integrating the Self-Invariants.'

So, what does Dolto's formulation of the interpersonal in the structuring of the child's subject bring to the sum of our knowledge, given that other schools have already focused so much attention upon it? A great deal, I would suggest.

Firstly, Dolto clarifies how the distinction between desire and need arises at the earliest stage of infancy. Dolto has desire deriving from the affective charge attached to 'the subtle' (smell, sound, touch of mother) that consistently accompanies 'the substantial' interactions of feeding and handling. This has implications for the construction of the primordial signifier, as it is 'the subtle' that becomes its transitional phenomena and carries the trace of desire. Dolto's infants' desire is for *the mother in communication with them*, even if their need at the beginning of life is still for feeding and cleaning, and this desire is far more important than need in the structuring of the subject as a unique human being – the Lacanian 'desiring subject' – as distinct from an animal representative of a species whose needs are instinctively and stereotypically satisfied. From the outset of human life, desire is coded in the subtle phenomena of mother–baby communicative exchange, and not in the phenomena of the satisfaction of physiological need. Lacanians struggling with his graph of desire and formula of fantasy may find that Dolto's ideas on these matters could resolve some questions.

Secondly, where the cornerstone of psychoanalysis in both its practice and its ideas of infant development is the communication and interplay of minds, Dolto takes this a step further into the purely physical realm of early infancy, even of foetushood. While it is a Lacanian truism that it is through language that the human subject is formed, she insists we broaden our ideas about language to include all attempts to communicate, whether by physiological functioning (e.g. infantile diarrhoea), physical gestures, facial expressions, sounds or later speech. Drawing upon her experience as a paediatrician as well as psychoanalyst, she describes case after case of childhood functional disturbance in which the body has tried, with varying degrees of desperation, to communicate what could not be formed into a thought.

Thirdly, the unconscious body image is a conceptualisation of self-representation unlike any other in its emphasis upon and detailed explanation of how it is grounded in the physical. It is not a body image in the familiar sense used so popularly today by young people who feel social pressure to look a certain way (although a Doltonian understanding may help elucidate these concerns); it is an unconscious and imaginary self-representation founded at the outset of life by perception, proprioception and interoception, then elaborated through the affective and communicative aspects of holding and handling, and finally by the more flexible and powerful tool of speech. Dolto points out how ideational representation in the form of speech can override even the limitations of the real body so that people born with a severe disability can have an unconscious body image capable of running, leaping, playing music and flying, if their parents always spoke to them about these things as if they could imagine what they felt like; and she contrasts this with able-bodied people who are functionally crippled because of pathologies in their unconscious body image. It is therefore in the pathology of the unconscious body image that we need to look for direction in our treatment of psychosomatic disorders, eating disorders, hysterical conversion disorders and certain sexual disorders. The section in Chapter 3 in which she distinguishes between psychosomatic disorders and hysteria is illuminating, and the argument here depends entirely on understanding *who the object of communication is in each case* – whether it is another person (or object in the British sense) with whom the subject is in communication via the symptom, or if the symptom creates an entirely narcissistic communication in which the ill body-part represents for the subject a constantly communicating, libidinally invested part object.

Fourthly and finally (though only for the purposes of this introduction, as I am certain that readers will discover many other ramifications of her theory), the second chapter of this book, 'The Body Images and Their Destiny: The Castrations,' illuminates the whole vexed question of how children come to accept the law and become socialised, as opposed to dissocial, human beings. In my view, this issue has been a kind of holy grail for psychoanalysis ever since Freud postulated the dissolution of the Oedipus complex as the mechanism by which the child comes to accept that he cannot marry his mother out of a fear of castration – literally having his penis chopped off. He says that although this renouncement of desire comes about firstly through fear, it becomes acceptable through an identification with paternal authority: 'The authority of the father or the parents is introjected into the ego, and there it forms the nucleus of the super-ego.'[2] This proposition has caused controversy since its publication, but few have argued very hard against the basic clinical observation that children do go through a phase of wishing to 'claim' partnership with the parent of the opposite sex and rejecting their same-sex parent, followed by an acquiescence to the state of affairs in the home; or that this is accompanied by an often stronger identification with the same-sex parent and usually ends the period of turbulence and heralds the onset of a more creative and productive latency phase. Because of these commonplace observations, it is hard entirely to dismiss the Oedipus complex as the gateway through which a child must pass in order to integrate social law into his or her mind.

Lacan took up the challenge of making the Freudian formulation work better, by treating the ideas of phallus and castration as purely imaginary and symbolic. His paternal metaphor and Law-of-the-Father are more satisfactory formulations of how the subject submits to a symbolic castration that in reality means accepting a language-based explanation for why he or she cannot always have mummy to him- or herself, but this still requires a certain suspension of disbelief and turning a blind eye to the practical realities of children and their families. There is something rather mystical about the idea of the castration as an initiatic experience that magically creates a barred subject submitted to the law.

2 Freud, S. (1924). *The Standard Edition of the Complete Psychological Works of Sigmund Freud*, vol. 19, 171–180.

With incredible observational common sense, Dolto demystifies this. Instead of castration, she writes of 'castrations' in the plural and shows us how every prohibition of the satisfaction of desire in a particular way that was once permitted constitutes a castration, which can be 'symboligenic' and lead to the 'promotion' (developmental forward-movement) of the child, or can be experienced as purely painful, distressing and pathogenic. She writes of well-delivered castrations as having an effect similar to that of the pruning of a plant, where by the snipping off of the early blooms of libidinal pleasure, the libidinal drive is redirected into the next phase of development. Every phase of development involves a castration, even the birth phase: there is umbilical castration, oral, anal, pre-Oedipal genital and then Oedipal castration. She is also clear that badly administered castrations are not symboligenic and may cause psycho-pathological outcomes, including perversions and the antisocial mindset. I will go no further in précising what is well set out in this book, but want only to say that when I taught Dolto's views on how a child integrates social law in his mind to a group of non-psychoanalytically trained practitioners working with disturbed latency-age children (teachers, teachings assistants and residential care workers), they showed an immediate, gut-level understanding of it and could relate to the theory with practical examples of their own. I can think of no higher recommendation of this piece of work than that.

Readers from the British and American IPA traditions unfamiliar with Lacanian ideas and use of words that they may understand differently may be inspired by this book to try to find out more about those terms of reference. I am just going to elaborate on one thing, for the sake of disambiguation. It is Dolto's neologism 'symboligenic' that is crucial to understanding her ideas about castration and the acceptance of social laws. I do not think this should be understood as 'symbol creating' in the sense that Kleinians speak of symbol formation.[3] Rather, it should be understood in reference to Lacan's Borromean knot of Real, Symbolic and Imaginary orders that structure the human psyche; it is therefore something that contributes to the development of the Symbolic realm in the child's mind.

Incidentally, in proposing a process whereby the castrations become symboligenic, Dolto illuminates also the mechanism of sublimation, which eluded Freud all his life (or at least is missing from his published work). By way of the linkage of drive and desire, she suggests that it is by the deviation of desire from the now-forbidden means of its gratification that the drive bound up with it becomes refocused and reinvested in other, more culturally and socially valued and valuable means of gratification:

> The drive thus repressed undergoes a dynamic modification and desire, the initial goal of which has been forbidden, and aims at its satisfaction through new means, sublimations – means which demand for their satisfaction a process of elaboration that was not demanded by the object first aimed at.

---

3 Segal, H. (1957). Notes on Symbol Formation. *International Journal of Psychoanalysis* 38: 391–397.

Dolto's writing style is discursive – at times she seems to be speaking out loud to students and talks around a subject (usually a clinical case) until her discourse brings her naturally to the next idea. The book is by turns an easy, fluid read or so dense with complex ideas that pause for a great deal of thought is required. I wish readers as much enjoyment, enrichment and satisfaction in reading this book as I obtained out of translating it.

Chapter 1

The unconscious body image

Bodily schema and body image

At the start of my child psychoanalytic practice (1938), on the advice of Sophie Morgenstern,[1] the first child psychoanalyst in France, I offered paper, colour pencils and a little later plasticine to children who wished to understand the unknown internal causes of their known and lived difficulties.

Drawings, smudged colours and shapes are spontaneous means of self-expression for most children. They like to talk about what their hands have translated of their fantasies, and to verbalise what they have drawn or modelled to those who listen to them. It is sometimes without logical connection (for the adult) with what the adult believes she sees in it. But what is most surprising has been imposed on me, little by little: that the agencies of the Freudian theory of the psychic apparatus – the id, ego and superego – are detectable in all free compositions, be they graphic (drawings) or plastic (models) etc. These productions of the child are indeed true represented fantasies in which the unconscious structures are decipherable. They are decipherable as such only by way of the discourse of the child, which, when spoken to the analyst, anthropomorphises and gives life to the different parts of the drawing. This is what is particular in child analysis: what in adults is deciphered from their associations of ideas upon a recounted dream, for instance, can in children be illustrated by what they say about their drawings and plastic compositions, which lend support to their fantasies and the confabulations of their transference relationships.

The mediator of the three psychic agencies (id, ego and superego), in the allegorical representations provided by the subject, showed itself to be specific: I have called it the body image.

Example 1

Two drawings of an 11-year-old child with serious tics.

---

1 Who committed suicide in 1940 when the Germans entered Paris.

DOI: 10.4324/9781003312499-2

The first drawing: a horse whose head could not fit into the frame of the paper, on which there was a rider who fought with an enemy who was not totally visible but whose sword could be seen arriving from the top left of the picture, threatening the rider's head, while to the lower right part of the picture a venomous snake could be seen, which (according to the child) was going to bite the rider's horse. In this picture, the horse has no head while the rider has one.

The second drawing, made at another session, was a variation on the previous motif. The head of the rider was not completely on the sheet of paper; the horse had a head but there was no space on the paper for its tail. The snake was replaced by the head of a tiger to the bottom left that was ready to attack the horse. The tiger's head is in fact on the side where the horse's head should be, but lower down.

At the invitation of the analyst, the young boy talked about his drawings, putting himself in the place of all the characters and, from the position of each of them, could imagine and talk about what they represented. Thus, what appeared successively was a head that signified oral devouring – the head of the tiger; a head that mastered the anal musculature, represented by the horse's head; while the mastery of the rider's head signified the human being. While the three heads could be present interchangeably, the child excluded the possibility of them all being present in the drawing at the same time. Also, there was always a danger for the rider, represented either as the orality inherent in a body (that of the tiger) or by the venomous snake that from behind shows the earthy and anal forces that could avenge themselves on the individual; and at the same time, the sword of a hierarchically superior human that takes aim at him.

Subsequently, in the last drawing of this child, the danger is represented by a lightning bolt that destroys simultaneously the rider, the horse and probably other animals that were there, and which found themselves in conflict with the living agencies, a conflict represented by the attack.

The explanation of these different dangers could be discovered through free association about enemies, storms, venomous or devouring dangers – figurative themes linked with a family drama.

This involved the death of the child's paternal grandfather, which was followed by family conflicts linked with inheritance, and the child's father being witness to a murder attempt on one of his brothers by the eldest of the sibling group. The child had learned about this by overhearing the conversation of his parents while sleeping in their bedroom at his grandparents' house. Everything had been telescoped in his mind – the oral greed of the inheritance, the murder taboo and the astonishment at his parents' connivance as they spoke in his presence in low tones in the conjugal bed, siding with the would-be murderer – who fortunately had only injured the other (in an apparent hunting accident) – and agreeing to hide it. The child's tics had begun on their return home after the grandfather's funeral.

Thanks to the sequential drawings, we can see how the analysis of the unconsciously represented memories and associations allowed the freeing of what seemed like irresolvable contradictions for the boy, who could not at the same time keep his head, his muscular vitality and control of his behaviour. He found himself a silent witness and therefore complicit in the parental conversation, which had a dehumanising effect with regard to the code of law. But, importantly, what allows us to see that the psychoanalysis of children is possible is that he himself brought the data for interpretation in what he said about his phantasmagorical drawings: he was the snake who thought like that, he the tiger's head, which represented the dangerous mother (whom his father called the tigress) with whom he identified, and who was dangerous to the horse, which in this case represented the father; and all the while, the sword of God, replaced by the lightning, comes to strike the child and injure his humanisation, as by judging his father, the accomplice of his murderous uncle, he too appears guilty in the eyes of the law. What he heard in their speech was that his parents, especially his father (as his mother was agonised about being in the secret), were in their desire also transgressors of the law. In addition, as the chance witness of the conjugal discussions in the house of his paternal family line, he became in the moment an incestuous child.

Example 2

Concerns a highly inhibited child of around 10 years of age who had almost no voice and a fixed, anguished smile. He could say nothing about himself and apparently didn't dream. When asked to express himself in drawing, he started to make graphic representations of 'tank battles.' In fact, all the drawings of his first sessions represented this theme in a way that showed clearly the magnitude of his inhibition in relation to others. For instance, in one of his drawings there was a tank drawn pale and tremblingly in the middle of the page, and only at the extreme right-hand side, the end of the cannon of another. That cannon fired nothing; the only shell discharged in the picture was from the visible tank, though directed away from the other so that the invisible tank could not be damaged.

Session after session, this impossible combat between two tanks continued like this until it was replaced by one between two boxers drawn in profile each with only one arm visible, keeping a respectable distance from each other. The problem of rivalry was thus confirmed in the form of the impossibility of body-to-body contact. From the start of this series of drawings, the boxers lacked either a head or feet, because both could not be accommodated in the space of the paper. Realising this, he re-drew the boxers on their knees before each other, but their arms, even when extended, could not touch each other.

When at last, after several sessions, he managed to make the two boxers stand face to face, what appeared in the drawing was that one had a stripy top, and in response to my question, if he were in the drawing, he would be that one. However, the associations he made with the striped shirt showed it was the shirt of a classmate, who having taken home a bad report, received a spanking from his father.

> I asked: 'You would like your father to give you a spanking?'
> 'Ah! That's not what I mean, but he has a dad who looks after him.'

In fact, this child had a father who was completely indifferent to him and who had never recognised the child as someone valuable. All the inhibitions of the child could be explained as the self-destruction of his virile libido by the absence of a possible identification with a father who did not recognise himself as such, and who did not recognise in his son a boy increasing in value, as he had no interest in him. There was even a reversal of the Oedipal situation: it was the father who was jealous of his son and would not allow him to construct his identity in reference to himself in elaborating the psychic agencies of ego, superego and ego-ideal, because he was not an interlocutor for his son, nor had he a superego that inhibited the non-observance of the law of work. He only knew how to say 'be quiet,' 'go away,' 'leave me alone.' This means he could not bear the ego-ideal of a phallic-oral boy who had the right to speak to his father and to be in a dialogue with him. The child therefore felt he was too big a danger for his father as he (the father) was scared of him; at the very least, the father, in negating him, behaved as if he was.

It was the interpretation by way of these drawings that brought to light the libidinal self-inhibition because of the insecurity of the father with regard to his child, which was resolved by the child in a puerile life of no competition and therefore no creativity, all libido blocked by the danger the child felt he posed to his father. The desired ego was to be the son of a strong father capable of controlling the inhibition of his son towards work and formative of a superego that inhibits laziness: a father who could be an ego-ideal. His dream was to be like the boy with the striped sweater, with a father who was interested in whatever interested his son (the father of the boy with the striped sweater also rewarded him whenever he got good school reports). It was the boy's mother who had herself knitted him that beautiful striped sweater, so there was in that family a mother who could love her child without making her husband non-existent, while he continued to be a father who controlled and at the same time supported the energy of his son, so that he becomes a social being, armed for life.

It is in these volumes of representation in space – volumes that express intentionality – that the child expresses himself. At the start, it seemed to be about drawing a scene, but in reality, by the ways in which he interpreted himself, in which he spoke of his drawings, he showed in these graphic stagings how he was managing the part instincts of his desire that were in conflict with the part instincts of his desire at another level. These levels of the psyche are what Freud described as the ego, ego-ideal and the superego. And the energy brought to light in these imaginary scenarios of the drawings and models is nothing other than libido expressed passively or actively by the body – passively in a psychosomatic balance or actively in relationships with others.

Let us give an example of a situation where plasticine modelling is the representational support.

Example 3

A young man in lycée class 3, a brilliant but 'very nervous' 14-year-old pupil, was brought to me for a consultation. The complaint was that at school, he was compulsively kicking the tables until they came apart. The mother who accompanied the boy herself had bruised legs with ulcers on her shins. She told me that aside from her own legs, his strange acts targeted the foot of her side of the conjugal bed and the family dining table leg on the side where she usually sat.

> During this first contact, all that the boy could tell me about his symptom was, 'I can't help it, it's stronger than me.'
> 'But how come this always targets your mum and not your dad?'
> 'I don't know. I don't do it on purpose.'
> Saying that he couldn't draw, he chose to make a plasticine model and created an old well, very artistically reproduced. I said, 'A well – what have you to say about that?'
> 'Well, there's water at the bottom, it's an old-fashioned well. Nowadays there aren't any wells.'
> 'Yes. And what can be hidden in wells?'
> And together, we came to talk about wells and the truth that is supposed to spring naked from them. As the session came to an end, we had to arrange the subsequent meetings, and the young man, who seemed quite capable to me, said, 'Ah, you have to ask Mum.'
> 'Why do I have to ask your mother? Don't you know when you are free?'
> 'No, you have to ask Mum.'
> Mother then came and sat on his left. While she talked to me about dates for subsequent sessions, the young man took his mother's right hand in his left and used her index finger to stroke the inside of the model well, apparently without her noticing this. Instead of letting him leave with his mother, I said to her, 'Please wait a moment, I need to speak to your son again.'
> She left and I asked the boy, 'What was the meaning of the gesture you made with the index finger of your mother in your model?'
> 'Me? What? I don't know . . .' He looked surprised, flustered, answering as if he had forgotten or had noticed nothing.
> I described to him what I had seen him do, and added, 'What does it make you think about – your mum's finger in the hole of the well?'
> 'Well, I can't go to the loo . . . Mum doesn't let me go to the loo at school because she has to see, she still supervises my poo.'
> 'Why? Have you got a long-term intestinal problem?'
> 'No, but she wants to, and she creates scenes if I have a poo at school.'
> 'Go and get your mother.'
> The mother returned and confirmed that she too had not noticed him playing with her finger in the well. I told her that her son, who was still present, had told me that she found it necessary to check his excrements.
> 'Well, Madame, is it not the duty of a mother to maintain the good functioning of her children's bodies? Even my eldest son [a 21-year-old boy] – I massage his anus every time he goes to pass a motion.'
> 'Ah, yes – and why?'

'The doctor ordered me to do that. When my eldest son was 18 months old, he had a prolapse of the rectum and the doctor told me to massage his anus after every motion, to push back the prolapse.'

It was around this problem – that the mother could not bear that the vegetative functioning of her sons become autonomous – that the apparently 'nervous' illness of the 14-year-old boy had been organised, first at pre-puberty and then at puberty.

The boy was also expressing his jealousy of his older brother, who had the right and prerogative to their mother's anal massage, while he only got his mother's visual inspection of his excrement – he had never had the 'luck' of having a rectal prolapse when he was small.

The well was the projection of a part image of the anal body: it represented the boy's rectum, with which he linked the 'truth' about a woman's sexuality in her enjoyment of excrement. Overall, he had remained stuck at an anal sexuality, fixed that way by the perverted desire of a mother, innocently incestuous towards her sons under the cover of 'medicine' and 'duty,' touching the 'good functioning' of the object-body of her children.

This also allowed us to understand the meaning of the motor symptom of aggression by kicking. The motor functioning that, when socially adapted, is an expression of the sublimated anal pleasure, was altered in this boy. His two bottom limbs came up and behaved in his symptom as a substitute for the third lower member – the penile member. His legs kicked the legs of his mother as he was not able to penetrate her vagina with his penis.

Finally, one can see played out the rivalry with the eldest son, an eldest son who could only imperfectly take the part of an ego-ideal, being more a regressive model that the younger, since earliest times, would have liked to supplant.

Example 4

This was also an example using modelling. An 8-year-old boy created an armchair during a session. I asked him, 'Where would this be?'

'In the attic.'
'But it looks quite solid, and very solid armchairs don't get put in the attic.'
'Yes, that's true.'
'So, who would it be, this armchair, if it were someone?'
'It would be Grandpa . . . because they say he is old and he doesn't want to die.'
'And is that annoying, that he won't die?'
'Well, yes, because we haven't got room at home and we have to be in Dad and Mum's bedroom, he doesn't want anyone to sleep with him in the other room.'

So here you have an inconvenient old person whom the parents had taken on in the hope that he would die soon, a paralysed old man who was always sitting in an armchair and whom they would have liked to put in the attic with other broken objects. The armchair represented the encumbering body of the overly well old man who was impinging on the lives of a family in a small dwelling. It seems certain that the child could not have told this story in any way other than by this fantasy, which illustrates an anal fixation with the seat, literally speaking, which had also made this child soil himself. It was because of his encopresis that he had come for the psychotherapy consultation.

There again, one can see how a child with the help of a plastic production anthropomorphises what Freud distinguished of the psychic agencies. The grandfather incarnated an anal superego (guilt about doing, about dynamic and progressive action). The problem was to eject this being while keeping and respecting him. This was probably the reason why the child had anal retentions that were evacuated by the non-control of the sphincter, at the same time as failing in the sublimation of oral and anal drives, the mental manipulations that represent scholarity for a child.

These examples are interesting because they show us how in all free composition the body image is represented and recounted: the associations supplied by the child come to actualise the conflictual link between the three agencies of the psychic apparatus.

With children (and psychotics), who unlike adults engaging in free association, cannot speak directly about their dreams and fantasies, the body image is for the subject a medium for expressing them, and for the analyst the medium for recognising them. It is, therefore, a 'said' – a 'said' to be decoded, and for which the analyst alone has not got the key. It is the associations of the child that bring the key; it is by this that he finds himself to be, at the end of the day, the analyst. For it is he who manages to apprehend himself as the lieu of the contradictions that inhibit the mental, social, sexual and emotional powers appropriate for his age.

Let it be understood: the body image is not the image that is drawn here, or represented in models; it is what is revealed in the analytic dialogue with the child. This is why, contrary to what one believes in general, the analyst cannot know how to interpret straightaway the graphic or plastic material brought to her by the child; but it is that, which in association with her work, can give the elements of a psychoanalytic interpretation of his symptoms; and there again, not directly but in association with the spoken narrative (e.g. the striped sweater of the boxer). This means that talking about the image – the body image – doesn't imply that it is only of the imaginary order, since it is also of the symbolic order, being the sign of a certain level of libidinal structure involved in a conflict that is to be disentangled by the narrative of the child. And the listener must receive it through the narrated events of the child's personal history.

The bodily schema is not the body image

The preceding examples allow us to focus on these two terms: one must not confuse body image with bodily schema.

All of the mentioned cases have been about children with healthy bodily schemas; it was only the functioning of these schemas that had been impaired by the
pathogenic body *images*. The tool – the body – or perhaps better called here the
organised mediator between the subject and the world, was potentially in a good
condition, without lesions; but its functional use adapted to the subject's consciousness was blocked. These children's bodies per se were the theatre of inhibition of the bodily schema in the first two cases (the tics, and the total inhibition
in ideation and motor functioning of the mute boy with the frozen smile), and of
the non-control of the bodily schema in the second two cases (the uncontrollable
kicking and the encopresia). The appropriate use of the bodily schema had been
cancelled, impeded by the linkage of the libido with an inappropriate, archaic or
incestuous body image – the libido impeded by the lack of castrations that should
have been given by adults to their archaic drives, and the lack of sublimations that
the responsible adults should have allowed them to acquire for their humanisation
(education).

This invalidation of the healthy bodily schema by a disturbed body image can
for instance be found in the case of the child who drew two tanks that could not
manage to have a proper fight. A non-invalided bodily schema *should* have produced a firm line and guns trained on the enemy; or in the subsequent drawings,
boxers who each had two arms and wouldn't need to be on their knees to box. One
could almost say that despite a healthy and integrated bodily schema, it was the
body image that lacked an arm, that was on its knees (showing the incapacity of
the boy to endorse the potential of the standing stature and situations of rivalry).
In the fourth case, it was the part or absent parts of his body image, forbidden to
be aggressive towards the inconvenient grandfather to whom the parents submitted, that stopped the child from identifying himself as a successful boy; whereas
he had a friend who had a mother and father not in conflict with each other, as
were his parents (because of the presence of the grandfather), and who contributed
to supporting the humanised existence of their son and his efforts at school. *The
bodily schema is a factual reality; it is in some ways our carnal life in interaction
with the physical world.* Experiences of our reality depend upon the integrity of
the organism or of its injuries, transitory or indelible, neurological, muscular or
skeletal, and also of our visceral and circulatory physiological sensations – also
called coenesthetic.

Indeed, early organic damage can provoke a disorder of the bodily schema, and
this, because of a lack or an interruption of language interactions, can cause some
transitory or lifelong modifications of the body image. Frequently, however, a
disabled bodily schema and a healthy body image cohabit in the same subject. Let
us consider children who have suffered from poliomyelitis, which causes motor
paralysis but no sensory deficit. If the illness happens after the age of 3, that is
after the mastery of walking, of sphincter control and of the knowledge of their
sex (primary castration), the bodily schema, while it can be partly chronically
damaged, stays compatible with an almost always intact body image, as can be
seen in the drawings of these children.

The bodily schema is however always damaged at least in part when polio-myelitis happens early, while the child is still milk-fed and in the cot, and mostly before s/he is able to walk. Even if these children do not recover a healthy bodily schema, intact from the point of view of motor functioning and neurology, their disability may not affect their body image: for this, it is necessary that until the ill-ness, during it and during the convalescence and rehabilitation, their relationship with their mother and human environment has remained supple and satisfactory without excessive parental anxiety; that their relationships are adapted to their needs, which should always be spoken about as if they could be met by the child himself while the muscular damage caused by the illness and its sequalae make him incapable of this. When a child suffers from a disability, it is indispensable that he is explicitly told of his physical deficit, in reference to his non-disabled past or to the congenital difference between him and other children when this is the case. He must also be able, in imitative language and speech, to express his desires and fantasise about them being realisable or not, in accordance with the disabled bodily schema.

So it is that a paraplegic child[2] needs to play verbally with his mother, talking about running, jumping, things that his mother knows he won't ever be able to do. In this way, he projects a healthy body image symbolised by his speech and drawings in fantasies of erotic satisfaction, in an exchange between two subjects. Speaking about these desires in this way to someone who accepts the projective game allows the subject to integrate these desires in language despite the reality of his disabled body. Language brings the discovery of a personal means of com-munication. A child with phocomelia born without lower or upper limbs has a disabled bodily schema; however, his body image can be quite healthy and allow a language of interhuman communications as complete and satisfactory as those of a person without disability. It is the case of Denise Legrix, trunk-woman, author of the book *Born This Way*, and who, crippled from birth, was loved by her mother and father and their social entourage. A child who has only one arm can with this arm manage to manipulate objects he needs. The fact that his mother has never wanted to talk to him about his disability, while he can see the difference between his body and those of other children, makes the child badly socialised and bad tempered, with an unhealthy body image, and in a relationship of dependency upon his mother, in a phobic or philic fixation, impossible to castrate at the time of weaning, and then at anal castration (autonomous action).

The healthy evolution of the subject, symbolised by a non-disabled body image, depends therefore on the emotional relationship of the child's parents with his per-son: that true information is very precociously delivered in words about his disabled physical state. These humanising exchanges, or on the contrary their absence – dehumanising – come from whether the parents have or have not accepted the disability of their child's body. Are they feeling guilty about their genetic

2 Neurological paralysis of the lower limbs.

transmissions? Are they anxious? Is this child narcissised[3] by being loved as he is? Or on the contrary feel de-narcissised in his value as an interlocutor, who as disabled is not loved, and whose disability is neither recognised nor spoken about? As a cripple, is he rejected by his parents, rather than being fully recognised as their son or their daughter in this ordeal, and considered as a legitimate human being with a disability? If he is recognised as the subject of his own desires – and the symbol of the Word that harmoniously united two tutelary[4] humans responsible for his birth and who love him in his own reality, which they do not try to make him forget – his parents (and then educators) will be able to give the structure of a healthy body image in response to his questions, through the mediation of language and in a fashion unconscious to them. 'If you were a bird, you could fly' . . . 'if you had feet, hands, you could do what this little boy is doing' . . . 'you are as smart as he is.'

And you can see children without arms or legs who manage to paint with their mouth as well as those who have hands; and those who have only feet managing to be as skilful with their feet as others are with their hands. But this can only happen if they are loved and supported in the means they still possess in becoming creative, and which are representative of their drives in exchanges with others.

A human being may not have structured his body image during the development of his bodily schema. This is sometimes due, as we have just seen, to disability or early neuro-vegetative or muscular illnesses; this could also be caused by neonatal illnesses, the consequences of obstetric accidents or infections that destroy some subtle zones of perception in early childhood (deafness, anosmia, cleft palate, blindness etc).

One can hypothesise that the non-structuration of the body image is largely due to the fact that the tutelary agents, disorientated by never having had the responses they might expect from a child this age, stop trying to communicate with the child in ways other than by bodily contact for the maintenance of his needs, and who abandon the attempt to humanise him. It is more than likely that such a human being, as his body survives, would sooner or later be able to develop a language of his own according to his particular body image, by means of sensorial relational markers or by his emotional complicity with someone who loves him and who

---

3 Translator's note: Dolto's use of the word 'narcissism' is positive rather than pejorative and refers to the subject's self-image and self-esteem – how he experiences himself at a deep and unconscious level. Her neologism 'narcissising' refers to the process of constructing this unconscious self-image and self-esteem – a process dependent upon the subject's experience of being loved as he is. Furthermore, Dolto names as 'de-narcissising' any processes that produce a damaged and unbearable self-image and self-esteem.

4 Translator's note: Dolto uses the terms 'tutelary adult' and 'tutelary agent' throughout her work when speaking of adults in the position of parents or guardians to the child, emphasising their role in bringing up the young human to be a fully socialised being, rather than simply as genitors, 'trainers' or 'owners' of the child. Tutelary agents are either true parents or those acting in *loco parentis* who have the trust of the child, who believes that they hold true knowledge of life and the world – 'tutelary' encompasses ideas of authority, trust and kinship.

introduces him to a triangular relationship and allows him to enter into symbolic relations.

In children who suffered early poliomyelitis, for example, and who have a more or less severely affected bodily schema, a perfectly healthy body image can develop on condition that they were not neurotic before the illness and have been supported during the acute phase of the illness by their mother and father in their relationships with others and with themselves. These children then draw bodies that present none of their own disabilities.

Body image and bodily schema – how to distinguish between them

Let us return to our essential distinction in another way. The bodily schema specifies the individual as a representative of the species, whatever the place, time or condition in which he lives. It is the schema that will be the active or passive interpreter of the body image, as it allows the objectification of an intersubjectivity, of a language-mediated libidinal relationship with others without which, without the support it constitutes, would remain forever a non-communicable fantasy.

If the bodily schema is in principle the same for all human individuals (more or less of the same age and in the same geographical region), the body image by contrast is specific for everyone: it is linked with the subject and his/her history. The body image is specific to a libido in a situation, to a type of libidinal relationship. The result of this is that the bodily schema is partly unconscious but also preconscious and conscious, while the body image is eminently unconscious; it can become partly preconscious only when it is associated with conscious language, which uses metaphors and metonymy referring to the body image, as much in facial as in verbal expressions.

The body image is the living synthesis of our emotional experiences: interhuman, repetitively experienced through elective erogenous sensations, archaic or current. It can be considered as *the unconscious symbolic embodiment of the desiring subject*. And this even before the subject in question is able to self-designate with the personal pronoun, I – before he is able to say I. I want it to be understood that the desiring unconscious subject in relation to the body exists from the moment of conception. The body image is at every moment the unconscious memory of all the relational experience and at the same time is present, alive and in a dynamic situation that is both narcissistic and inter-relational: it can be camouflaged or revealed in the here-and-now of a relationship, through any expression – linguistic, in drawing, modelling, musical invention, in plastic creations but also in facial expression and gesture.

Our body image, held by and interwoven with our bodily schema, allows us to enter into communication with others. Any contact with the other, be it a contact through communication or the avoidance of communication, is underpinned by the body image; as it is in the body image, which underlies narcissism, that time is interwoven with space, that the unconscious past resonates in the present relationship. In the present moment, something of a past relationship always shows itself, like a watermark. The libido is mobilised in the immediate relationship but an archaic relational image can be awakened, resuscitated; the image that was repressed returns.

Let us here underline that the bodily schema, which is the abstraction of an experience of the body in the three dimensions of reality and is structured by learning and experience, while body image is structured by communication between subjects and the trace, memorised from one day to the next, of frustrated, repressed or forbidden enjoyment (castration in the psychoanalytic sense of desire in reality). This is why the body image relates exclusively to the imaginary, to an intersubjective imaginary marked from the start in humans by the symbolic dimension.

Put another way: *the bodily schema relates the body in its current state and place with its immediate experience. It can be independent of language* understood as a history of the subject's relations with others. The bodily schema is unconscious, preconscious and conscious. The bodily schema evolves in time and space. *The body image links the desiring subject with his enjoyment, mediated by language memorised from the communication between subjects.* It can free itself from the bodily schema. It is connected with narcissism, which originates in the carnalisation of the subject from the point of conception. The body image is always unconscious, constituted by the dynamic linkage of a basal image, a functional image and an image of erogenous zones where instinctual tensions are expressed.

The role of the couch in psychoanalysis

In psychoanalytic technique, it is precisely because the patient's bodily schema is neutralised by lying down that the body image can be given free rein. One finds that the body image comes into play at the same time that it is impossible to see the analyst's body and especially his facial expressions, which provokes in the analysand an imaginary representation of the other instead of the perception of his visible reality. There is, therefore, an absenting of enjoyment of the scopic drives and the frustration of enjoyment of auditive drives (as it is the analysand who speaks, and the analyst very little). In a way, without knowing it, Freud used the body image even more than we do today, as he was frustrating his patients of all genital satisfaction for the duration of the treatment.

The search for desire and defence against desire are language-based processes that construct the body image, aiming to protect the integrity of narcissism and of the bodily schema – that is, the body itself as a cohesive, carnal ensemble that has to stay whole to be able to perceive. When exposed to excessive pain, the whole organism (the whole psyche?) anticipates that the meeting between an obstacle and his suffering body, wounded or in pain in this or that area, might provoke a feeling of non-security, and protects himself by keeping a distance from others. This is in the realm of the bodily schema consciously imagined; this is not about the body image.

It may happen that the process of negation of the affects of pleasure–unpleasure, or ideational processes of negation of the erotic object through body language or verbal language, is aimed at protecting the subject from a repeated experience from which he can only expect displeasure.[5] It is interesting for the psychoanalyst to capture the dynamic of unconscious desire at different levels: firstly at the level of the body-thing, then the level revealed by the body image at each stage in its three unconscious aspects: the language of facial expressions, the language of the viscera and that of unconscious gestures. In the modelling of the well mentioned earlier (p. 33), we have seen how the partial anal body image could be actualised in a relational experience. Let us give the example of a girl who during her first session, while on her own with me, drew a very beautiful vase with blooming flowers, indicating the water level in which the stalks dipped. Next, I have an interview with the mother while the little girl is present; while this is happening, she draws a second picture of a miniscule flower pot without a water level and inside, a miniscule bunch of wilting flowers. There one can see the difference in the girl's body image as experienced unconsciously, according to whether mother is present or not. Relative to her mother, she feels pathetic and wilted, while when she is the only interlocutor of the analyst who listens to her, she feels authorised to bloom and to be in her narcissistic seductive beauty.

The bodily schema of this girl is not modified by the presence of her mother; this presence involves a modification of her body image and its projective representation. This modification allows us to understand in the here-and-now the disturbance in the relationship between mother and daughter. The symptoms – the reasons for the consultation – are hereby illustrated. The child expressed by way of her drawings what she felt of a wounded narcissism in relation to her mother, and that could only be unknotted and decoded through psychoanalytic work. This decoding had to take place with regard to not only the desire of the little girl in relation to the desire of the mother and vice versa, but also the desire of each in their triangular Oedipal relations – current for the girl, in the past for mother – that is, with the object of their genital desire; for the girl, the father, which is to say the partner of her mother.

The triangular situation that the presence of the analyst caused to appear – the triangular situation in which the mother was talking with the analyst – put the child in the situation of the sad flowers, wilting and losing their vitality[6] – while the binary situation of child and analyst had 'narcissised' her. (The analyst, although a woman, seems to have been in the position of the father). The drawing expressed the painful experience of genital castration in the girl, who because of her mother's presence, imagined herself to be non-desirable to her father.

---

5 A banal example of this is shyness, its body language: blushing, sweating. Erythrophobia is its neurosis, but shyness is not neurotic.

6 Flower: a projection of the erogenous zone of the passive oral-anal body image, a place where plants bear fruit, individualised living creatures but not autonomously mobile or animated.

Thanks to the observation of children in their real relations with family and friends on the one hand and on the other in their transferential relations during analytic sessions, I could understand the major role of the patient's body image, both in itself and in its projection onto others, in every existential fantasy of being himself and of being in the world.

Analytic technique adapted for children

Letting the child draw or play with plasticine during the analytic sessions is not playing with him. The rule for the analyst is to not participate actively in the child's game, meaning that she doesn't mix her own fantasies with those of the child in treatment; by implication, the analyst does not eroticise her relationship with the patient, nor attempt any form of reparation. The work is about putting into words the fantasies of the children, who at their first session often express themselves only in looks and not games. Children do not come to analysis to distract themselves or to have fun any more than do adults. They come to express themselves truthfully. Many children who have had the chance of psychoanalytic treatment have not been able to benefit from it simply because the sessions had been presented to them with these words: that they are going to play with a man or a lady who likes children. The result for the child is an eroticised relation submitted to, a continuation of 'being the plaything of the other.'

The role of the psychoanalyst is not to substitute a supposedly 'healthy' desire in place of the supposedly pathological desire of the parents, nor to 'kidnap' the child from his biological parents or carers, who theoretically have been, are or will be 'bad' for him; on the contrary, it is to let the child know through gestures and linguistic signs, to which are added words addressed to him (whether the parents are present or not), that the analyst has the confidence of his parents who remain responsible for his upbringing, so that he comes to his own understanding of what makes him suffer. He can thereby rediscover himself as the desiring subject in the initial triangle of his primal scene, and if he does suffer, he can accept, at least on trial, the contract that is offered: not to play just for fun but to express himself to the analyst in play, as he cannot yet express in words his thoughts, feelings and fantasies. The destiny of his drawings and plasticine models is to be spoken about – they happen within transference in the way dreams, fantasies and free associations do in adult psychoanalytic technique. I would add that as a rule with children who have not reached the Oedipal stage, even if they are not major autists or major phobics, and whatever their age, I see them at the start with their parents, then I see their parents alone frequently, and whenever the child wishes it, I let them attend the child's sessions and even to play a part in them.

I have always refused to play with a child during analytic sessions; in the same way that with adult patients we don't start a conversation, similarly with a child, we shouldn't mix our fantasies with theirs, but be there to listen to what they have to say by means of their behaviour, what they experience and think, and which is a priori totally accepted by us.

From his drawings and by the association of ideas, the child gets to talk about his mother, his father, his sibling group and his entourage, about myself in relation to him and of the interpretations that I offer. These 'interpretations' being, as with adults, questions regarding the re-experiencing of this or that fantasy and mostly of a rapprochement between his associations regarding this or that past period of his life.

However, drawings and models are not suggested with the aim of making him talk about his mother and his father; they are like the dreams and fantasies of adults – testimonies of the unconscious. Any drawing, any representation of the world, is already an expression, a mute communication, a statement to oneself or to another. During a session, it is an invitation to communicate with the analyst, to which we must add that when the child talks during a session (just as with adults), if he talks about his father, mother or brothers, he doesn't talk about these people as a reality but of his father 'in himself,' his mother 'in himself,' his brothers 'in himself' – that is to say, he brings a dialectic of his relationship to these real people, who in his speech are fantasised.

Believing that he talks of these people in their reality, in fact, in the way he represents them, he talks of these people in relation to his own subjectivity; these experiences are the product of super-positions during his history within his relationships with adults. From this comes the possibility of projecting these lived relational experiences onto the plastic representations that we have described in terms of anthropomorphism. To my question 'who would be the sun?' – a question that put in the conditional the possibility of associating about the sun, the child can answer: 'the sun, that would be dad, the grass, that would be so-and-so.' I could also ask, 'if you were in your drawing, where would you be?' – not forgetting that the small child can only get into a relationship through projection. It is indeed only with Oedipal castration and the entry into the symbolic order of the law, the same for everyone, that a direct real relationship will become possible. Until then, a man is referenced to the father, present or absent, a lady to the mother, present or absent. It is therefore through the observation of his projective interpretations – 'grandmother would be the cup,' 'grandfather would be the armchair' – that we can see to what extent a child can loan a part or the totality of his body image to objects, animals, people etc. And it is at the moment where the projection is made that he communicates his unconscious life.

A child of 17 or 18 months is at the window. He looks at the sky. For the first time, his attention is attracted by the vision of a star in the twilit sky. His mother comes to close the shutters. 'Wait, wait, look!' he says. His mother explains, 'That's a star. It's the evening star, the first star you see in the sky,' and she adds, 'it is cold, we have to shut the window.' Regretfully leaving his place, the child says, 'Goodbye, Princess,' waving at the star. One doesn't say goodbye to fairy-tale princesses, but one does say goodbye to a star that shines like the gaze of the mother, in reference to the princess of the child's heart, the princess that she is for him. Plucked from life, this example allows one to get an idea of what the sky in the drawing of a child can represent. You just need to observe that the small child who looks at an adult from bottom to top sees the head of the parents profiled against the sky, when they are outside, and therefore associates their face with the imaginary occupant of the sky, his god or his king in the spatial reality of their drawing, that is to say his king in the 'imaginary reality' (the fantasised parental omnipotence), that of the cosmic or divine omnipotence and the omnipotence that reigns over his behaviour, symbolised by the words 'king' or 'queen,' a way of finding in the childish sky the superego or the ideal-ego.[7]

The body image before the Oedipus can be projected in any and all representations and not only in human representations. This is why a drawing or a model of a thing, a plant, an animal or a human is both the image of the one who draws and the image of those whom he is drawing, as he would like them to be, true to what he allows himself to expect of them.

All these representations are symbolically connected to the emotional turmoil that has marked his being in the course of his personal history, and take into account the erogenous zones that successively gained primacy. We know that the primacy of choice of erogenous zones modifies itself and is displaced through the growth of the subject and the development of his bodily schema as allowed by the child's neurological apparatus (incomplete at birth and only mature towards 27 or even 30 months). This evolution of erogenicity is not only the unfolding of a physiological programme, but is also structured by the content of the inter-psychic relation with the other, in particular the mother, and it is this to which the body image is testimony.

The term 'inter-psychic relationships' signifies that need is not the only thing in question and that contact is not only between bodies. For example, when a child asks his mother for a sweet, the anticipated pleasure is linked with the vanished pleasure of his mouth in contact with the nipple or teat, but it is removed from the nutritive value of lactation as well as from the maternal smell. Getting the sweet is proof that the person who gives it loves him, that he can feel loved and his desire recognised – it is a gift of love.[8] Moreover, if you refuse to grant the demand for a sweet while recognising that the child is asking someone for a relationship, and if this person is interested in the person of the child, talks to him and communicates with him, this proves to the child that he is loved while a bodily gratification has been refused. This love given, even if his demand for an oral pleasure was not responded to, accords to him the pleasure of human value that largely compensates for his not getting the sweet.

---

7 The ideal ego is an agency that takes a being from reality (a you) as an idealised being (model) for the pre-subject that is the ego (me) in reference to the you – the master model with the right to say 'I.' After the Oedipus, the subject is himself the subject I, assuming me, his behaviour marked by the genital law as much as adults are, and the ego ideal is no longer in reference to someone but to an ethic that serves as an imaginary support to the ego for the accession to adulthood.

8 Unfortunately, this does not always practically prove he is loved as the sweet is often a way of despatching with his request for a relationship – one is trying to shut him up by giving him a sweet.

It will only be with entry into the symbolic order through Oedipal castration that the subject will be able to express himself clearly in a true relationship with speech as responsible for the acts of his ego, as manifested by his body. Until then, the child's own desire – be it olfactory, oral, anal, urethral (in boys) or genital (in boys and girls) – cannot be directly and autonomously expressed in language, as it relates to and depends upon the tutelary agents who, in focusing the desire, define the relational world of the child. The child can only express his desire via partial desires, by way of the projected representations he gives of them – wherefrom arises the theoretical and practical importance in psychoanalysis of the notion of the body image for pre-Oedipal aged children. The desire of the child expresses itself to any man or woman, including the analyst, with the defensive caution necessary to preserving the ongoing structuration. He doesn't mobilise in a relationship with someone outside the family the erotic drives that must stay engaged in the secure emotional situation given by the family space – a situation unconsciously erotic vis-à-vis his two parents. These parental figures are in reality the respondents of his narcissistic cohesion, situated in time at his primal scene and in space in his present relationship of dependence upon them to survive. The structuring aspect of his incestuous desire (obviously unconscious) – homosexual and/or heterosexual – is and has to remain engaged towards his father and mother. Since then, emotions caused by his current erotic situation in the course of evolving towards the establishment of the Oedipus upon the parents cannot without danger to the narcissistic cohesion of the child be transferred onto the psychoanalyst or onto any other person, masculine or feminine. The danger comes from the risk that the child could only projectively transfer non-castrated, non-symbolised emotions linked with archaic drives: and the risk is increased if, as is frequently the case, the parents themselves also regress in the face of the treatment of their child to archaic libidinal positions – for example, to an attitude of unconditional trust or of irrational suspicion towards their child's analyst. The child is therefore engaged in a no-win situation, where he has to face his parents' archaic unconscious behaviours, eroticised and eroticising. They, while still responsible for his upbringing, cannot be the representatives of a masculine or feminine ideal-ego, as behaviours falling to an archaic libido start to dominate their behaviour as adults, animated by a genital desire towards each other. When a child is in treatment, even more than for any child evolving towards the Oedipus and the castration of genital incestuous desire within his family, it is important that the parents assume their place as responsible for the child and his castration by affirming their autonomous desire as adults, feeling confident in themselves as they feel themselves to be adults among adults of the same age – in short, they need to preserve their narcissism. The possible regression of adult guardians faced with the archaic desire of the child explains why *it is unthinkable to train psychoanalysts who would only be child psychoanalysts. A child psychoanalyst has to be first and also an adult psychoanalyst.*

This is what makes it necessary for an analyst to accept in certain cases to listen to the discourse (or the silence) of a child and to work in the presence of one of the parents, as long as he desires a protective presence with regard to the adult that we are. As the child agrees to come to the analyst and to stay during the session, it means he agrees to be helped – but not to the detriment of his relationship with his parents, so long as he doesn't feel totally secure towards us, that is to say while he is not sure that we respect him as his parents' child, and through him those parents that are his, as they are, without trying to separate him from them while he is still stuck to them, nor to modify their behaviour towards him.

The requirement to be an adult psychoanalyst is imposed in relation to the decision whether or not to accept into treatment a child brought for symptoms that worry his doctor, his parents and his educators, while the child himself so far suffers from nothing, no doubt precisely because of these symptoms. The preliminary sessions with the parents, together or separately, without the child present, can in themselves improve considerably the state of the child, which leads us to understand that one or other of the parents, or both within their relationship, are anxious because of a personal neurosis and, by not speaking of their anxiety, provoked the reactional syndrome in the child. Eight out of ten times, the subject for treatment is not the child but the parents or someone older than him in his entourage for whom the child is, unbeknownst to them or him, the 'reactant' that alerts the family.

In the case where a child is indeed personally affected by an irreversible disorder of which he suffers, it is important that his parents remain his main educators, animated from day to day by a pedagogic project and a desire for the child to find his way. The role of the psychoanalyst is different – he does not deal directly with reality but only with what the child perceives of it, related in the present to his past libidinal history.

The point of decoding the body image through the plastic and graphic images produced by the child is to understand how he can start a language-based communication, and truly express himself with an adult without talking to him. Adults often react when faced with a child who does not talk with an 'oh, you've lost your tongue?' – without understanding that precisely, this child cannot give tongue with him or her. Even without distrust (if the parents do not experience it), the child here does not yet feel safe with an adult who is an unknown quantity with regard to whether he/she knows and respects the free game between the parents and their child, and the parents' relationship with each other and the child's relationship with them.

A person who demands that he (the child) talk, although he doesn't know her and is still engaged in the primacy of his relationship with his parents – this person is experienced as violating and kidnapping with regard to the child's desire and words that the child doesn't have to give. She would be even more so if, through seduction, she wanted to 'play' with the child or if, without the child being aware of the profession of this adult to whom his parents take him, she behaved as if she had rights over his person – under the pretext that his parents wish that he starts a relationship with her, while still a stranger to him, and while he still hasn't understood why and how she is to help him.

Body image and life and death drives

For a human being, the body image is at any moment the immanently unconscious representation wherefrom arises his desire. Following Freud, I think that
the drives that aim at the satisfaction of desire are both life and death drives. Life
drives are always linked with a representation and may be active or passive, while
death drives – the resting place of the subject – are always lacking representation
and neither active nor passive. They are lived in a lack of ideation. Death drives
prevail in deep sleep, dissociative absences and coma. This is a desire not for
death but for rest.

Death drives are characterised as being without representations that contain the
residual representations of erotic relations with an other. They are a fact of a body
that is not responsive to desire. Death drives often incite the subject to retire from
all erotic images, as in deep sleep, or the fainting fits that follow a very strong
emotion, and also as in the secondary enuresis or encopresia that appear in a child
who has already become continent, and in whom the bodily schema has acquired
the continence natural to all mammals. Such a child, confronted with an emotional state that he cannot assimilate into his body image and the ethos[9] that goes
along with it – a state that cannot be represented within his narcissism – resorts
to putting to sleep either an image of the body's functioning or an image of an
erogenous zone, here the urethral or anal zones.

And so he sleeps not like the 3-year-old child he is now, but like the child
he had been before acquiring the diurnal and nocturnal continence of the bodily
schema of a 3 year old. Thus, he can lose, by the death drive, in the course of
his waking and sleeping life, this continence which is after all as I say acquired
spontaneously by all mammals; he can lose it because of a desire he forbids himself, which causes him to return during his sleep to an archaic body image. It is
during sleep that his continent bodily schema can be neutralised by the revival of
a libidinal period characterised by subject-to-subject relations, in which the baby
human (man-cub)[10] was for a long time neurologically immature and therefore
incontinent. Sleep is marked by the prevalence of death drives and the putting to
sleep – literally – of life drives (except in dreams[11]).

The body image is always, at least in fantasy, an image of potential communication. There is no human solitude that is not accompanied by the memory of

---

9 Translator's note: Dolto uses the word *l'ethique* quite frequently, but those who worked closely
with her have confirmed that she used it without any moral connotations and that it should not
be translated as 'ethic.' Her use of *l'ethique* is much closer to the English *ethos*, and describes
a prevailing set of behaviours, attitudes and 'givens' of an entity endowed with intentions and
capabilities.

10 Translator's note: Dolto uses the term *'petit d'homme'* to emphasise the specificity of human
babies, as compared with young animals. 'Man-cub,' borrowed from Kipling's *The Jungle Book,*
conveys this idea.

11 In dreams, the subject does not communicate with the real object but with the fantasmatic or introjected object. Dreams are the guardians of sleep.

past contact with an other, who is anthropomorphised if not real. A solitary child is always present to himself by way of a fantasy of a past relationship, real and generative of narcissism, between himself and an other with whom he had in reality a relationship he has introjected. He fantasises this relationship, as the baby in its cradle made present its mother by his babbling, believing he was repeating phonemes he had heard from her and thus deceived, no longer feels alone but that he is for and with her.

The small child's world view conforms with and depends upon his current body image. Therefore, it is by way of the body image as intermediary that we can enter into contact with him.

From birth, words and phonemes have accompanied contacts perceived by the child's body. The words with which we think originate from the words and groups of words that accompany images of the body in contact with the body of another. These words are heard and understood by the child differently according to the stage he has arrived at. It is therefore necessary that we psychoanalysts understand that the words used by children are words that correspond with a sensory experience that has been or is in the course of being symbolised. It is obvious that the word 'love' does not express the same thing to a 6-month-old baby in its oral phase as it does to an adult who has arrived at the genital phase. The child whose body image is at the oral phase can only understand words relating to the pleasure of the mouth and the held body, those that relate to oral functioning and eroticism, and to a body whose bodily schema that is not yet autonomous.

A little girl of 5 or 6 years came to a consultation having for two years held nothing with her hands: partial death drives had made her upper members absent from her body image. Whenever an object was presented to her, she would curl her fingers into her hands, her hands into her forearms and her forearms to her chest, so that her hands would not touch the approaching object. At the same time, this child could eat from plates when she saw food she liked. I held out to her some plasticine and said, 'You can take this with your mouth-hand.' Immediately, the plasticine was seized by the child's hand and conveyed to her mouth. She could understand 'mouth-hand' because it used words that fitted with her oral eroticism. She did not react when I just held the plasticine out to her. She would not have reacted either if I had said, 'Take the plasticine with your hand,' or 'Make something with this,' as these words would imply a body image at an anal phase she had lost. For her, these words no longer connected a body image with a bodily schema and would have remained empty of meaning for her. In a way, I invoked for her the fantasised mediation of the mouth, the erogenous zone kept for taking in and surviving, which allowed her to use her hand. While the only hand she had was her mouth, I used words to evoke a mouth in her hand, which gave her back an arm that relayed her hand of mouth-arm to the hand-mouth of her face, also lost to her. Her bodily schema and her body image having regressed when it had to do with 'taking' (but not with walking) to a time when it was not yet interwoven with action and doing, which belongs to anal eroticism. Her ethos was based on edible/inedible, containing/contained, pleasant/unpleasant, good/bad. The notion of a palpable form was dominated by the tactile, labial, auditive, visual and olfactive perceptions of the oral phase; the perception of volume only comes at the anal phase.

Inscribed in the body image are relational experiences of need and desire, valuing and/or devaluing, which is to say narcissising or de-narcissising. The valuing/devaluing sensations are shown as a symbolisation of variations in perception of the bodily schema, and more particularly of those that induce interhuman encounters, among which the contact and speech of the mother is predominant.

The body image and the id

Let us underline this: *the body image is on the side of desire; it does not relate only to need.* As the body image can pre-exist, but does coexist with all the subject's expressions, it bears witness to the lack of being that desire seeks to fill, where need seeks to satisfy a lack of having (or doing) in the bodily schema. *The study of the body image insofar as it is the symbolic substrate could contribute to clarifying the term 'id'* – on the condition that one adds that this is about an id that is first and foremost in a relationship with a part object necessary to the survival of the body, a relationship linked with a former relationship with a whole object, and one that has been transferred from this object to another, either part or whole.[12] The body image is an already-relating id, an id that is not foetal but already taken up in a body situated in space, given autonomy by dint of being a space-occupying mass, an id a part of which constitutes a pre-ego – that of a child capable of surviving temporary separation from the body of an other. The drives, emanating from the biological substrate structured in the form of a bodily schema, can in effect express themselves in fantasy, as in a transferential relationship, only by means of the body image. *If the place and source of the drives is the bodily schema, the place for their representation is the body image.* However, the elaboration of this body image can only be studied in children in the course of the structuration of their bodily schema in relation to their adult carer – *as what we call the body image is later repressed, in particular because of the discovery of the scopic body image and then by Oedipal castration.* In the course of the first three or four years of life, the body image is constituted in reference to olfactive, visual, auditory and tactile experiences that have the value of communicating with others at a distance without body-to-body contact – firstly with the mother and then with others present in his entourage. When nobody is there, when there is a new sensory experience in the absence of any human witness, it is theoretically only the bodily schema that is affected. But, in practice, this sensory experience is for the subject recovered by the memory of an already known symbolic relationship.

---

12 What I call a 'whole object' is a living being in its entirety – tree, animal or human being. What I call a 'part object' is a part that represents this whole object by which the subject can enter into a mediated relationship with the whole object.

Fantasy, desire, reality, need

For example, a child who bumps himself against a table believes it to be wicked, and expects the table to console him for the hurt it has caused. He projects onto the table a body image. It is only because of his mother's speech that he comes to discriminate between things and people. Up until then, people are to him just masses against which he could bump himself but that then console him, while a table is a mass against which he could bump but that doesn't console him and doesn't react, however much he howls at and hits it. On the other hand, as soon as there is a human witness, real or memorised, the bodily schema (place of need), which constitutes the body in its organic vitality, links up with body image (the place of desire). It is this interweaving of relations that is going to allow the child to structure himself as human. Later on, the human relationships thus introjected will allow the narcissistic relationship with himself (secondary narcissism).

To return to the previous example, when the same child later bumps against a table, it is his own hand that touches and caresses him, and it is he who comforts his hurt body – he no longer expects that things behave with intentions. He introjects the experience of the difference between a thing and a living body, in this case his own – the thing, his mother's body and the table object. He has transferred into his own hand the capacity of a salving and comforting action that only his mother could have performed when he was small and hurt himself against things. This introjection allows him to self-mother.

It is in the measure in which the body image is thus structured by intersubjective relations that any interruption of this relation and communication could have dramatic effects. The nursling who waits two weeks for his mother's return expects her to be just the same as when she left. When she returns after 15 days, he sees her as 'other,' and he too has become other in his reality. This is where autism can set in, because he cannot re-find with this other the sensation of the him of 15 days ago; he doesn't retrieve in his mother either the same mother as before nor the same 'himself.' It can also be this kind of change that is traumatising in his view of his mother returning from having a baby: she no longer has a baby in her tummy, as she did when she left; and although this is what the child expected without knowing that he expected it – he did not expect that she would return with a nursling. From what he had been told – that he would be getting a little brother or sister – he expected her to return with a child his own age.

His fantasy of the expected is not what happens in reality. The sometimes-pathogenic effect of the discordance between the imaginary and reality is what psychoanalysis operates on. All children have constantly to adjust their fantasy, deriving from past relations, to the unpredictable experience of what happens in reality, which differs either completely or in part from the fantasy. This constant adjustment accompanies the continuing growth of the bodily schema in the face of the reality of adults whose form appears to him perfect, immutable (all change in them is to him bizarre) and desirable. As we have said, the body image is about desire and not only about need.

The constant repetition of the ways in which need is experienced, followed by the almost complete forgetting of the tensions that came with it, underlines the fact that the human being experiences more narcissistically the feelings of desire linked with his body image than the sensations of pleasure and suffering linked with the excitation of his bodily schema (except, it is true, in limited cases where life is in danger or where, in children, the region in which there is tension is narcissistically over-invested by fantasies shared with the tutelary adult, especially if they remain unexpressed by either party).

Only desire always seeks satisfaction, without ever achieving it, by theoretically limitless expressions in speech, images and fantasy. Need can only be 'stalled' by speech for a little while; it has to be satisfied in the body. With or without pleasure, it has to be effectively filled so that the life of the body can continue. It is by these two processes – the tensions of pain or pleasure in the body on the one hand and on the other the words of an other that humanise these perceptions – that the bodily schema and the body image relate to each other.

Constructed in the language relationship with others, the body image constitutes the means, the bridge for interhuman communication. It is this that explains, conversely, why living in a bodily schema without a body image is living mute, solitary, silent, narcissistically insensitive, at the limits of human distress – the autistic or psychotic subject remains the captive of an incommunicable image, an animal, vegetal or thing-image that can only manifest itself as an animal-being, vegetal-being or thing-being, breathing and pulsing without pleasure or suffering. One observes this in children who, mute about themselves, seem to ignore their sensations or thoughts, and can only express themselves by lending their voice to a doll, a cat or a puppet.[13]

It is through speech that past desires could be organised into a body image, that past memories could affect zones of the bodily schema, which become by this fact erogenous zones, even while the object of desire is no longer present. I wish to emphasise the fact that *if words have not been given, the body image does not structure the subject's symbolism, and he becomes a relational idiot.*

In this case, there is all the same *a* body image but a very archaic one – a fleeting, hazy image without words to represent it so that it cannot be communicated to anyone. Such a subject is awaiting symbolisation. He can express nothing of his body image; he cannot express it in his facial expressions. He can only express a silly or alert stupefaction, awaiting meaning. Meaning is given by language, which forms a bridge for the sharing of emotions between two subjects of which at least one speaks of his feelings, is a person. These two subjects communicate by their body images, which are in a complementary relationship. If this is lacking for any reason, the subject remains apparently retarded, because his body image is without the mediation of language.

13 See '*Cure Psychoanalytique a l'aide de la poupee-fleur*' – *Au Jeu du Desir*, ibid.

Retardation in question; schizophrenia[14] in question

Perhaps it is too much to speak of learning disability, as we are not sure in effect that learning disability exists. What exists is the interruption of communication for reasons that in each case remain to be deciphered. Even when there is speech or sounds, if they do not signify for the child subject the communication of a person with his person, there can be a sort of breach in symbolisation that could result in schizophrenia.

In cases of apparently clinical learning disability, the potential for symbolising the body image is asleep. In the case of schizophrenics, this potentiality for symbolising the body image has been interrupted at a certain point, and as there were no words coming from the person with whom there was a love relationship with a structuring effect, the child symbolises for himself everything he experiences in a code that is no longer communicable. And that derives from what was never addressed to his person, or because what was said or what he heard were words that were not felt – I mean, words not in conformity with the emotion they were supposed to express, noise-words, without true emotional value, not humanely charged with intention, capable of communicating life and love (or hate) of the subject who was talking to the child and to whom the child spoke. All other perceptions, be it of words, examples, communications, not coming from a known accomplice, are experienced as noises of words, sensorial perception deprived of meaning for his body image, and again he is reduced as before the dawn of knowledge to a bodily schema – that of the moment at which he becomes schizophrenic. This bodily schema, separated from the body image, creates a rupture in space and time – one could say a fault-line at which the child tips over into the imaginary of a desire dissociated from its possible realisation. His desire no longer has a representation that is credible and aimed at comforting the narcissism of a subject in communication with another subject.

Thus, a noise coming from outside seems to him to be a response to a present bodily experience; the whole world of things is in a conversation with him but not the world of humans. The relationship with the other has become a danger because the other let him go – or did he let go of the other? Whoever started it, he is lost and cannot understand himself. He withdraws into himself and establishes within himself a code of language – delusional for us – which for him gives

14 Translator's note: Dolto uses the word *la schizophrenie* to mean what today in the English-speaking world is usually called autism. In France during her time, clinicians distinguished between two forms of severe developmental pathologies: autism and infantile schizophrenia. Autistic children had no or very little communicative language while the others had. In the 1970s, the term schizophrenia was replaced by *psychose infantile* (early childhood psychosis), but the distinction between that and autism continued to be made. Dolto's use of the term reflects the period at which she practiced. Because of these two possible English translations of *la schizophrenie* (autism and early childhood psychosis), I have chosen to retain the word schizophrenia.

meaning to what he experiences; he 'unspeaks' producing phonemes that are not a meaningful assembling of words.

One can understand why a troupe of mime artists who performed in a psychiatric hospital before an audience that included psychotics felt better understood than when performing before the general public.

Body image and the intelligibility of the language of gestures and words

The mime artist who translates body images is immediately intelligible for the psychotic or schizophrenic, who does not read the mime show linguistically. He does not, like the general public, put words to what he sees. The mime show speaks directly to his body image.[15]

Generally, the comprehension of a word depends on both the individual's bodily schema and the constitution of his body image linked with the lively exchanges that accompanied for him the integration, the acquisition of that word. Indeed, words have a symbolic meaning in themselves, beyond time and space, that reunites human beings, who even without any shared experience can transmit in a spoken, recorded or written communication the fruits of language acquired by them in the interweaving of their body image and their bodily schema. But he who has neither the body image nor the bodily schema that corresponds with the uttered words hears the word without understanding it, due to the lack of a relationship of body image to bodily schema that gives it meaning.

Someone blind from birth can, for example, talk about colours, pronounce the words 'blue,' 'red' and 'green' – words that make an image that take on meaning for a sighted interlocutor (as, for him, the scopic perceptions have contributed to the constitution of a body image); inevitably, the person born blind knows nothing of the meaning of his words. More precisely, the signifiers for colours cannot bring together for him the body image of a sighted person with the bodily schema of a blind one. Every one of us has, thus, a narcissised relationship (bound up with narcissism) with sensorial elements that resonate with words in our vocabulary.[16] Nobody can know, even among sighted people, when someone says blue, of

15 Let's observe that mime is not always interesting for healthy children, while clowns are. This is because the mimed behaviours of the clowns are connected with archaic images of the body, oral and anal, while the behaviours mimed by mime artists are often linked with feelings and behaviours of a human eroticism post-anal and genital castration, i.e. connected with a post-Oedipal body image and with an ethos in tune with social morality. This is not the case of clowns, who wait for a signal from the ringmaster to stop their playful anal and oral erotic fantasmatic elucubrations.

16 Thus, may we understand how an analysand reacts to an interpretation of the analyst by resisting it, saying it is incomprehensible. It is true that the terms used by the analyst may refer to body images that the patient has repressed, obliging him to dismiss an explanation, a question or an intervention that refers to it, and this even if the analyst has taken up words already used by the analysand because these terms do not evoke the same mental links or affects as for the analyst. This is sometimes the cause of an abrupt rupture in the transference relationship that is irrecoverable and necessitates a change of analyst.

which blue he is speaking. It is only when the interlocutors seek among the blues, the blue of which each is speaking, that they can notice whether they are indeed talking of the same blue.

The person born blind has no body image formed by his eyes – he has a bodily schema, he knows he has eye-organs, but he has no relational image formed by vision. This does not stop him from using signifiers of vision. I have had such blind people in analysis who often say, 'I saw him' or 'I didn't see him.'

> 'What do you mean by "you saw him"?'
> 'Yes, he came to the house.'
> 'But you heard him. Why do you say "I saw him"?'
> 'Because everyone says that!'

Although he has never seen a colour, the blind person has heard others talking of colours, of cold colours and warm colours, of the intensity, beauty, sadness and gaiety associated with colours by those who see them; he can make an auditory and emotional connection with colours in his relationship with other people. Auditory and also tactile, calorific.

It is the same for the child, who when speaking about his teacher, says, 'She is not nice, she is green! The other class has a blue teacher, I'd rather be with them!' (while both teachers are wearing white gowns!).

The case of the person born blind allows us indirectly to understand what it means for a child who cannot, because of his immature bodily schema, register the affect underlying certain words spoken by adults by means of the encounter between the sensory experience and his body image. He hears and repeats these words at their invitation. While resembling an adult in his language, the child does not, unlike the adult, possess in relation to what he says a fantasised body image, an afterglow of personally lived experiences, corresponding in meaning to these words as for the adult.

To become meaningful, the words must first be embodied, be metabolised in a relational body image. This is the case for the adult, who has in principle passed through the phase of genital castration, and speaks of a field of experience relating to his sexually adult body, his bodily schema and inter-relational perceptions as he knows them – all unknowable for the child. When the latter takes into his language words he has heard from an adult, they are for him representative of an erogeneity other than that to which the adult might allude.

Body image and the particular case of the given name

Of all the phonemes, of all the words heard by the child, there is one that is of primordial importance, ensuring the narcissistic cohesion of the subject – it is his given name. From birth, this name – linked with the body and to the presence of the other – contributes in a deterministic way to the structuration of the body images, including the most archaic images. The given name(s) is/are the phoneme(s) that accompany the world of the senses of the child firstly in his relationship with his parents, then with others, from birth to death. Even in a deep sleep, it is the speaking of the given name that can awaken a subject; if he is in a coma and is called by his first name, he opens his eyes. The given name is the first and last phoneme connected with his life, and which supports it because it was from birth the signifier of his relationship with his mother, on the condition obviously that she did not call him sweetums, munchkin, boo-boo or poppet for a long time. While the given name accompanies the subject beyond Oedipal castration and is reprised by everyone in society, the nickname that might be given by the mother to her baby should be abandoned at the time of weaning or sphincter control.

All this explains why one cannot, without serious risk, change the given name of a child.

The case of Frederick

I had in treatment a child who, having been abandoned after birth by his biological parents, was placed in a residential nursery and adopted at the age of 11 months. At the time, the adoptive parents gave him a new name – Frederick – different from the one he had had until then, but this was not mentioned by his mother during the meetings preliminary to the therapy. Frederick was 7 years old when I saw him for a session, and came with symptoms that appeared psychotic. The start of the psychoanalytic treatment led to the discovery that he had a hearing difficulty. He was fitted with hearing aids, and with the help of the psychotherapeutic work, his intelligence awoke and his sphincter incontinence was resolved.

He began to become a perfect fit with the rest of his age group, but at school refused to read and was unable to write. I observed however that he used letters, and in particular the letter 'A,' which he distributed everywhere, written in all directions in his drawings.

> 'Is this an A?'
> He nods, yes.
> I repeat the question: 'And this one?' (an upside-down A).
> He answered with a yes, breathing in while he always talked with the sound emitted when breathing out.
> The teacher wrote to me to say that he was taking part in all activities but was refusing to learn to write or read.

I researched who could have been designated by these 'A's because there was no one in his family whose given name started with this letter. The interpretation that it could be the matron of the clinic, whose name started with an A, had no effect. The adoptive mother then revealed to me what I didn't know: that the child, when she had adopted him, bore the given name of Armand. This allowed me to interpret to the child that it could be Armand that he is signifying in his drawings with all these As; that he has possibly suffered from this change in given name at the time of his adoption – an adoption of which he had been informed very early. But this interpretation didn't give any result.

It is then – and this is testimony to the importance of the analyst's body image, because what follows was not thought through by me – that after a moment of silent waiting in which the child was drawing or playing with plasticine and I was thinking, it came to me to call out, without looking at him or addressing his physical presence in front of me, in a high pitched voice with different tones and intensity, turning my head in every direction, to the ceiling, under the table . . . as if I was calling someone whose location in space was unknown to me: 'Armand! Armand! Armand!'

The witnesses at this public consultation at Trousseau saw the child listening, his ears pricked up, towards every corner of the room. With neither of us looking at the other, I mimed this search for an 'Armand' and for a moment, the child's eyes met my gaze and I said, 'Armand – this was your name when you were adopted.' Here, I perceived in his gaze an exceptional intensity. The subject Armand, de-nominated, could reconnect his body image to that of Frederick, the same subject so named at 11 months. What had taken place was an unconscious process: he needed to hear this name not spoken in a normal voice – mine, a voice he knew – which addressed him in his body, here, now, in the space of present reality, but said by a placeless voice, a falsetto voice, a voice 'off,' as they say today, calling out to him. It was that kind of unknown mothering voice that he had heard when people talked to him or called him when he was at the residential nursery. It was this reunion in the transference onto me, his psychoanalyst, of an archaic identity, lost since the age of 11 months, that allowed him to overcome in the following two weeks his difficulties in reading and writing.

The enormous significance of the most archaic phonemes of which a given name is the typical example, shows that *the body image is the structural trace of a human being's emotional history. It is the unconscious lieu (and where to be found?) whence every expression of the subject is elaborated: the place where interhuman language-based feelings are received and given out.* The durability of its cohesion is drawn from the attention and the style of love lavished on the child. It goes without saying, therefore, that the body image depends on an emotional trade with the mother and relatives. It is a structure that results from the intuitive process of organising pre-genital affective and erotic relationships and fantasy. Fantasy here means the olfactory, gustative, auditory, visual, tactile, baresthetic and coenesthetic[17] memorisation of subtle, weak or intense perceptions, felt as the language of desire of the subject in relation to an other: perceptions that accompanied the variations of substantial tensions in the body and notably among the last, feelings of satisfaction or tension due to vital needs.

17 Translator's note: Baresthetic refers to the sensation of external pressures on the body, and coenesthetic to sensations generated internally within the body.

The three dynamic aspects of the same body image

As the body image is not a natural, anatomic 'given,' as may be the bodily schema, but one that on the contrary is elaborated in the history of the subject, *we have to study how it is constructed and reshaped in the course of the child's development*. This is what leads us to distinguish three modes of functioning of the same body image: *the basal image, the functional image and the erogenous image, which together constitute and assure the living body image and the subject's narcissism at each stage of his development*. They are permanently connected with each other and their cohesion is maintained by what we call the dynamic image (or rather substratum), designating by this the subjective metaphor of life drives that, springing from biological sources, are continuously held in tension by the subject's desire to communicate with another subject with the help of a sensorially signified part object.

Basal image

The first component in the body image is the basal image. The basal image is what allows a child to feel a sameness of being, a narcissistic continuity or a spatio-temporal continuity that stays and expands from birth, despite the changes in his life and the displacements imposed on his body and in spite of the trials to which he is subjected. This is how I define narcissism: a 'sameness of being,' known and recognised, and the 'going-on-becoming'[18] true to the essence of his sex for each person.

It is from this perpetual sameness, strong or weak, that the notion of existence arises. The feeling of existing of a human being who moors his body to his narcissism comes from this conviction, probably illusory, of continuity. This is why, conversely, eclipses of narcissism open up a number of aberrations for the balance of a human being. This is where functional disturbances and dysregulation are located that we may interpret as real 'drops' or flaws in narcissism, prone to causing injury to organs by way of heart attacks or sudden ulcers at moments of emotional shock by means of death drives localised in regions of the body.

But if narcissism is continuity, it has nonetheless a history and is nonetheless susceptible to rearrangement, which obliges us to distinguish different phases in it. And as I am at the moment talking about the basal image, I have to add that it is fundamentally 'in reference to' and 'constitutive of' what I call primordial narcissism; by this, I mean the 'narcissism of the subject' – *the subject of the desire for life, which pre-exists his conception*. It is what animates the call for life in an ethos that supports the subject in desiring. It is what makes the child the symbolic

---

18   Translator's note: Based upon Winnicott's concept of 'going-on-being,' Dolto developed her own idea of 'going-on-becoming' to describe the continuity of the processes of development.

heir of the desire of the progenitors who conceived him. This ethos of the foetus is linked with the enjoyment of the daily growth of the fleshly mass; it is an ethos of vampiric addition, an ethos of amassing, of taking; and because this ethos is about placental blood, it appears later on, in phantasmatic memory, as a vampiric[19] period.

In a way, this primordial narcissism constitutes a lived intuition of being in the world for an individual of the species, although deprived of all means of expression, as is the child in utero. The signifier is what gives a sense of social identity, which is symbolic. In this resides, as we have underlined, the value and the importance of the given name that, at the moment of the transition from foetus to nursling, is received by the subject from his responsible adults, linked with the body that is now visible to others, and that certifies for him, in reality, his existential permanence; *proof, while he can recognise himself in the phonemes of this word, of the dominance of his life instincts over his death instinct.*

Damage or alteration of the basal image must immediately give rise to a representation, a fantasy, that threatens life itself. This fantasy is not however the product of death instincts, which are about vital inertia, and especially are without representation. When the basal image is threatened, a phobic state appears, which is a specific defence mechanism against a danger felt to be persecutory, the representation of this persecutory fantasy being itself linked with the erogenous zone prevalent at that time for the subject. He therefore reacts to whatever is threatening his basal image with a persecutory fantasy that may be visceral, umbilical, respiratory, oral or anal – of being punctured, of bursting – according to the moment of the first trauma experienced in his own history.

This means that each stage modifies the representations that the child may have of his basal image; otherwise stated, *there is a basal image that belongs to each stage*. Thus, what appears after birth is firstly a respiratory-olfactory-auditory basal image (cavum and thorax) – the first aerial basal image. This is followed by an oral basal image that includes not only the first respiratory-olfactory-auditive image, but also all of the buccal zone, the pharyngeo-larynx zone – from the nasopharyngeal zone to the thorax – that links the image of the stomach, the representation of fullness or emptiness of the stomach (which may be hungry or satisfied) and that could resonate with foetal sensations of hunger or satisfaction of the stomach.

The third basal image, which is the anal basal image, adds to the first two a retentive or expulsive function of the lower part of the digestive tract and also the body mass around it constituted by the pelvic girdle, with a tactile representation of the buttocks and the pelvic floor.

19 Vampiric of a pretended other on which the foetus would be a parasite; however, the placenta is his, elaborated by the fertilised egg itself, as are the amniotic envelopes. Expressions like 'taking it upon yourself' to get out of a state of weakness or 'turning in on oneself' to retrieve a cohesive peace are unconscious references to this time or epoch.

We will keep returning to what is a truly relational architecture, but that is only a relational architecture if the nurturing mother talks while giving care to the child: an architecture centred on the localities of erogenous pleasure (in particular but not exclusively the orifices of the body), which are always linked with a functional place where perception is expected, sometimes called for by screams, and expectations are satisfied or refused by the nursing mother.

Nowhere better than at the level of the basal image and of primordial narcissism can the conflict between life and death drives[20] be grasped, the latter of which could prevail for a long time in a baby, when the mother (or human environment) treats the newborn as a package, an object of care, without talking to him as a person.

I would like to illustrate the above with an example.

The case of Gilles, the restless child

The principal symptom of an 8-year-old enuretic boy, Gilles, was an extreme restlessness – he found it impossible to stay in one place. His family and school had difficulty tolerating him. He was not a bad child; he had no friends and no enemies. All remonstrations and punishments seemed to slide off him.

In sessions, he never stopped looking around every corner of the room. His restless eyes hardly stopped moving while he was drawing, and as soon as he moved, he resumed looking all around him. As the treatment had much improved him and his enuresis had stopped, I told him that we would be stopping the psychotherapy. It was in what was planned to be the last session that he said to me: 'Now, I can say where the danger is' – 'Because you are leaving?' – 'Yes.'

He explained to me, with the help of his drawings, that the salient and re-entrant angles, the angles of the walls and furniture, were in his fantasies like shooting arrows. The bisectors of the angles were the arrow shafts, and the problem was that if he was at the meeting point of three arrows, at their intersection, he risked being pierced from all directions and would die on the spot. Before his treatment, the danger was everywhere; afterwards, it was only in his analyst's office.

We were able to understand later, as we decided to continue for a few more sessions, that this haunting by murderous angles was linked with the signifier 'English' – *anglais*. This Parisian child had been 3 years old during the evacuation of 1940. It was at this moment that his bodily schema underwent its first

---

20 I take this opportunity to suggest it is a mistake to mix up death drive and aggressive drive, active or passive. In death drives, no aggressive drives can slip in, be they active or passive. These drives, active and passive, whatever the body image in which they are experienced, are always serving the libido, and therefore the desire to live of a subject in a relationship with the external world, which aims to satisfy the sexual drives of the current stage until their complete satisfaction. All through existence, some death drives compete with life drives, as night follows day, and they triumph precisely during our natural sleep when all and sundry are submitted to the primacy of death drives, thanks to the body, anonymous, resting from the demands of the desire of the subject.

real test – he was in an accident with his family in a car driven by his father who was taking them to refuge with his relatives in the Midi. And soon afterwards, at the seaside, he had almost drowned after escaping from his father, who had been trying to teach him to swim (he was resuscitated by artificial respiration). The psychoanalysis of the child thus brought back memories forgotten by all, but of which the parents, surprised by his recollection, had to confirm the accuracy. Following these events, Gilles could no longer bear to be separated from his mother and was always 'stuck' to her, constantly between her legs. And he was there in reality in a phone booth during a telephone conversation between his mother and her brother, a dramatic conversation in which the brother, after the call of the 18 June said that he was leaving for England to join up with De Gaulle in London. This created in his mother a heavy load of anxiety; she was very attached to her brother and there were grave risks ahead for him. In addition, she was afraid that her son, having been able to hear the conversation, would be able to repeat the content, while his father's job required him and his family to return to the occupied zone. In fact, from that moment, all the unspoken things within the family and the preoccupation of the parents revolved for the child around these words – 'English' and 'England': 'Angle-taire' – 'angle' plus 'unsaid' equalling 'lethal danger,' if the Germans who used two rooms in the house and whom the child often met, learned about it.

It was thus at the session planned by both me and him to be the last one, that all these elements, unknown to me and totally forgotten by the parents, could reappear: the basal body image of that child, so phobic and anxious, had been eroticised as far as the olfactory sense, under his mother's skirt, by the odour of her anxiety while she was talking to his godfather, whom he adored; he perceived the emotion that this separation caused in his mother, while the mother, leaving the phone booth, thought it best not to say a word to her son about what had been exchanged between her and her brother and that she hoped that the 3-year-old child had not understood.

That moment had left to him the words 'Anglais,' 'Angle-taire' as the signifiers of great emotions and of danger, as much for the body as for 'what is said that must not be said.' Because at this time, two successive incidents with the father spelled danger (car accident and risk of drowning), the child's ideal-ego had regressed towards the mother – then the only safe and protective adult image – and towards a secondary loss of sphincter continence.

This intense moment of his childhood history during its Oedipal organisation, threatened by his mother's two men – the father and the maternal uncle – had remained encysted under the shape of the threat coming from the bisector of angles, which were armed with the arrows of vectors (images of anal and urethral sexual zones), fantasmatically persecutory for the basal body image of the child. His body in its spatial mass (anal functional body image) was trying to master the phobia due to the sexual drive through motor instability, the erogenous urethral–anal zone being represented in space by the *anglais* and their supposed arrows rather than being located first in the anus and then in the penis, master of continence of the urinary flow and assuming erections, which had become forbidden as nesting in his mother was his only refuge, at least in imagination (in almost hallucinatory fantasies of living inside the earth and sleeping in a country named by him 'La Lifie').

The functional image

The second component of the body image after the basal image is the functional image.

While the basal image has a static dimension, the functional image is the highly energetic image of a subject that aims to achieve its desire. Desire is aroused when a specific lack is felt through the mediation of an erogenous zone in the bodily schema. It is thanks to the functional image that the life drives can, after having been subjectified in desire, manifest themselves for the obtaining of pleasure, and objectify themselves in relations with the world and others.

So, the functional anal body image of a child is first of all an image of expulsive emission, at the start in relation to the defecatory need to which the child submits and passively feels, and which may or may not acquire the status of language with the mother; and then secondarily, it takes the form of an image of an energetic expulsive expression in relation to a not always substantial part object, which can be transferred by displacement onto a more subtle part object. For example, the expulsion for pleasure of the pulmonary air column by modifying the shape of the opening and the emission of sounds, which allows the sublimation of anality into what is said in speech and in the modulation of the singing voice. One must understand that in contrast with just the activation of the erogenous zones, the elaboration of the functional image allows the enrichment of the possibility of relations with others.

The hand, for example, which is first a prehensile oral erogenous zone and then anally rejecting, has to integrate a brachial functional image, giving the child the skeletal-muscular freedom needed to reach his goals when used for the satisfaction of his needs and the expression of his desires through play. Conversely, when the functional image is wholly or partially denied, for example during a physically repressive or verbally castrating intervention that goes against the actions of the child ('don't touch!'), the child can choose as a way out a withdrawal response so that the erogenous zone does not enter into contact with the forbidden, dangerous object, and nor does his desire come into conflict with the desire of the tutelary adult.

Let's return to the example of the young girl with a phobia of touching, who could retrieve the grabbing function through my saying, 'Take this with your hand-mouth.' By these words I had 'feinted' around the tactile image; the child took the object, kidnapped it and immediately conveyed it to her mouth with her arm, which rather than staying folded against her body was able to extend itself to allow the hand to take – something she hadn't been able to do for months, as if she didn't know she had hands. I gave her back the possibility of an oral-anal functional image and some oral interest in anal things, which the body of a 20-month-old child would have. This child was nearly 3 and a half and according to what was said by those who knew her had been a playful and communicative child until the age of 2 and a half, when she experienced a series of derealisation-inducing traumas.

The erogenous image

The third component of the body image is the erogenous image.

Just in terms of presenting it, I would say that it is linked with a functional body image in the place at which is focused erotic pleasure and unpleasure in relation with an other. Its forms of representation may be circles, ovals, concavities, spheres, palps, lines and holes, imagined to be actively producing or receptively accepting of emissive intentions, to a pleasant or unpleasant end.

What is important is to describe how these three components of the body image may be metabolised, transformed and reshuffled, taking into account the trials and limitations confronting the subject, notably in the form of the symboligenic castrations[21] imposed upon him; to describe, therefore, how the vicissitudes of his history allow, in the best cases, that his basal image guarantees his narcissistic cohesion. For this, it is necessary:

1   That the functional image allows the bodily schema to be used in an appropriate way.
2   That the erogenous image opens the subject up to the path of shared pleasure, which is humanising in that it has a symbolic value and may be expressed in not only facial expressions and action but also words spoken by others, memorised in situ by the child, who may then use them knowingly when he speaks.

As we have previously indicated, the body image is the living synthesis, constantly coming into being, of three images – basal, functional and erogenous – linked by life drives, which are actualised for the subject in what I call the dynamic image.

The dynamic image

The dynamic image corresponds to the 'desire to be' and to persevere in becoming. This desire, being fundamentally marked by absence, is always open to the unknown. The dynamic image *therefore does not have a representation specific to it: it is the tension of intention*; its representation would be the word 'desire' conjugated as active, present and participant in the subject, as the incarnation of

---

21 See following chapter, p. 78 in original French text.

the verb 'to go' (in the sense of 'going-on-desiring'[22]) attached to each of the three images in active or potential communication. *The dynamic image expresses in each of us Being, wanting a Becoming; the subject in its right to desire, I would like to say 'in desiring.'*

If we want to decode a representative schema of this dynamic image, it would take the virtual form of a dotted line that leaves the subject by way of an erogenous zone of his body and goes towards the object; but this representation is very approximative. The dynamic image corresponds to an intensity of the expectation of reaching the object, and it appears indirectly in the ballistic images created by children with guns and cannons, which show these little dots leaving the guns or cannons that reach towards the targeted object. It is the trajectory of desire endowed with meaning, 'moving towards' a goal.

It appears again in another virtual form, very precociously in children's development (9 to 10 months): when interested in an image, they take a whirlwind 'tour' (later represented by them as a snail) around all the parts of the graphic representation interesting to them, before turning the page and looking for other things. And that is the image of the (enlivened) subject who feels dynamic, in a desiring state. These graphic traces punctuate its rhythm.

That we can find it in one or other of these two graphic forms makes it no less true that the dynamic image is that which is unrepresented and is, therefore, inaccessible to any castrating event. It can only be subtracted from the subject by a phobic state, the phobic object coming to obstruct the desiring trajectory of the dynamic image, threatening its very right to exist.

We can speak of an oral dynamic image that is centripetal[23] in relation to need and both centrifugal and centripetal as regards desire. We can speak of an anal dynamic image centrifugal in relation to need and both centripetal and centrifugal with regard to desire (the last being accomplished in the sodomy of another or in being sodomised by another in homosexuals).

The genital dynamic image is in women a centripetal image in its relation with the penile part object and in men a centrifugal dynamic image. In the act of giving birth, there is an expulsive centrifugal dynamic image in relation to the child, which is a subject and thereby the total object, while the newborn foetal body is a part object in the genital channels of a birthing woman, who will soon be vis-à-vis the subject and from the moment of its birth, the accepting or rejecting mother.

Let us refine what we mean by returning to the case of the oral–anal dynamic image. The complete image of the digestive body should conform with the bodily

22 Translator's note: Dolto uses an invented concept – '*allons-desirant*' – which is, like her '*allons-devenant*,' based upon the Winnicottian concept of 'going-on-being.' I have therefore translated it as 'going-on-desiring.' These new-minted expressions emphasise the continuity of development that Dolto sees as a fundamental aspect of being human.

23 Translator's note: Dolto uses the words centripetal and centrifugal to indicate movement towards a point of focus and away from a point of focus respectively – inwards or outwards.

schema, an always centripetal image in the sense of the peristaltic path from mouth to anus. When there are reversions of the peristaltic movement – as in the case of vomiting – it is the oral and not the anal image that is reversed, which means it is 'analised,' rejecting the ingested part object. It is reversed in relation to the other, the real or imaginary person present, or in relation to an object felt to be dangerous in the stomach.[24]

Such an example reveals the vitality of the dynamic image, which, in its linkage with desire, may go so far as to reverse the trajectory of the part object of need. Add to this a case of regressive damage to a genital dynamic image: this is about an adolescent who, feeling impotent and unable to have relationships with girls, became an obsessional masturbator. The desire for the object is substituted by a regression to the functional body image (the hand masturbating his penis), which becomes for him sufficient as a desired fantasy object that has nothing to do with the reality of an existing person. So, he enters into a sort of 'autism' connected with the genital relationship, which in reality makes him more and more inhibited and phobic with regard to encounters that would get him out of his isolation. The dynamic image is always that of a desire looking for a new object. In this way, it utterly contradicts auto-eroticism, which only happens to palliate the absence of a real object that fits with desire.

It can be seen at another level at the beginning of thumb-sucking, which happens at three months in children who are not chatted to by their carers after their feed; because if one talks to the child after the milk feed, puts objects to his hands and names them as he brings them to his mouth, if the mother – total object – names for him all these oral and visual tactile sensations of things he touches, tastes and throws away, the child has an experience of real pleasure shared with his mother and then, tired, falls asleep. After a few bottles, he doesn't suck his thumb any more. The thumb was only the tactile substitute for the nipple, part representation of the mother, the total object with whom the child wished to communicate the desire he had for her. Because the child has many dynamic potentialities for his libidinal drive, which searches for an encounter with an other who makes him feel his existence and his coming into being, he may, when experiencing a mother who disappears too quickly as an object of desire after the satisfaction of his need, put his hand in his mouth and in so doing satisfies those potentialities for his drive in the masturbatory lure of sucking his fingers. As the place of lack and its expression through cries has been cancelled, the child does not warn his mother by calling and, little by little, reaches the point where he does not expect anything from the presence of others. Every time he experiences a libidinal surge in the absence of an object, he contents himself with this transference, rightly called auto-erotic, onto a part object – his fist the stand-in for the breast, his thumb for the nipple; a part of his body becoming the illusory support of the decoy for the other. Thus, he

---

24 'He vomited his bottle, he threw up all I gave him.' (What mothers say). 'A performance to make you sick.'

enters into a compulsive symptom of an obsessional style, where his desire uses the body image, functioning for the sake of it. This symptom provides the repetition of the same bodily sensation through sensorial relationships with different part objects in reality, accompanied by different fantasies but without relational contact between subjects, and even less emotional, inter-relational and language relationships to be discovered anew every day.

Chapter 2

The body images and their destiny

The castrations

The evolution of the body images

Of the evolution of the body images, one could say that the difficulties they encounter are always reducible to the same scenario. *Desire, acting in the dynamic image, seeks fulfilment by way of the functional image and the erogenous image,* upon which it focuses to reach pleasure through the seizing of its object. But, in its quest, desire encounters obstacles to its realisation: either because the subject hasn't got enough desire, or because the object is absent, or again because the object is forbidden.

However, it must be said that it is first in the game of presence-absence of the object of desire, while this has not been exhausted, that this or that zone is instituted as erogenous.

In fact, desire always overwhelms need; the subtle places of perception – of the cavum, of hearing, of seeing, and later of the anus, vagina, penis – become erogenous zones, either from the fact of their contact with an appeasing part object relating to the mother (later a sexual partner), or from absence mediated by language in cases where the part object is lacking. Hence, the primordial and eminent importance of the mother, total object and subject, who expresses herself verbally, by gestures and by facial expressions and sounds, in communication with her child (while he elaborates his basic functional and erogenous images).

It is the mother who talks to her child about what he wants but that she does not give him, mediating for him the absence of a part object or the non-satisfaction of a demand for partial pleasure, while validating through the very fact that she recognises and talks about it, the desire for the satisfaction of which is being denied – a situation with which she sympathises. The erogenous zone can only be introduced in the language of speech after it has been totally deprived of the specific object by which it had been initiated into an erotic communication. And this is only possible if the same total object (the mother) vocalises the phonemes of words that specify this erogenous zone: 'Your mother's breast is now forbidden to you,' 'No, that's finished, no suckling' – words that allow the mouth and the tongue to regain their value in desire. This takes place because the erotic part object is evoked by the total object (mother) who deprives the child of the breast

DOI: 10.4324/9781003312499-3

he desires – but a child whose hunger and thirst has already been appeased by another means and who no longer 'needs' it.

Speech, because of its symbolic function, causes a mutation of the level of desire: from partial erotic satisfaction to a love relationship that involves subject-to-subject communication, or rather from a pre-subject (the infant) to the subject that is the mother, total object for her baby, who only knows the world and himself through her.

This is to say that in normal processes of the subjective elaboration of body images, words are exchanged, and this is what allows the symbolisation of objects of past enjoyment. As a result, the pre-linguistic transitional phonemes have something paranormal. Because the transitional part object, whatever it is, substantial or subtle, is both a perennial thing and the confused language of the child–mother or child–father relation – materialised language, a ghost of unspeakable words,[1] unconsciously conjugated with a sensorial Having that seems to vouch for the existence of Being in a passive state that would lead passively to the subject being.

The transitional object may be the lexicon of the words for which the child has no vocabulary, but it is indecipherable and promoted to represent the whole subject who has an intuition of his relational self as a potentially erogenous body-object and, in his functional relationship, is still fused with 'the mother' (the adult upon whom his survival depends).

Children who have sufficient expressions of love and playful freedom in motricity have no need of transitional objects. Whatever their desire for security, they have enough motor inventiveness associated with their mother and enough of verbal exchanges with her – she is sufficiently present – that they can renew their stock of language – audible transitional objects, perhaps – before linking up with situations and actions to become real words that he will keep in mind in moments of solitude and sleep.

The transitional object is an object that links children with the tactile images of the oral and olfactive basic, functional and erogenous zones; and with anal functional manipulative images of the time when, before becoming autonomous in walking, they were moved around by the adult. They displace onto these transitional objects the past relationships they had with adults in which they felt themselves to be part objects for these adults.

They need the transitional objects when in danger of being separated from the place of maternal safety, and while they are losing their anal functional image, that of motricity and walking, that is to say when they are put to bed (sometimes when they move house).

---

1 Translator's note: Dolto refers to transitional objects here as 'materialised language' and 'a ghost of unspeakable words,' suggesting that the transitional object is a materialisation (concretisation) of concepts already symbolised in language, which reverses, or perhaps mirrors, the original Winnicottian idea of the transitional object, which pre-exists full symbolisation and is a material object in which qualities are concretely represented as a step in the child's journey towards abstract symbolisation.

They then need an object, said to be transitional, one chosen among others, that represents the recollected relationship of themselves with the adult that made them feel safe when they were little – the adult whose potentially omnipotent role is had by the child vis-à-vis the thing that is the transitional object, an anti-danger fetish; a fetish that represents for the subject his communication with the security-giving other, in space, for the time it takes to fall into a deep sleep when the desire to communicate vanishes, as the drives of desire are taken over by the death drives.

Let us say in a very general way that if the mother attends to her child, his anxiety is humanised by her subtle perceptions and speech. This security-building exchange with his mother is for him proof of a lasting human relationship, beyond the wounds of the functional image or the threat of attack upon the basal image, and beyond the feelings of disturbance in the exchanges involved in the servicing of substantial needs that when disturbed leave the child feeling ill. He rediscovers with this perennial object his oral and anal body image, in its olfactive, tactile etc. aspects – a rediscovery of a primordially narcissistic knowledge of himself, which is the very basis of his health. The imaginary constant reciprocal communication between child and the biological and nursing mother is re-established and rediscovered, linked with the fantasmatic remnants of the first symbiosis – 'me–mum–the world.'

The child's body image thus re-established in its integrity keeps of his past suffering a symbolised experience of his life drives, as a subject co-existing with his body, which prevails over the death drive (falling asleep, illness). During a trial, the child, when helped by the mother and by the fact that he feels like the chosen object in her re-found arms, is vaccinated against anxiety so that he will find in subsequent trials that he is better armed than a baby who has never been so tested and helped. 'Medicine' takes into account the organic disorders of the child and allows the evaluation of the material and health conditions of the good physiological functioning that are in play for every human individual (educational, paediatric etc). Psychoanalysis has allowed us to discover that these interactions are the subtle supports of a narcissism that is indispensable to the recovery of emotional health, upon which is founded the prognosis of the psychosocial future of each particular child, borne of particular parents, and saved from physical dangers. As we can see, narcissism, which at the start of life appears to be linked with the euphoria of good health, is since birth interwoven with subtle language relations that are creative in the human sense, that originate from the mother and are maintained by her – a relationship that from the start of life cannot be interrupted for any length of time without danger.

The case of Agnes

Thus it was for this little girl, breastfed for the five days since her birth, whose mother had to be hospitalised when she became highly feverish due to a gynaecological intervention. In the days that followed, the baby wanted nothing that her father or aunt (who had been present in the home since her birth) could give her – neither water from a teaspoon nor milk from a bottle; her eating refusal was total. On the advice of the paediatrician, who was at a loss in this situation and who knew me, the father rang me up. I have to add that all this happened in the provinces during the war, and bringing her to see me was out of the question. I simply said to the anxious father: 'Go to the hospital, bring back the blouse that your wife is wearing in a way that keeps her smell on it. Put it around the baby's neck and give her the bottle.' The bottle was accepted at once!

It was my work on the concept of the body image that allowed me to have this idea and to make this suggestion. What was lacking for this baby in her mother's absence, for her to be able to swallow? She wasn't ill but had lost weight – she was hungry. Having suckled for three or four days, it could only have been the olfactory image of the mother, suddenly absent, that she missed. The subject's fundamental narcissism (which allows it to live) is rooted in these first repetitive relations that accompany respiration, the satisfaction of nutritional needs and of partial desires – of smell, sound, vision and touch – that illustrate the mind-to-mind communication of the baby subject with the mother-subject.

On the basis of the indifferentiation of the bodily zones in the real place that is the body of the baby, primary narcissism comes to be centred around certain bodily functions and the sensations derived from them because of their repetitiveness. These are the parts of his body in which the infant recognises, from day to day, the movement from tension-lack to relaxation-satisfaction, by way of thirst-hunger followed by fullness, a repetitive sameness he feels as a re-finding of being and of functioning. But together with these functionings involving body substances – contributions of substance to and deductions from the body's erogenous zones of cardio-respiratory, oral and visceral-anal functioning – there is at the same time sound, smell, touch and vision that accompany the satisfaction of the infant in his erogenous zones and flesh out his narcissism. When an infant and his nursing mother are separated, his desire is frustrated; the infant only realises the separation when need linked with desire reappears, and anybody can satisfy the need, while his desire cannot recognise the sound, vision and smell of the person who had previously accompanied the satisfaction. The place in which the tensions of need and desire are confused becomes the place of promised and expected enjoyment, whether satisfied or not. And this place in which a lack is felt, this place of a quest for not only substance (for the survival of the body, or need), but also subtlety (the quest for a heart-to-heart union, of the other self in love, that is to say of desire) – this place in the body is an erogenous zone. But the place in which is repeated, in time, the encounter that responds both to needs and desires, becomes the safe space for the child. For instance, the child can hear further than he sees. His auditive safe space is larger than his visual safe space. And his tactile safe space is still more reduced than his visual safe space. The ensemble created by the place of safety is the space in which the link with the mother can potentially be re-found. We understand that the breast and the nipple, when linked with the smell of the mother, the suckling mouth of the baby and its pituitary mucosa, as he nestles in the crook of his nursing mother's arms – all this forms a *pattern* of desire confused with the pleasure of being and the satisfaction of living and loving, in this simultaneous satisfaction of need and desire. At each satisfaction, sleep follows, and each time the child grows hungry, a re-finding occurs that makes him continue to find erogenous the place and the ensemble of places he links with his mother. The part instincts of desire continue to be focused in the mouth and the cavum of the baby in the expectation of these re-findings. Each time the infant feels a state of tension, whatever the reason – need or desire – he seeks a way of accessing this goal of nirvana that is the maternal presence and the safety of her lap. The temporary privation felt by the baby in a state of tension elicits all the potential substitutions of which he is capable, linked with the substantial sensoriality of the part object, the breast, for an encounter with the other that he fantasises with any associated sensoriality, that can be linked with past encounters and that could be taken as a promise of the other. Likewise, the sound of the maternal voice in the distance promises a meeting he awaits with pleasurable tension that causes him to develop auditory recognition of this voice.

We could therefore say that beyond the body-to-body distance between the baby and his breastfeeding mother, while she is outside his visual field, it is the subtle perceptions of her smell and her voice that continue to be for the child the place within his spatial environment in which he watches for the return of his mother, that is to say the place of his narcissistic link with her, and the continuation of this lively feeling of safety that he feels with her. Similarly, defecating in his clothes brings him the excremental smell and the tactility of toileting contacts with his mother, the excrements present at his bottom are for him a promise that she will return shortly; and from this, the meaning of later encopresia – in a situation of anxiety, it is the unconscious way in which an older child may try to re-find a safe maternal space. The baby's new ways of humanly relating – subtle ways across time and space and no longer a body-to-body relationship involving substances – will have to be preserved so that the subject does not experience too many ruptures in his narcissism: that is to say, his relationship with this primary other, the known total object, his breastfeeding mother who makes him recognise himself as human and love being alive, is necessary to ensure the safety of his continuity of being, found and re-found as being in a relationship with this first other. The fact is that in his early childhood, a continuum of perceptions, repeated and recognised as present or absent, is indispensable for the image of the body to organise itself, while other perceptions, unknown and new, raise questions for the child. While the child recognises some perceptions, others surprise him. Faced with these surprising perceptions – colour, shape, perception, person, unknown space – it is necessary that the witnessing adult gives him in sound a response to his surprise. It is thus that his range of tolerated subtle perceptions, experienced in safety, can expand. First, the perceptions that feel strange but are linked with the presence of the mother, who keeps her known ways and names things, and then the experience of mother's absence followed by her return, allows the child to memorise the link that, integrated into his sensorium, unites him with her. When she is not there, everything around him that she has humanised during her presence by her mediation through her speech, her motor functioning, her manipulations and her moving around, becomes the spatial guarantee of the child's existential security – his being, fantasies and actions – through his trust in the coming return of the one who loves him and whom he loves.

It is in the place given by this relational link, interrupted and retrieved, that the child finds himself as a whole pre-person in the process of structuration. The first person and himself find themselves a little different at times, but she always recognises him; for the child, it may take a little while, but then the link is re-established even if the child takes a while to find the link. This is what makes me talk about 'motherised'[2] objects, which is to say objects that bring to the child the secure, memorised presence of his mother by means of the association of fantasies. Among these, we can count the common objects of the spatial framework of the child, the toys she has named for him, the familiar animals, and especially the people in his entourage, with whom the mother communicates in language and who by this fact can be recognised by the child as humans other than the first, elected other that is the mother. The child, thanks to this introjected link, the symbol of his fundamental narcissism, is thereby at all times and in his entire body 'cohesed.'

His body image, unified by the continuing symbolic relation, assumes perceptions that, if this relationship did not exist or came to be missed for too long a period, would become fragmenting for him. The fantasmatic fragmentation of himself and of the ambient world arises from the (metaphoric) image of the alimentary and excremental functioning (jaws and anus) that are conditions of the human bodily schema; this conditioning is at the origin of the discrimination between need and desire and. It has been the common reference of the relationship of communication with the mother, the mind-to-mind communication, contaminated by the perceptions of communication of the substance of the oral part object and the excremental part object, the pleasure of tenderness that accompanies body-to-body contact during the care of needs – changes, feeding and toileting. The more the relationship with mother continues in a lively way outside those moments of needs-based manipulation of the child's body, in subtle relations that may be vocal, visual, olfactive, through facial expression, play and playfulness, the less such fantasies of fragmentation will become established and persist.

That narcissism assures that the continuity of being of a human individual does not mean that this narcissism need not be redesigned as a result of the trials with which the child's desire collides. These trials, these castrations, as we call them, will allow symbolisation and at the same time will contribute towards the forming of the body image throughout the history of its successive re-elaborations.

---

2 Translator's note: Dolto invents a word, *mamaisés*, to emphasise the infantile nature of the feelings imbued in the objects.

If we start with the idea (which we will develop further later on) that castration is the radical prohibition of a satisfaction sought after and previously experienced, it implies that the body image is structured by way of painful feelings linked with erotic desire, a desire forbidden after its enjoyment and pleasure have been known and repeatedly tasted. This path, one day, is definitively cut in the pursuit of 'more and more' pleasure provided by the direct and immediate satisfaction felt in the body-to-body contact with mother and the appeasement of substantive need. The results of this rupturing operation allow the possibility for the child to collect, in the *après coup*, what could be called 'the fruits of castration.'

To make explicit what we mean by this, we will give a first idea of the successive castrations before re-examining them in detail.

The 'fruits' of castrations

THEIR HUMANISING EFFECTS

The fruit of *oral castration* (weaning from body-to-body nursing) is the possibility for the child to access a language that is comprehensible not only by the mother; this is going to allow him not to be exclusively dependent on her.

The fruit of *anal castration* (or rupture from body-to-body tutelage of mother to child) deprives the child of the pleasure of manipulation shared with mother. While he does not need the adult any longer for washing, dressing, eating, wiping his bottom, moving around, his desire suffers from being deprived of the return to intimacy shared in pleasurable bodily contacts. It is thanks to verbal language, the fruit of weaning if castration has been tolerated, that the development of the bodily schema allows the linkage of facial and gestural language to acrobatic and manual physical abilities. Having delivered anal castration to the child, the mother continues to provide security with verbal, technical and anxiety-free help, so that the child can assume selfhood within the tutelary space and have his own experiences, and acquire an expressive motor autonomy with regard to his needs and many of his desires.

For many children (not to mention certain mothers), this 'being dropped' by their mother is as unbearable a trial as weaning: the physical separation, the forbidding of the joint bodily pleasure of child and mother in the so-called anal castration, is nonetheless the condition of the humanisation and socialisation of the child of 24 to 28 months.

The total deprivation of the mother's physical assistance is also the beginning of autonomy for the child, as compared with when he needed her as a prop and was dependent upon mother's desire – a desire that prevailed over all other relationships. This decision, seen as a promotion, and prepared by the mother through helping the child to acquire the technical means of dealing with the maintenance of his body, the cautious use of his freedom of movement, his progressive initiation to knowledge through true answers to whatever puzzles him – we could say this decision opens the child to communication with all other children of his age and to anybody else, in verbal exchanges, playful or utilitarian acts shared with the familial and close social environment, in which he feels promoted by association.

The fruit of anal castration, which ends the parasitic dependence upon the mother, is also the discovery of a lively relationship with the father, other women and preferred friends; it is the entry of a boy or girl into socialised acts and deeds, including knowing how to master their own actions, discriminating between saying and doing, and between the possible and the impossible, and of not giving in to the pleasure of an act that could be detrimental to oneself or to the one that one loves.

Thanks to the autonomy conquered through anal castration – the autonomy of the child with regard to his mother and moreover of his mother with regard to him – the girl or boy child feels human and can put themselves in the place of the other, mostly children or animals, and of the weak with regard to the strong, and thus develop the underpinning of human ethics: 'not to do to another what I would not want done to me' – with unfortunately also this frequent impulsive, infantile corollary – revenge.

It is language that allows this to be no longer 'training' – a word that should be banned when speaking about human beings – but learning, right from the first hours of the child's 'upbringing' and already an education.

The child cannot do anything but imitate what he perceives and then identifies with the humans around him. These human models upon whom his survival depends are for him invested with the right to limit his aggression or passivity to the benefit of his belonging to the familial and social group, providing cultural, utilitarian and playful goals towards which he strives with those like or unlike him. In speaking with those around him about his observations and desires, he receives responses of agreement, negation and judgement. It is during these verbal exchanges with father, mother and close companions that the child hears interdictions spoken again and again. This is how symbol-creating castration is given repeatedly, one way or another, by someone trusted by the child because of his belonging to the group. By means of his acceptance of these interdictions, the child acquires the value of a living element of the group.

At this time, what becomes irreplaceable for the child is his attendance of the extra-familial world without being torn from the group and mostly from his mother, who is the guarantor of his continuity of being. Particularly in the case of an only child, it is being with other children that allows a healthy entry into the Oedipus, with the child's knowledge of his sex, masculine or feminine, according to the comparisons he can make by observing other children of both sexes. He needs then accurate answers with regard to his observations, both of sexual differences and of social or racial differences, concerning what he observes of the appearance and actions of boys, girls, men and women he meets.

He develops an identification with older children of his sex, and experience shows that when these, and also the adults he sees, have themselves received the castration of archaic drives, he develops in a healthy way towards an Oedipus that fits with the current morality of his culture. In contrast, he shows immediate signs of anxiety before adults and elders whose archaic drives are badly castrated, therefore badly sublimated, and who because of that are attracted to children, as they are not done with their own childhoods. The pleasure these adults expect from the encounter with children and that these children, trapped, let them take or exchange with them, not only does not bring an education to the children in the sense of an initiation to the sublimation of the drives in the direction of adult creativity, but 'seduces' children by trapping them in their narcissistic pleasure, which does them no good – and this not only for the individual, but for the social group to which he belongs. A lot of child neuroses come from the fact that these children are not informed in time of the limited rights over them of all the adults – including their parents, familiars, teachers and society in general. Everything is different for a child if he can speak trustingly and receive information that an adult has been guilty of a transgression of his rights. This very affirmation is enough to return to the child the natural order of human ethics, which is never to stop itself in its search for the repetition of known pleasures. The human ethos is the constant quest for advancement. After anal castration, the child is open to attending society outside his family and has begun seeking the affirmation of his sex and competing with his elders. He aspires to the rights and pleasures of the adults of his sex – parents or teachers – of his mother and father relative to their preferential object (the other parent or the loved one of the teacher).

It is only because the taboo of incest is spoken (and if he is raised by other than his parents, the taboo of sexual relationships between adults and children), and also and mostly because of the experience of the real impossibility of succeeding in his seductive tricks towards both the parent of the other sex and the rival adult of the same sex, that the child receives Oedipal castration. The fruit of that castration is adaptation to all social situations. In addition, the oral, anal and urethral drives, which have already been castrated at the time of weaning, and then when the body is becoming autonomous, will be metaphorised in the manipulation of subtle objects that are words, syntax, the rules of all the games (this does not mean that the child accepts the loss involved and does not attempt to cheat). In the end, the signs representing phonemes – writing, reading – the signs representing numbers, are sublimations, that is to say the fruit of all the previous castrations, and get their meaning from the orientation of the boy and the girl towards a future genital life, expected as a promise and prepared by the pleasure of acquiring knowledge and power, techniques, curiosity and pleasure. At the end of the Oedipus, the child no longer lives to please father or mother but for himself and for his peers.

After Oedipus

It is the latency period into which he enters with all the promise of a future when at puberty, sexual maturation occurs. A castration that has every chance of success (in the symbolisation of castrated instincts that will follow) is the one that is given on time – neither too early nor too late – to the child by an adult or an elder whom he values and who loves and respects the child in such a way that through him, the child feels that his progenitors also are respected.

Let's suppose that for a child, each castration has been given in a timely and non-erotised way by someone whose prohibitions are credible from the very fact that the behaviour of the prohibiting man or woman fits with their discourse.

After this trial, at first always hard to accept, the fruit of receiving the castrating discourse is the renouncing of forbidden acts, through which the child was aiming to access a pleasure even greater than the one he had already tasted, even if only in his imagination, his projects. It is the mourning, in reality, of dreams of pleasures that the child recognises as unrealisable for him, because of his love of the adult who forbids and his wish to identify with him or her. It is the renouncing of cannibalistic, perverse, murderous, vandalising instincts.

If I want to summarise what I call the 'fruits of castration' in one or two sentences, it is the destiny of the drives that cannot be satisfied directly in body-to-body satisfaction, or by the satisfaction of the body with incestuous erotic objects. These drives are maintained in a prohibited state by the model of identification who decreed in speech the prohibition with respect to the humanisation of the child – there is here an element of reality that promotes the child's humanisation. After a period of silence, of repression, these drives enter into what we call a process of sublimation by means of the wish to imitate the ways in which others who are valued in society employ their drives – that is to say, in culture. For the body-subject, this comes in ease, in grace, in poise, in sporting ability and in total autonomy; for the mind, it is in communication in language and knowledge of things life. At the age of 3, the sign that the child has received a good oral and anal castration is that with regard to sexual things, outside of his interest in the pleasure derived from erogenous zones and sentimental sexual attraction, he takes pride in his name, his sex, in belonging to the family group, and takes pleasure in joining in with other children of his age.

The sublimations of the genital drives, which will happen after the Oedipal castration, received between 6 and 9 years of age at the latest, develop during the latency phase (from 8–9 to 12–13 years old) with extra-familial objects in social relationships of exchange according to the law and within the child's effort to promote himself in view of puberty, which will open the way to adolescence: when all the conflicts of the failed castrations of the subject and of his archaic models – his elders and parents – are remodelled. Then, after a time of adolescence, when all the castrations have been considered and accepted because they are the price to pay for the blossoming of the sensual and creative potentialities without pathogenic decompensations, adolescents who have assumed responsibility for their symbolic speech, their person and their acts, their love and social life, become adults, the equals of their progenitors, those entering or not into old age, with at times its serenity but also at times with decrepitude and requirement for support.

This presentation, this form of panorama that we have just laid out of successive humanising castrations, probably allow us better to understand that we were talking about 'symboligenic' castrations. It is to this important notion that we now turn our attention.

The notion of symboligenic castration

Of the word 'symboligenic'

Linking the adjective 'symboligenic' to the word castration seems important to me. It gives to this last term the sense it has in psychoanalysis. In effect, the word 'castration' signifies in French the mutilation of the sexual organs and therefore a physical damage that makes the castrated individual irreversibly sterile. However, the word castration in psychoanalysis accounts for the process that accomplishes itself in a human being when another human being signals to him that the gratification of his desire in the form that he wanted to give to it is forbidden by the law. This signification is transmitted by language, be it gestural, in facial expressions or verbal.

The prohibition of actions that he had energetically pursued comes as a shock to the subject receiving it, reinforcing his desire in the face of the obstacle, sometimes provoking a rebellion, as he feels the total hopelessness of pursuing his object threatens to annihilate his desire.

He secondarily experiences inhibition leading to depression. It is the result of the repression of the drives in question: a repressive pressure that, in going beyond the renouncement of the object of desire and the modes of satisfaction, damages the value of this desire in itself and can lead to a definitive mutilation (of the psychic order) of the sources of the drives. We then need to talk of a traumatic invalidation – hysterical mutilation – and not of castration in the psychoanalytic sense. The confusion of the subject between the trial to be endured and the imaginary risk of mutilation of his body and the erogenous zone involved in the interdiction incites us to maintain, in French, the name of 'the castration complex' to this complex.

An illustrative example would be to compare the individual to a very young plant that has just put out its first flower, believing this to be the only one it will ever have. And then the gardener cuts it off. We know the flower is the sexual organ of a plant. If the plant could think, it would then consider itself to have been mutilated in its reproductive destiny. In fact, if the gardener cut this first flower, it is because he knows that the strength in the roots will make the plant grow better, and that if on the contrary he had allowed the branch to flower, it would have been to the impoverishment of the plant's vitality. The education by humans of the developing human child corresponds to what the knowing gardener does, when he supplies the plant the trial of the nullification of the glory of that first flowering, which it (if it could think) imagines to be its only chance of promised fecundity. As for the flower, castration has to be repeated over and over again for human beings. When the conditions of the emotional relationship between the child and the adult are rich in reciprocal trust, a humanising meaning is born by example and by what is said. The child, in imitation of the adult who represents for him the image of his completed future being, accepts what the adult imposes on him because he wishes to emulate the example of someone who appears credible to him, who is in charge of bringing him up, who has by law rights over him – in order to increase his own value.

The verbalisation of the prohibition given to the object of his desire helps the child to bear the ordeal *provided that he is clearly aware that the adult is also subject to this interdiction*, and the child can still trust in his right to imagine the goal of his desire that the adult has forbidden. It is therefore through this prohibition that the desiring subject is initiated into the power of his desire, which has value, at the same time as being initiated into the law, which gives him other ways of identifying other human beings who are also subject to the law.

This entails a process of mutation for the subject and of reinforcement of desire. The law in question is not only a repressive law but also a law that, even if it seems in the moment repressive of action, is in fact one that promotes the subject in his ability to act within the community of humans. It can never be the law of this or that adult who utters it for his own profit against the child. It is the law to which this adult submits as much as the child does.

The drive thus repressed undergoes a dynamic modification and desire, the initial goal of which has been forbidden, and aims at its satisfaction through new means, sublimations – means that demand for their satisfaction a process of elaboration that was not demanded by the object first aimed at. It is only this last process that bears the name of symbolisation, flowing from a castration understood in the psychoanalytic sense.

This is not to say that castration equals sublimation. *Castration can lead to sublimation, but it could also end in perversion or repression with a neurotic outcome.*

Perversion is a symbolisation, but a symbolisation that does not correspond with a law for all – the law of the progression that, from castration to castration, drives s/he who experiences it to a humanisation in the sense of creativity as much as of ethics. There could be a hijacking of the drives towards a satisfaction that does not introduce a progression of the subject towards the integration of the law. Thus, when castration drives the individual towards the negation of vital processes, the outcome is masochism.[3]

Let's suppose a little girl reacts to the aggression of a little boy by freeing her aggressive drives in a scream. If the mother intervenes to counter this oral manifestation of her daughter's aggressive drives by making fun of her, as if she, as a mother, was complicit with the boy, the daughter, for whom the mother is an identificatory model, may end up experiencing the aggression as what her mother effectively desires for her – that is to say enjoying a physical suffering supposedly approved by the completed image of herself that the adult represents.

This is how the superego becomes perverse, masochistic, hypochondriacal (when introjected) or masochistic in its relation to the other, self-destructive (repetitive accidents) or deprived of defensive immunity in the face of pathogenic

---

3 See the case of Leon, chap. 3, p. 189.

attacks.[4] Depending on the adult that gives the castration, the child who receives it and mostly upon the parental couple as the example of life and what the future promises, castration can sometimes be understood as the prohibition of any desire that has pleasure for a goal and as a negation of the child's accurate intuition with regard to the enjoyment of his physical, mental and affective development. There is here a perverse symboligenic effect of castration, often completely unconscious on the part of the parents and educators from whom it originates. *Castration that induces the desire to satisfy itself in suffering rather than in pleasure is a perversion.* This is also the case when there is a homosexualising effect of this interdiction regarding the accomplishment of incestuous genital desire. The forbidding of the woman who is the object of the boy-child subject (i.e. his mother or his sisters) could be said to him and heard by him as the forbidding of any woman, all women being the property of his father. The behaviours and pronouncements of his father forbid him to try to attract the attention of any woman in his family and social milieu. Thus, the castration the father imposes on his desire causes the boy to direct his phallic centrifugal drives towards the search for a man and not a woman.

Let us say again: *castration is not exactly synonymous with sublimation. If there is sublimation, it is because there has been a castration*, which has supported the symbolisation of drives towards the search for new objects in conformity with the laws of the close family group and of the social group, and because the subject found a greater pleasure in the interplay and satisfaction of his drives that avoids the prohibited field of action. That there has been a castration given and received does not ensure that the process will end in a 'healthy' sublimation, a source of new symbolisations excluding a symbolisation that becomes stuck and that we must call 'pathogenic.' Pathogenic symbolisation elicits a perverse direction in the satisfaction of desire. The subject can then be lured by the pleasure he has discovered, for example in the fixation upon an object that brings an intense and repetitive pleasure, where narcissism becomes trapped because the quest of his desire stops in the body, the partial or total lieu of enjoyment, but an object of death.

All my research regarding the precocious disorders of human beings can be applied to decoding the necessary conditions so that the castration given to the child during his development allows him to access sublimation and the symbolic order of human law. It is this symbolic order that promotes a human specimen borne of a man and a woman, given a masculine or feminine body, to become a responsible subject within a given ethnic group while at the same time being a representative of his culture and an actor within its development in a given place

---

4 Translator's note: the original French states *'de defense humorale devant des aggressions pathogenes'* – invoking the archaic idea of the humours (sanguine, bilious, etc). This would evoke the purely bodily (as confirmed by the mention of pathogens) as well as deep-seated psychological defences against aggression. While Dolto's clinical experiences may have led her to this observation regarding children whose physical immune system seems unusually weak, it is also a valid metaphor for psychological weakness in the face of attacks.

and time. Throughout the development of a human being, the symbolic function, castration and body image are tightly linked. The symbolic function with which every human being is endowed allows a newborn to differentiate itself as a named and desiring subject from an anonymous representative of the species (to which, however, he is going to be reduced in his deep sleep at a time where the subject of desire is not relating to an object in reality).

It is due to castration that subtle and creative communication between subjects at a physical distance from each other comes about, involving the image of the actual body and language, and occurring throughout each phase of libidinal evolution.

Castration generates a new way of being in the face of a desire that becomes impossible to satisfy in the way in which it had been satisfied up until then. Castrations – in the psychoanalytic sense – are tests of symbolic partitioning: they are an irreversible signifying statement or act that becomes law, and therefore has an operational effect in reality, always painful to admit in the moment when the aforementioned castration is given. But they are as necessary to the development of the individuation of the child with regard first to his mother, then to his father and then to those close to him, as they are to the development of language.

Weaning from the breast for example, in separating the mouth of the child from the lactating breast, separates the child from his mother as the substance of nourishment. But weaning – the first oral castration – aims only at one modality of the satisfaction of desire, which is partial. The tactile sensations, the smell, the body-to-body contact while bottle-feeding or spoon feeding or drinking from a cup remain. The mother remains the total object of her relationship with the child. It is true that the maternal breast at the point when the child suckles it for the last time, this breast, which is a part object of his desire (and at the same time a mediator of his need), this breast which is part of the mother, is felt by the child to belong to him. He is therefore separated from a part of himself, obviously illusory, but his survival of this ordeal is a symboligenic experience, the effect of which depends upon the way, during weaning, his mother promotes their relationship in language, in tenderness and inter-comprehension.

And so, the 'short cut' of desire from mucous membrane to mucous membrane – from the mouth to the nipple – transforms itself against a background of tension, suffering, discontent or lack, into a long circuit of communication from psyche to psyche; a communication more extended in space and time and more subtle than had been the repetitive body-to-body communication of needs linked with desire. One could say that the child, weaned of the breast and suckling (a system of communicating vessels – phantasmatic anthropophagy) erogenises[5] even more the

---

5 Translator's note: Dolto uses a neologism '*erogeniser*' that I have translated as 'to erogenise' rather than 'to eroticise.' This is to make a distinction between the physicality of the relationship between mother and suckling infant and the more complex forms of interaction between a weaned baby and its mother that ultimately lead to the child's development of the capacity to symbolise.

subtlety he perceives from his mother. The erogenisation of subtlety – olfaction, audition, sight – is already symboligenic in a way that favours language development better than does the pleasure of swallowing milk and suckling, because the substantial is linked with repetitive need in its modality of pleasure without surprise. In the subtle, the interweaving of the voices of mother and of others when heard by the child introduces him to new relationships, while in the relationship between mouth and breast, nobody comes between them. The successive castrations are separations with a symboligenic effect of this kind and it is through these that the erogenous zones, linked with touch before the ending of bodily contact, will become zones of desire and pleasure received and given to another, signifying alliance.

The pleasure given is henceforth felt to be a discovery, an invention, a creation by two people, for the conjugation – through the body – of the minds of the mother and her nursling. The enjoyment becomes symbolically the fruit of an encounter both imaginary and real, in time and space, linked with the body of the child in its partial sensations and also with the whole body, thanks to the subtle and expressive presence of the mother: a presence of which the modes of perception are retained in memory and are not eliminated, as is the case for the substantial.

This is not about the disappearance of the maternal object, but about a modification that has a symbolic value, renewed daily, of the maternal presence: it is a refinement of the knowledge that the child has of her and of himself in the pleasure of remembering her, of waiting for her and of re-uniting with her, similar and surprising and different in some way. However, if the object disappears forever, castration is no longer a valorisation of desire, nor does it support life as the child knows it, nor does it open or call for interhuman communication. It is, after a period of expectancy, a wearing out of desire and a cessation of the dynamic of desire, a mutilation of the body image that had developed in the relationship of the nursling with his mother. What follows is the impossibility of symbolising a disappeared link, and therefore of its sublimation in subtle language-based relationships that other people could share. As a consequence, these drives, abruptly unbound from the relationship with the only person through whom the child knew he existed, return to the body of the child, which has become anonymous in relationship with his desire. The child regresses to being as 'one before its birth' but no longer having pre-birth references.

This is autism

By comparison, in symboligenic castration the mother who has weaned her child and witnessed through his screams his difficulty in living and accepting this ordeal devises ways of consoling him – all the more so as often, she too suffers from this change in the relationship with her own body and with her baby. She initiates the child into feeling as close to herself and even more pleasantly than before the loss, through human exchanges with her. In language communication between baby and herself, she initiates him into relationships with others: father, brothers, sisters, comforters and replacement interlocutors, allies of the mother, who reveal the social world to the baby. When a child smiles, opens his arms and another person is there and says, 'Isn't he lovely, your baby? Isn't he smiley?' – this person introduces him to an other than his mother and he enters into communication with society, bouncing from person to person who recognises that he is communicating. This is how weaning as oral castration becomes symboligenic.

The eighth-month anxiety

This is why, for instance, what is called the eighth-month anxiety, which has been observed and described by certain psychoanalysts, is neither fatal nor necessary, and happens because sometimes the child is not carried enough or helped to move towards what attracts him, what he wants to touch (because of course his desire for motricity in his imagination is precocious to the capacities of his real bodily schema). The eighth-month anxiety comes from what the adult has failed to mediate spatially between the objects the child sees and, upon seeing them, wants to have access to with his touch, his body. It is a feeling of impotence that arises from the lack of mediation by the mother, a lack in the socialisation that the baby needs at this time; and so, he gets bored, something perishes from lack of being exercised, something in the language of his desire is not understood.

Let us take this opportunity to remark that for the castrations to have their symboligenic value, it is necessary that the bodily schema of the child is able to bear them. The events of birth, weaning and separation from the two-headed agency – feminine and masculine – formed by the two parents must respect the most tenuous integrity that from the origin specifies the narcissistic continuum of the subject's body image.

Without special care, a child who has not reached seven months of foetal life cannot bear birth, cannot symbolise through respiratory exchanges the umbilical castration. A child who has not had sufficient time with the body of his mother is not able to bear weaning without regressing to the most precocious stage of the first day of his life. There is a right moment for each castration to be imposed; this moment is when the current drives have brought some development of the bodily schema that makes the child able to rearrange his pleasures in some way other than in the satisfaction of total bodily contact, which is no longer absolutely necessary to this specimen of the human species represented by the physical body, in order to survive as a being of need. It remains that this physicality, which makes the child a being of need, is linked with a subject of desire.

The subject, who may be present from fecundation, shows itself only through desires. These desires cannot be separated immediately from their conjunction with needs. It is language, in the widest sense of the term and in the more precise sense of words, that mediates these evolutions, which are castrations that have been overcome.

For example, a child who has reached motor functioning, the ability to move around within the family setting near his father and mother, if he knows the person with whom he is going to change his setting, can continue to develop his motor functioning and *joie de vivre*; thanks to this human mediator between the past space and the new space, he is in imagination still with his parents, in particular if she speaks of them to him. But if he is suddenly transported to another place by someone who does not know his parents and does not talk about what he is experiencing and of the meaning of this change, who does not link him with past memories, the child experiences this as a psychic trauma. He stops his motor development and only re-grafts himself onto the new milieu in which he is fostered and brought up by regressing, losing acquisitions and re-establishing an archaic relationship with the new setting. The separation – which is the castration of desire engaged in the love of the people in the previous setting – has not been symboligenic; the separation has been traumatic, there is regression and symbolisation will restart later. For the time being, it is a trauma.[6]

Another condition is necessary to ensure the symboligenic dimension of the castration process. It depends on the quality of the adult whose role it is to give the castration. A child accepts a limitation and a delay to the satisfaction of his desire and even a prohibition that it will never be satisfied, if the person who gives the prohibition is beloved by the child, who knows also that he has the right to access his/her power and knowledge. This adult can only make the child access the symbolisation of his drives if, at the time the castration is given, he is motivated by the respect and chaste love for the child to whom he offers momentary limitations or definitive prohibitions as to such partial enjoyments as the child was seeking.

On top of this, the adult must be for the child the example of human success and the promise that these very drives could be satisfied by the obtaining of a far greater pleasure, in the image of the one who talks to him and directs him. He is therefore a model that the child can follow and listen to if he wants both to develop – to be on the path to accessing the symbolic phallus – and to be certain that his desire is valued, that pleasure is accessible and approved of by the adult. The child doesn't yet know how he should find the way, but because his guide found it, why should he not find it himself in listening to and in trusting him (and not in submitting to him)?

Thus, the castration suffered leads the individual to a greater confidence in themselves and to a more and more differentiated communication with others, and this inasmuch because of an increasing ability to use vocabulary and language in general, as because of increasing manual abilities that allow the child to do things. Thus, the child may gradually leave behind his dependence upon the adults who bring him up by acquiring the know-how by which he comes to be appreciated by others and able to engage in exchanges with them. Progressing from castration to castration is the means of leaving behind puerile impotence and moving to being

6 It is a castration that mutilates the dynamic image of the body, i.e. not symboligenic.

a pre-citizen in the process of accessing all his rights: on the condition that these rights are paid for through the acceptance of the laws that regulate those in whose tutelage the child has put himself through love – i.e. his parents, his teachers, his peer group and his older friends. This feeling of promotion allows the child to leave behind the enjoyments of early childhood, to access a greater enjoyment – the enjoyment of those older than he is. This desire to grow up is naturally present in children, a project included in their organic growth. This hope – to not remain small – supports their courage in the face of many disappointments due to their impotence in reality compared with their creative initiatives. Alas, many adults do reproach or express in a pejorative way their displeasure at the child's failure, devaluing them as a subject because of their physical incapacity, which is vexatious for the child. One can easily understand that the growing child can at times fear a return to a pre-castration phase, as this would entail losing the acquisitions he has just made by means of the castration. Until he is absolutely sure of himself in these new modes of cultural functioning, it is dangerous for the child to look back and identify with his past self.

This is what the phobic attitude of small children is connected with; when put in a new space, they hide in the skirts of their mother with anxious faces and may become very anxious, to the point where they lose the ability to speak – precisely because it is language that uses the oral drives in a civilised way, while phobia projects these drives into the idea of a danger in space, which could have the shape of a jaw aiming to devour all or part of the body that was looking for enjoyment.

When on the contrary the child has reached the stage of anal castration, he is able through his bodily schema to use sublimated motor drives, as seen in the ease with which they use their body, an ease in all the modulation of the drives in a cultural way. At that point the child is no longer scared to identify with himself as he was when he was small. It is the age at which children are not afraid of looking after smaller ones, of laughing at their funny ways, and are no longer jealous of the liberties permitted to babies by people who love them.

Conversely, when anal castration is badly accepted, either because it has been badly given by the adult or because the adult who gave it in words is not a model the subject wants to imitate (if the adult himself is anxious about his own desires), the one being educated will never be able to sublimate enough, i.e. to talk, fantasise (for fun) his anal drives. The tutelary adult mistakes the imaginary and the real; he is neither tolerant nor indulgent, nor permissive with regard to his own fantasies of his oral or anal drives, which have to stay unconscious, split off or repressed. It is a sad fact that many adults are unable to give a symboligenic castration of archaic stages because they themselves regret not being children anymore, or regret that their child is growing up and wishes to be autonomous from them. They prevent the child from reaching a level that would allow him to overcome this archaic ethical stage in which he had to be for a while, and from which age will extract him in an almost spontaneous way if he is with happy parents, by which I mean parents who live their genital libido in a way other than at the libidinal level of consumption and work (oral and anal sublimation). In a family dynamic, it is far more the unconscious that is the agent of education, successful or not, than learned knowledge about parenting. (Outside the family dynamic, the incestuous trap is no longer directly present.)

Now that I have explicitly stated what I mean by symboligenic castration, I will study in more detail how it realises itself in the child's developmental experiences.

Umbilical castration

That birth constitutes, in fact, the first castration, with the meaning we have given this term, may be surprising. This is, however, what I am going to show here. Birth is apparently firstly a fact of nature, and its symboligenic role for the new-born leaves as a blueprint the first ways of feeling he experiences in coming into the world as a human being, man or woman, received according to the sex displayed by his body for the first time, and according to the way in which it is accepted, frustrating or gratifying for the narcissism of each parent.

What separates the body of the child from that of the mother and makes him viable is the cutting and ligature of the umbilical cord.

From the umbilical severance and in separating from the placenta and the membranes that he leaves behind in the uterus to which they belong, the bodily schema comes into being within the limits of the skin envelope. The body image, which in part originates in rhythms, warmth, sounds, foetal perceptions, becomes modified by the sudden change of these perceptions, in particular the loss for the auditive passive drives of the double beating of the heart heard by the child in utero. This modification is accompanied by the appearance of the pulmonary bellows and of the activation of the peristaltic movement of the digestive tract, which when the child is born produces the meconium accumulated during foetal life. In the light of what follows in human destiny, the umbilical scar and loss of the placenta can be considered as a prefiguration of all the trials that we will name later as castrations (adding to it the adjectives oral, anal, urethral and genital). This first separation will therefore be called umbilical castration. It is concomitant with birth and, in the terms of joy and anxiety that accompany the birth of the child, constitutes a founding element in his relationship with the desire of others. The terms of the birth, this first mutative castration, form the matrix of terms of later castrations.

Thanks to the physiological modification that operates in the child's body, birth is accompanied by a sonorous cry by which he manifests himself while, at the same time, he reacts by the evacuation of the substantial intestinal content at the cloacal end, while before he had been a foetus only centred by the umbilical passage, by the swallowing of the amniotic liquid and urinary miction in the amniotic liquid.

Along with his respiration and the scream that he hears coming from himself, the coming into play of olfaction (the maternal smell) is unconsciously the first impact for the newborn of a specific marker of his relationship with his mother.

The dulled prenatal sounds disappear, to be replaced by the intensified hearing of already known voices – those of father, mother and those close to them.[7]

This loss of familiar perceptions and surge of new perceptions constitute what has been called the 'trauma' of birth, which is an initial mutation in everybody's life and marks with a more or less memorised style of anxiety the primary sensation of asphyxia experienced by each foetus in its introduction as an aerial life-form, linked with his being discharged from the warm aquatic element and appearance into the aerial world of gravity. Thus, our birth is marked by cataclysmic modifications, our first mutative partition, by which we leave behind an important part of what constituted in utero our very organism, amniotic membranes, placenta, umbilical cord: parts that allowed us to be viable in another space. These modifications, with which we are welcomed into the aerial world, make it forever impossible to return to the preceding space and to the forms of life and enjoyment we knew there.

We could say that instead of the placental blood that passively fed the symbiotic life of the foetus in the maternal organism, the fleshly life now grafts itself upon air, a new element common to all terrestrial creatures, the flux and reflux of which is maintained by the pulmonary bellows. With these bellows appears a modification of the pulsating cardiac rhythm, which is no longer pendular but rhythmic, as was the undulating heart rhythm of the mother during foetal life. Yes: the newborn child has, in being born, lost the sound of his own cardiac rhythm as he knew it; the sensation of body weight submitting to gravity also appears, and the forms of manipulation of which he is the object in the hands that receive him, and the surface of the bed or of the mother's body on which the child rests. Light dazzles his retina, the smell of mother fills his cavum, the voices of those present and noises make themselves heard clearly, while up until then the sounds of the world had only been perceived through a wall of water and flesh, against a background where the rapid pendular rhythm of the foetal heart mixed with the two and a half times slower beat of the maternal heart. At different times of day this syncopated rhythm alternated with that of the walking of the carrying body and with the noises of its industrious activity, sometimes marked by the sonorous vibrations that the words, mostly spoken by low voices – masculine – transmitted in a muffled way to the egg from which the child was developing. At night, it was the resting double sound rhythm to which were added the snoring of maternal sleep and the grumblings of the digestive visceral movements of the sleeping mother.

Thus, suddenly, forcefully, he discovers perceptions of which he had no notion until then: light, smell, tactile sensations, sensations of pressure and of weight,

---

7 It is to be noted that recent studies found evidence that in utero the child hears low-pitched sounds, i.e. men's voices and that what he hears of the mother is the beating heart and a noise that sounds like the noise of waves crashing on the beach. He only hears the maternal voice if it has low frequencies. The strangest thing in that this is reversed after birth, when he then hears mostly higher frequencies.

and the sounds, strong and clear, that until then he had only dimly perceived. The most striking auditory element is going to be, through its repetition, his given name, signifier of his being in the world for his parents; also the signifier of his sex, as it is the first thing he has heard: 'It's a boy!' – 'It's a girl!' – the words that immediately gush from the mouths of those present and the voices of those close who welcome him, voices that come nearer, that grow distant, but are perpetually heard, the phonemes of the words 'boy' or 'girl' accompanied by the name by which his parents designate him thenceforth. This given name and this designation, the designation of his sex, are thrown about by animated voices in joy or in reticence, declaring (or not) the satisfaction of the entourage, and we discover everyday how much newborns keep 'engrammed,'[8] as with magnetic tape, somewhere in their cortex, these first expressions of what is already narcissising joy, or of the reticence or even distress or anxiety that is for them de-narcissising.

It is language, therefore, that symbolises the castration of birth, which we call umbilical castration; this language will repetitively strike the baby's hearing as the effect of his being, and he intuitively perceives in the modulations and affects borne by the sonorous syllables his emotional impact upon his parents, without us knowing exactly how he perceives this. It is as if all these affects accompanied by phonemes were the incarnation of a primary narcissistic mode of being.

The first syllables that have signified us are for every one of us the auditory message that symbolises our birth, synonymous of the present (in the double-meaning of 'current' and 'gift') that is the veritable life of this child who, from out of the imagination of his parents, becomes real: an irreversible reality, feminine or masculine, as is and will be, as he appeared to us, to his parents and to the representatives of society who welcomed him. It is as boy or girl, named this or that, that he is given from his father to his mother, received by his father from his mother, both receiving not only from one another but also from the previous generations who brought them into the world, and from the destiny that does or does not bear for them the name of God, but which anyway has put a signature on this existence. It is inexorable, it is girl or boy, that's how it is, a fact outside of the power of the parents. And in this sense, they too suffer a castration in this affair. Their castration lies in the registration of the child in the register of births, which seals his status as a citizen, whatever happens to his parents. Whether they protect him or are unable to protect him, he is from now on their responsibility, if they can assume it; but it does not entirely belong to them as he is a legal subject of society over whom their rights are limited – and their duty unlimited!

The fantasmatic project of giving a name and gender are stopped by the fixing of this in the births and deaths register, including his belonging to whomsoever recognises him as legitimate or illegitimate, or who refuses to give him legal, or

---

8 The French 'engrammés' is also a neologism, drawn from the concept of engrams, a word from neuroscience that denotes the means by which memory traces are stored. The meaning here is of a permanent recording.

even more so, emotional recognition. Fantasy is no longer possible once this act has been accomplished at the registry office; the child has entered a reality from which he cannot disengage except according to the law. Symbolisation for the newborn as for the parents of this castration of the foetus and with him of his parents with birth and registration is his full and complete adoption, affective and social, or its reticent adoption signified by the way his genitors have decided to register him. This writing of which a trace is left at the registry, jointly with a patronym, gives him for life the major signifier of his being in the world, that which his body will carry until death.

One may be surprised, but this is how it is: psychoanalyses always find the impact on the newborn of his hearing and otherwise perceiving the upwellings of joy in the heart-to-heart conversations of his parents, or on the contrary of the depression in which his birth has put one or both parents, because he is of this or that sex or presents this or that aspect. However this umbilical castration has been symbolised, we now have the formal proof that it could deliver to the child a greater or lesser symbolic power according to the way in which the mother has experienced the physiological fact of the afterbirth – that is to say the expulsion of the placenta – usually around half an hour after the birth, and how the parental couple have experienced the promise kept by reality in the boy or girl child, relative to their fantasy of fecund and viable genitality. They can feel fulfilled; but the baby may not conform to what they hoped for in fantasy.

There are therefore two forms of vitality promoted by the symboligenic aspect of umbilical castration: one due to the organic impact of birth on the equilibrium of the psychosomatic health of the mother, and through this of the parental couple in their genital relationship; *the other is the affective impact that the viability of the child adds to or subtracts from the narcissism of the two birth parents*, who accordingly will adopt him with the characteristics of their emotions at that moment and introduce him into their lives as the bearer of the meaning he had for them at that moment.

These two sources of symboligenic power resulting from the *umbilical castration of the child* and of the *imaginary castration of the parents* are clearly visible when one or the other has dried up at the moment of birth. The death or illness of the mother marks in an indelible way, in an unconscious guilt in living, any child who has seemed to their father to have been, by their birth, responsible for a pathogenic or deadly effect on their birth mother. Similarly, when the sex and the appearance of the child have profoundly disappointed consciously or unconsciously, one or other parent (or worse, both) living is for him fundamentally linked with guilt, together with his given name; language inculcated in the subject about living or about living his desire in his body. It is what we find in cases of early infant psychosis that we have to treat, where we can see that the deterioration of the means of communication of desire is due to a precociously disturbed symbolic order.

Contrary to what one may think, it is not the fact of a death or of a post-natal haemorrhage, for instance, that by causing an indelible organic impact on the child, leaves him in a psychotic state. In fact, it is the psychogenic element that has caused a prohibition of the baby's psychological development, and this can be seen in reality and is what the psychoanalytic treatment proves. The analysis of this birth and the re-living of this ordeal can be accurately spoken of by the parents and by the child, and these are what frees him definitively from the toils that trapped him in an interdiction of living of his own account.

It is to a catastrophic birth that one used to impute the early disturbances of bad somato-psychic development of a psychotic child, and that some may attribute to an undetected encephalitis. However, the fact that analysis can help the child out of psychosis proves that the disturbance does not originate from physical injury – of early lesional disturbances having affected the body of the newborn. The developmental difficulties have in themselves been the expression of early feelings and affects shared with the entourage without having been given meaning in words said to the child at the right time, even if these were words that nullify the child's symbolic life.

Thus, in the triangulation of parents and child in which the dynamic vitality of the unconscious circulates, it is from the point of umbilical castration that anxiety or joy mark the psyche of a human being in a symboligenic way, whatever its organic state. It is about the switching on of the unconscious dynamic source that is going to sustain the development of the child in a rich or impoverished way. This power is largely or poorly delivered to the subject, according to the peaceable or conflictual narcissism of the parents; this is what sustains or impedes the child in overcoming the trials of the transformations of birth and of the first days of adaptation to aerial life.

It is through the openings, the holes of the face – open to subtle communication, centred and converging towards the cavum – nostrils, ears, linked with optical perceptions – that these encounters are possible and symbolic of his being in the world.

With this symbolisation, the foundation of being, masculine or feminine, that follows the birth and naming of the child, the baby enters the oral period. And so, those who have been hurt in their symbolic life show early disorders regarding these very holes that opened to exchanges of substance with the outside world at birth, that is to say, the entrance of the digestive tube connected in the head to the cavum, and the exit of the digestive tube in the pelvis, where the excrements in their solid and liquid forms are closely related through tactile contiguity to the development of genital sensations.

We would be ignoring clinical reality if we did not add that the child's older siblings are also affected by the child's birth and its conditions, the impact on the mother's health and the joy or sadness that the baby's sex brings to the household; all this also brings joy or disturbance to his older siblings, and that from this fact, the baby receives in return a greater power to or reduction from his desire for life. We know how much the parents' disillusionment in the sex of a younger brother or sister can cause a destructuration in the confidence that an older child has in his parents, when he hasn't yet reached the age at which he can understand that they are not omnipotent to the point of being able to master the realisation of their desire with regard to the sex of the child they bring into the world.[9]

We also know how much sibling rivalry can invalidate the symbolic power of the baby because of the drives of an older sibling who refuses to accept the existence in the home of a younger sibling. From the point of view of the older sibling, all the drama he experiences at the event of the birth of a younger sibling is to be replaced in the Oedipal situation. The sex of the newborn brings into play what he has not got and for which this little newborn, girl or boy, is responsible, is to be blamed. The birth of a baby in a family awakens the castration of the older siblings.

The separation from the placenta, the symboligenic moment of birth, is important for all humans. Until now, this has passed unnoticed; but since medicine saves numerous newborns, we observe how much this moment of being received into society, how it happens and is experienced, is important for the future somatic and emotional development of the child.[10]

This is how real dangers experienced by a child because of an infection of the umbilical cord, of the umbilicus, or of the anxiety of medical staff about a ligature of an umbilical cord that is too short and fear of a haemorrhage in the newborn, leaves indelible traces in the psyche and the propensity to anxiety in the baby, even when these have only been anticipatory anxieties and there has been no event in reality to confirm the anxiety of these few days. We could say that any psychogenic morbidity arising from neonatal anxiety manifests itself in children, and sometimes later, by the fact that any anxiety provokes a sudden pallor around the nose and the mouth, at the same time as visceral trembling, often accompanied by an episode of emotional fever: emotional fever, because it appears without any other reason in these patients – children or adults – and disappears when, through analysis, one has been able to put words onto the umbilical anxiety experienced during the first days, the first 15 days of life before the appropriate dropping of the umbilical cord has reassured medical staff and the family and therefore the child himself.

Oral castration

The second of the great renouncements typically imposed on the child is the oral castration imposed on the baby regarding what is for him cannibalism towards his mother (in other words, weaning) and also the stopping of him from eating

---

9 See the case of Pierre, page 162.
10 The importance of umbilical castration seems to be better understood these days, when studies on the physiological delivery of mothers led to research into delivery without violence, the aftermath proves that delivery without violence, when some children in a family have been able to benefit from it, protects them from newborn existential anxieties experienced by most other newborns. These studies are ongoing in many countries. It is Frederic Leboyer who in France is at the origin of this research into delivery without violence and the statistics of the long-term effects on children of this style of delivery. (See also studies on this question in the *Cahiers du Nouveau-Né*, published by Stock.)

what may be deadly poison for his body (the forbidding of eating non-food items dangerous to health or to life). This castration (weaning), when judiciously given, leads to desire and to the possibility of talking and therefore to the discovery of new means of communication within different forms of enjoyment, with objects whose incorporation is no longer possible. These objects support transference from the milk-producing breast or from suckled milk (suckled at the breast or from the teat of the bottle) to an even greater pleasure, shared with the tutelary power, the mother, father or close relatives.

Weaning, as castration of the baby, implies also that the mother accepts the rupture of the bodily contact in which the baby was totally dependent on her physical presence, as he moved from the internal breast to the milk-producing breasts and to being carried. This *oral castration of the mother* implies that she is able to communicate with the child in a way other than that of giving him food, taking away his excrements and devouring him with kisses and cuddles: she needs to communicate through words and gestures that are language. The fact of the oral castration of the weaned baby and of the mother (weaned of the erotic relationship of giving to the child's mouth and also of a tactile and grasping relationship with the baby's bottom) is displayed in the mother's taking an even greater pleasure in talking to the child, in guiding his phonemes until they become perfect in his mother tongue, as well as taking pleasure in his motor functioning in the seizing and throwing of objects that she gives and fetches – actions that constitute the beginning of motor language. The child can then symbolise the oral and anal drives through language because his mother is happy to see him able to communicate with her and with others; he perceives the pleasure she experiences in witnessing his joy in identifying with her, within his playful verbal exchanges with other people. These are possibilities of symbolic relationships in the unconscious and the psyche of her child promoted by this castration.

One should not forget that mother's bodily contact with the baby is eroticising. It is necessary, however, that it is that way: it is part of the mother–baby relationship. But weaning needs to occur to mark the start of a new phase, of a change, towards communication for pleasure and away from bodily contact: communication through gestures shows that she does not own the baby anymore and allows him to identify with her, in her relationship with others and the environment.

It is important that she lets her child be as happy in other people's arms as he is in hers, that she lets him engage in smiling and talking (experimenting with phonemes) with those other than herself. From the point of view of instinctual objects, oral castration is for the child a separation from a part of himself that was in the body of the mother – the milk that he caused to come into the mother's breast – he separates himself from the part object, the mother's breast, but also from this first milky nourishment in order to open and initiate himself to a varied a solid diet. He renounces the illusion of cannibalism vis-à-vis the part object that is his mother's breast. For a while, he might displace, if his mother is not vigilant, his cannibalistic drives onto his own hands, sucking his thumb or his fist with the illusion that thus, he continues being at his mother's breast. There is a partly failed weaning in the child who maintains an illusion of a relationship with the mother in establishing an auto-erotic connection between his mouth and his hands. We need to understand that the milk is first the child's milk, with which he is in communication, while at the same time he makes it come into the body of his mother because of his suckling.

When he is weaned, he is weaned of nourishment that he had responsibility for bringing forth in the mother and was his, at the same time that his mouth is deprived of the tactile relationship with the nipple and the breast, part object of the mother, but that he thought was his. He fills the gaping holes created by the absence of the breast in his mouth by putting his thumb in and finds in this a pleasure outside of feeding, which is also the pleasure of ensuring his mouth is still there.

This is precisely what I ask older children who suck their thumbs to study when they want to give this up. I ask them to think hard: 'Suck your thumb and pay attention to what you feel. Is it your mouth that needs your thumb? Is your mouth more happy to have the thumb, or is it that your thumb wants to take shelter in your mouth?' It is extraordinary to see how they concentrate on their feelings and think about it. They understand that it is the thumb and not the mouth or the mouth and not the thumb, and from there we can start talking precisely about the thumb replacing the maternal breast, and that when they were small they did not accept being deprived of suckling their mother, while being at that time big enough to talk and to put in their mouth anything that was at their disposition, that their mother did not think they were big enough to understand everything and not just share with her the pleasure of being at the breast, and this illusion has sustained what now irritates them but that they cannot give up when tired or worried.

On the other hand, when the weaning separation is progressive and the partial pleasure that links the mouth to the breast is driven by the mother to be distributed onto the successive knowledge of the tactile qualities of other objects that the child puts in his mouth, these objects named by her introduce him to language. Then you can see that when alone and in his cot, the child practices 'talking' to himself, first in babbling and then in modulating the sounds in the ways he has heard his mother do with him and with others.

It is at this point that you can see symbolisation at work: if from that time (around three months) the mother is attentive in giving something to the child in the minutes following the feed and before sleep, something that he can grab and put in his mouth instead of the breast. If she gives the child the words that signify what he is experiencing in tactility – for example 'it's the rattle, it's cold, it's metal, it's bone, it's your fluffy bear, it's cloth, it's your fist, it's dad's finger, it's wool from your jumper . . .' – then when she's not there, all these words make him remember her, and he tries to repeat the sounds that came with her and he can train himself to act like her with the small objects of their common life, and to celebrate with phonemes, cries, gestures and happy smiles the arrival of the father and of the family of people, without provoking in the mother feelings of jealousy or abandonment. This is how language becomes symbolic of the body-to-body relationship, the short cut of baby to mother becoming a long route by the subtlety of vocalisations and the meaning of words that recover different sensory perceptions, all of them 'motherised' by the mother's voice, the same voice he heard when at the breast.

The symboligenic effect, therefore, of oral castration is to introduce the child, now independent of the absolute need for mother's presence, to relationships with others. The child has arrived at language-based ways of behaving that cause him to accept the help of anyone with whom his mother is on good terms, and with whom he himself develops possibilities of communication, sketched out with his mother or father and developed with others.

Let us underline that it is only after weaning proper – the separation from bodily contact – that the assimilation of the mother tongue begins to happen, with groups of phonemes coming to accompany sensations and emotions – tactile sensations owing to the nearby presence of mother's body, emotions owing to her approaching or moving further away.

This is a period of imprecise language, of which the child cannot show the fruits straightaway. He will only be able to show this later, at the point when he discovers the pleasure of mastering the anal primordial object, that is to say his excrements, in playing with his urethral and anal sphincters, in playing with retaining or rejecting his excrements, especially if it is at the request of his mother, and producing sounds or not, that too at the request of his mother, in their face-to-face games, and then in naming his parents with phonemes and then his excrements, often before he can name his food.

The repeated words of two syllables by which language first appears, which correspond with a feeling of existing for the child, while he is still joined with mother as an alter ego and is the double of her sensations: ma . . . ma . . . poo . . . poo . . . It is always him-the-other, the same, 'paired' that provokes the start of speech in these two repeated syllables. Babies almost always start speaking in this way.

I believe that the double that he is of the mother, and this symbiotic relationship followed by a dyad, all makes this period one of a two-beat rhythm. Clearly, this has its roots in the heartbeat, but above all in the fact that he has to exist paired, so that uncoupling brings displeasure when mother leaves, and reunification with her brings pleasure in finding himself a double again, and the symbolic comes into being with the notion that sensations feel different depending on whether one is with or without mother – pleasure that is the remaining sensation after the subtraction of one of the sensations, taken away along with her by mother, and the reunion is accompanied by an additional joy also expressed by mother. It is the ensemble of the metaphorisation of the presence of part objects doubled by the presence–absence of the mother that seems to me to explain the double syllables that constitute the first signifiers between children and their nurses.

This is where the mother's role as initiator of language is primordial – a point not well enough known by mothers and carers. It is important that after each breast-feed, at the moment where the child, quite animated before falling asleep, likes already to 'exchange conversation' – which for him is manipulation of objects, and the illusion of watching himself in the mirror of his mother's face – the mother names for him all the objects he puts in his mouth, designates their name, taste, tactile quality and colour. The child learns to give these objects to his mother as if he would give her a spoonful of food. And the mother, in giving them back, takes pleasure in the game that consists in sometimes suddenly throwing the object overboard: exactly as in his mouth, after a certain time of manipulation, of chewing by the jaws and the tongue, the object disappears into the stomach by swallowing; the metaphor of the stomach here is displaced in throwing overboard, making things disappear out of the cot. It is a great joy for the child if the mother then picks up the thrown things, precisely because they are things, and not part objects of consumption. We are not here in the anal order of throwing away; this can arise, but the throwing away starts with the swallowing mode – causing something to be swallowed up by space.

Thus, we observe in a child weaned for two or three weeks – he is between 6 and 8 months and starting to cut teeth – the advent of the symbolic fruits of an oral castration that happened in happy partnership with mother. It is the language of facial expressions, modulated variably according to the people around and to the perceptions and feelings of the child. We observe in the child the advent of a modulated language, not yet grammatical, which reaches its highest intensity around eighteen months. The child becomes able to manipulate the people around him at a distance. His mouth has inherited some of his manual dexterity that had been valued by the parents; his tongue manipulates phonemes that are for his parents and his entourage signs of feelings, sensations and desires that he wants to communicate to them. What happens here between diverse erogenous zones is very interesting. The first language in which the words are not yet recognisable but where the intention and the intensity of desire are recognised by the entourage promote in the child, if he is not constantly with his parents, an inventive manipulation of distant and sometimes very close objects to make them come. He knows very well, for example, that as soon as he is bored because of his mother's absence, that if he causes things to tumble, if he makes noises or screams, it is going to make the adult return. And he does this as you pull on a rope to ring a bell! For him, this is language.

If the mother has exchanges with her child at a distance, both verbally and in facial expressions, the child truly enjoys it and claps with his hands: either one against the other when he has been taught to do this, but mostly by taking objects in his hands and banging them up and down with joy, arms outstretched, onto a fixed support such as a table. He screams with joy; he is all happy if the mother adds a song to modulate with him the joy that he experiences and that he shows by hitting what he is holding to a rhythm of his own. He hits according to his rhythm, which mother plays at following by putting words to it, sometimes modulating them, and so making a song: it is fantastic, everything makes sense.

This is what a baby is capable of that cannot yet walk but who doesn't get upset if his mother, or whoever replaces her, is present or not, on condition that she is not too far, within earshot. He does not get bored because the symbolic fruits of oral castration have already made of him a human individual who has an inner life in relationship with his mother's delight linked with his own delight; the delight of his mother in him also creates in him the certainty that his father and the adults in mother's entourage are proud of him; and if he has older siblings, that he is in the process of climbing the ladder that will make him equal to them.

I would forget an element that can sometimes play a capital role if I did not mention here *the olfactory aspect of everything in play around oral castration.* At the same time as breastfeeding, which fulfils a need, the child experiences an erotic satisfaction both olfactory and pseudo-cannibalistic because of the grabbing of the breast between the jaws. The weaned child who is given a bottle finds himself subject to the absence of the olfactory erotism that accompanied his imaginary cannibalism, even if the grabbing and suction during the weaning from the breast and move to the bottle continue to provide in another way the satisfaction he already knew. The cavum and the mouth of the child will, obviously in an unconscious way, play a part in the subtle communication with the mother, away from bodily contact, that is to say with the mother as a whole person and no longer as a substantial part object.

It is electively through olfaction that the mother can come to be singularised from a mammary part object to a whole object – because smell does not refer to a precise place for the child. The subtlety of smell spreads in the surrounding space; the child bathes in it, in the vicinity of his mother. The smell is no longer assigned to this or that part of the maternal body, and as the pituitary erogenous zone is always linked with breathing in through the nose, the smell left by the mother can only be lost to the child if he suffers from anosmia. It is important to understand that, as the need for breathing is not amenable to delay, olfaction accompanies each nasal breath. Thus, desire and discrimination of the pleasure caused by the mother's presence occur through smell, while the need to breathe is satisfied by any sort of air however it smells coming in as much through the mouth as through the nose.

Weaning could be an event that causes euphoria for baby and mother if on a known background of substantial communication (now, suckling the bottle) and of the functional image of suckling (swallowing of milk or liquid or semi-liquid food before solids are introduced, all having a taste different from mother's milk), the child and the mother keep together what remains specific of their psychic bond, alive in their combined presence. For the baby, the mother's body when she is close, her voice, her image, her gaze, her rhythms, everything that she gives off for him when she holds him and that he can perceive in their bodily interactions is a sensory-psychic link; at the same time, for the mother, nothing is changed in her baby who no longer suckles the breast but whose grace and development she admires every day. Conversely, it has to be said that a mother who does not talk to her baby while he is suckling, but who strokes him continuously or, while giving him physical care, seems to be totally indifferent because of depression, does not promote in the child a weaning favourable to ulterior socialisation, to correct verbal expression and motor functioning.

Still less a mother who, having weaned her child, cannot stop herself from constantly devouring him with kisses and oppressing him with pawing caresses. She was herself the wounded child of a disturbed mother–daughter relationship that she is desperately trying to heal. The child is for her the fetish of an archaic maternal breast from which she had been weaned in a traumatic way.

Anal castration

There are two aspects to the term 'anal castration' – the first, defined as a second weaning, is synonymous with the separation of the child, who is now capable of independent and agile movement, from the auxiliary assistance of his mother in everything that needs 'doing' in order to live within a family group. It is the acquisition of autonomy, 'I can do it – me, by myself.' This castration, taken on by the child, depends of course on the parents' tolerance of the child's day-by-day development of his autonomy in the safe space in which he is given the freedom to be useful, to play and have pleasure. The child, in becoming a subject, stops being a part object held in the dependence of the caring adult, submitting to the adult's possessiveness and to his/her total surveillance (feeding, dressing, washing, going to bed, moving around). The other aspect of anal castration is – between the child, newly autonomous in action, and his adult carer – the prohibition signalled to the child of all harmful action, 'doing' to another what he would not like done to himself. It is the access to speech that gives value to the relational exchange between people recognised as being masters of their actions and whose pleasure must be reciprocal and free. This is why this second meaning of the term anal castration is closely linked with the first one.

Any child whose parents have not been anally castrated from their child and who want to inculcate in him through what they say and do the prohibition to commit harm (while they themselves are harming his humanisation by considering him as an object to be 'trained'), convey in words the opposite of the example they give. They do not give anal castration. They 'train' a domesticated animal. The subject is denied, instead of the child's desiring impulses being partly forbidden and partly supported by the entry into language in playful and socialised exchanges between subjects that bring pleasure to them.

Therefore, we cannot speak of anal castration except where the child is recognised as a subject, even though his body is still immature; and his actions are not to be confused with the expression of the subject in him, as long as he has not acquired the total autonomy of his person within the family group.

Anal castration is therefore the interdiction of damaging one's own body or the animate and inanimate world surrounding the initial triangle of father–mother–child, by dangerous or uncontrolled rejecting motor actions. In fact and in origin, it is the interdiction of murder and vandalism in the name of the safe harmony of the group; at the same time as the initiation to the pleasure of the freedom of motor functioning shared with others, in a communication by speech and body language in which each person takes pleasure in agreement with others. This control of harmful motor drives, this initiation into the pleasure of communication in language and control of motor functioning, in the measure and mastery of strength applied to useful and pleasurable activities – all this allows the subject to be present in his own maintenance, preservation, movement through space, and then in creativity in both work and play (and not only utilitarian activities). At the same time, the path remains open to other pleasures to be discovered at the later stages, urethral and vaginal, which bring the boy or girl to the genital phase.

Human beings, whatever their age, are capable of giving this anal castration to younger ones, as much by example as by speech.

Why do we call this 'anal' when all I have just said seems to be about the privation of the pleasure of aggressive action that could be harmful to self and others, and the initiation into the pleasures of controlled motor functioning as well as of exchanges with others? It is because for the still immature child, this is the place of the first motor act in which the child sees proof that motor functioning is pleasing to him and in general gives satisfaction to his mother, because she comes and changes him and takes away what he has produced. After the suckling and swallowing, the urethral and anal expulsive motor functioning always provokes a modification perceptible by smell and often a variation of sensations in relation to the mother. With his excrements, the child expels the imaginary mother incorporated in the form of an oral part object, which after the swallowing that made it disappear and its path through the digestive tube, announces itself before externalising itself at his bottom. He has eaten from mother with a pleasure linked with imaginary cannibalism and now he expels of mother what dis-incorporates itself from him in liquids and solids. It is an imaginary mother he takes in and rejects, that he receives and gives, while the real mother gave him an alimentary part object and removed from him the excremental digested object. For the child, it is an object of which his mother seems fond, as he has no logic or ethos other than that he takes in good things; the child values his excrements as objects supposed to be food and pleasure for the mother. While the motor system develops and oral castration has been symboligenic, mother's care of the infant's bottom is accompanied by speech, games, a whole affective relationship with the mother during which the bodily schema develops day by day. *The bodily schema cross-develops with the body image*, which is attached to the erogenous excremental gift and to the pleasure of using his motor muscular strength. This pleasure is expressed by the happy kicking of his limbs, his body, his mouth, his smiles, his gurgling, his dreams, his babbling and screaming, all of which signal his distress or joy to his mother.

It is during the child's crawling motor games and his moving of objects (which he tries out with everything in his environment that can be moved) that the child's motor functioning becomes a problem that mother tries to solve by reducing his freedom or, on the contrary, by creating possibilities of exploratory displacement of greater and greater reach, which are possibilities of exchange with the child, a source of words, pleasure, upset and joy, and of restrictions and permissions orchestrated and signalled by language. *Anal castration is thus delivered little by little. It guides the child towards the mastery of his own motor functioning, and not only excremental.* This is to say he becomes continent when he has mastered his own motor functioning, in harmony with the code of motor language of animate beings in the external world. *Anal castration can only be symboligenic and conducive to the child's industriousness when he can observe and identify with the intentional motor activity displayed by the total objects represented by parents and elder siblings.*

When the symbolisation of motor functioning in useful or playful acts cannot happen, because it is not initiated, supervised or spoken about and has no part in the playful gaiety of his human entourage, the child cannot sublimate the anal-rectal drives in the exercise of motor functioning for greater communication with the people upon whom he has transferred his relationship with his mother; the anal-rectal motor functioning becomes the only pleasure left to him, and he goes back to it out of a lack of displacement of the anal drives, passive and active, onto other part objects elsewhere than in his body. *He returns, lacking in symboligenic anal castration, to the initial communication with the internal mother*; i.e. playing at withholding through constipation or at exteriorising the faeces, potentially in diarrhoea, in any way, in an incontinent, uncontrolled way. And then he gets bored, sometimes excites himself over any nonsense and, then again, gets bored. The mother remains imaginarily internal, instead of being unconsciously represented by all the external objects that she should have named and allowed him to manipulate.

Constipation can therefore be a sign of the inhibition of the motor relationship with the external world: because the child has not been initiated into this relationship by the mother, his relationship with his mother in regard to the excremental function is disharmonious. But he can also become diarrhoeic when the effects of a motor excitation cannot be expressed in another way and are repressed with regard to the action of his skeletal-muscular body on the objects of the external world. The anal impulses play upon the premier body image, that is, upon the peristaltic movements of the digestive tube, which becomes hyperactive, and thus its hyperfunctioning produces diarrhoea. This initial diarrhoea is non-infectious, but as the digestive tube is subject to over-activity, the tube lining that is no longer manipulating the contents of the digestive tube that have been too quickly expelled works upon itself and provokes an infection through the effect of peristaltic movement upon nothing, which causes a degradation of the mucosa. This is what was discovered by Madame Aubry's researches into the 'Parents of Rosan' – a nursery for adopted babies. When the nurses were quarrelling over the cots of the abandoned babies, whose body image, in the absence of parents, had already been reduced to the thoracic-abdominal bubble and digestive tube that runs from one erogenous pole to the other, and having no language addressed to them as people, they tried to bring themselves into unison with the violent language being exchanged between strangers that caused them anxiety, and their reaction was hyper-peristaltic movement that caused diarrhoea – a diarrhoea that Mme Aubry found to be absolutely amicrobial, and which she stopped by giving the infants two or three meals back to back, to fill the space of the digestive tube – which having something upon which to exercise its peristaltic movements, no longer gave any pathogenic consequences.

Diarrhoea is a way of rejecting an imaginarily incorporated maternal danger. It perhaps signifies, from the child's point of view, that if he expels a lot, the oral mother will 'top him up' – bringing oral part objects to the entrance of the digestive tube, while what he expels below is the 'bad mother' (and this because of what is said about the smell: 'that smells bad'), this could cause him to hope that what arrives at the top is the good mother – milk, porridge – 'that smells good.' It is anyway what happened in the experiment conducted by Mme Aubry. She had the children suffering diarrhoea given one or two meals in rapid succession where before, they would have been put on a diet. Of course, this shouldn't be done if the diarrhoea is already infectious, the digestive tube having been injured by the intrinsic rubbing due to exacerbated peristaltic movements. But all this proves, at least, that when diarrhoea begins in a child placed in an ambiance of great nervous tension, it is because he has no means other than digestive with which to show it. If he could cry, that would already be another means – the cry is an expression of tension, of extra tension looking for a way of communicating with another. If even the cry is heard by nobody, if it doesn't bring someone who comes to reassure the child and to enter into language with him, then it is towards the archaic, imaginary mother of the digestive tube that he directs the tension – because he suffers inside and what is in the digestive tube is linked with the external mother who makes him suffer through anxiogenic nervous tension.

The better to understand this dynamic, one could consider the child's digestive tube in the same way as those worms one sees at the seaside that, as they advance, swallow sand and then leave it behind them as if they nourish themselves with the environment they are crossing. Regarding the child, it is the mother that passes inside of him, from the mouth to the anus, the imaginary mother in the form of the part object he absorbed. And it is the real external mother – she who nests and nestles him and keeps him safe – who in an alternative fantasy gives to the mouth and takes from the anus. When the child violently expels the contents of his digestive tube, it is as if he is saying, 'fill me up from the top' – he is calling for a communication. He wants speech, but prefers food to nothing at all, and this is what he is expressing. It is the presence of the symbolic mother that he calls for. And if the mother does not understand that it is her he wants, her calm tenderness, if all she gives him is stuff to digest, to drink and eat, which is not language, then such a child – seen by her as a digestive tube whose needs she looks out for and which expels poo, which she whips away without accompanying speech – is inevitably inhibited in his initiation into language in the future. And this comes into play very early. When the child starts to talk, there have already been nine months in which he has been potentially talking, because he 'swallows/gobbles phonemes.' He swallows them with his ears and he must regurgitate them with his larynx, and this is for the subtle the same thing by analogy as for the substantial – it is a metaphor for what happens in the digestive tube.

Therefore, I say that motor castration that carries the law of the prohibition of murder, of vandalistic harm to both oneself and others and to the objects invested by others as their possession is part of anal castration. And I say that all human beings, whatever their age, are able to give this anal castration to younger ones on the condition that, being more developed than the subject to be castrated, they are models for him of what he will become, through the wish that the smaller one has to imitate them in order to gain narcissistic value in reaching a more developed and harmonious image, better adapted to the group than he presently is. This wish goes in the direction of his social development towards the adult pattern of a boy or a girl because he has, through language, the knowledge of his sex, and he also has it intuitively through his desire to imitate those he experiences as sexualised alter-egos (although we don't quite know how).

The case of François

Receiving castration from an older sibling of another sex without reference ever being made to behaviours of his own sex can cause a deviation in what the child will become.

'The first stage of becoming like my father was to be my sister,' said the child who had been driven to a suicide attempt. He was an intelligent 13-year-old boy who took two days to emerge from a coma. He had tried to kill himself with a kitchen knife, opening his belly. He terrified the surgery unit in saying, when he regained consciousness: 'But why, as I am going to have to do it again!' That is when, disgusted, they thought of the psychoanalyst of the unit and I was called.

I only knew that he had two sisters, one a bit older than him and the other one younger, and that he was the only boy. This is the first thing I told him. His eyes were shut, I waited for him to open them. He felt my presence, opened his eyes and looked at me, I told him my name and that I was a psychoanalyst and that the people from the unit called me, 'Because it took them two days to resuscitate you and your first words were, why do you resuscitate me because now I have to do it again. So, if you put yourself in the shoes of the doctors and surgeons who sorted out an almost dead child who then tells them, "I want to die," they don't understand and that's why they called me – me, a psychoanalyst, to see if you if you really want to die or if you want to live but you don't know how to do it. So if you want to talk to me, you will . . .' – he had re-closed his eyes – 'you will make a sign with your eyelids as you cannot talk.' (He had tubes everywhere). 'And if you don't want to see me, well, I would understand that very well. Don't make any sign and I will go away. You have the right to want to die, but I believe that it would be interesting that you understand that there may be for you, perhaps, a possibility of living if you understand the reasons for which you believe that you are not allowed to live.'

And so he made a sign, repeated this twice (opening and closing his eyes).
I told him: 'My name is Madame Dolto, your name is so-and-so and I come to the hospital on Tuesdays. We will be able to talk, but could you tell me, as you can talk a little, why do you have to do it again?'
'I have never been like the others.'
'Well, I am not surprised, as the others are girls and you are a boy!'
He opened his eyes wide as if amazed by my answer.
And me: 'See you next Tuesday.'

It was an extraordinary treatment, a lightning treatment, in five sessions at weekly intervals. It was impossible for this boy to reach maturity – a child whose claim was to identify with a man, but while being all the time enmeshed with his sister who was 14 months older than him. He reached the point of suicide shortly after the moment his sister reached puberty. In six months, she had changed from a child into a young woman, having periods and transformed as compared with him. Also, all the boys were interested in her, they were calling her on the telephone and he, her brother, always answered, 'She's not here.' If he answered the phone and it was a guy calling, she was never there.

These two children would never talk about each other in any form other than 'us' – 'us two – Christine,' he would say, 'we want this . . . we think that . . .' And she would say, 'us two, François . . .' – never any 'I' either from one or the other; they were always 'one and the other.' He was anorexic from the age of 7 but nobody worried about it in the family. He was slender, very lean, sporty, active, very academically advanced and the parents said: 'Yes, he never eats fat or bread, never any sugar, however he has been eating like this since the age of 7' – the age at which his younger sister was born. And with this, he gave me the key.

He told me that it was since his mother expected 'the ghost' . . .
I asked him: 'But what is the ghost?'
'Well yes, you understand, babies when they are born stand up in their cot and shake the veils. So I called her the ghost.'
'Who is the ghost?'
'Well, it was a girl.'
'Yes, then it's your sister?'
'Well, no. You see, if it had been a boy I could have been brother, but as it was a girl . . .'
'So if it was a girl, what were you?'
'Well, it is my sister (he was referring to Christine) who was "sister".'

In his absurd idea, he would have been brother if the younger sibling had been a boy, but here he was nothing. It was Christine, falsely twinned with him, who was 'my sister' and the young one was the ghost. In fact, it was he who was becoming a ghost.

He told me that when his mother was expecting 'the ghost,' the family doctor explained: 'You should take this opportunity to put your husband on a diet because he is fat and this could have an impact on his heart.' So much so that while she was pregnant, her husband, François' father, had followed a weight-loss diet and François added, 'You understand, the bigness of women makes babies, but the bigness of men suffocates their heart.'

It is amazing what he managed to tell me in a few sessions and while putting on 12 kilos! At the last session, he told me, 'What is your profession . . . what studies do you have to do for that profession? I would like to do the job you do.'

> 'You have to be first either a doctor or a psychologist and then you do a psychoanalysis and you learn the trade.'
> Then he said, 'Yeah, psychoanalysis, I know, It's the history of the Oedipus complex. Dad told me that.' It was the last session, a goodbye session. He had wanted his father to be present.
> 'Yeah, it was the story of a guy who was bothered by another one who was always talking[11] and whom he pulverised.'
> I said: 'Yes, that's more or less it, but there is something else.'
> 'Yes, you know,' intervened father at this point, 'I told you that it is because the father was in love with the same woman as the son.' (sic!)

In any case, returning to the difficulty of his identifications, if he had stopped eating fat it is because he wanted to become a man and did not want to have fat that would become a baby. From this stemmed the anorexia that brought him to the point of fainting. A few weeks before attempting suicide, he had been chosen class prefect at his lycée. About this, he said: 'When the guys chose me, I told myself, but I'm not a girl, why do they want me?'

When he talked about his total loss of appetite, which led to him fainting, I told him: 'How did it start? Did it start with the impossibility of eating or with the impossibility of pooing?'

'That's it – the impossibility of pooing. You have to understand, I was full of these bread rolls in the shape of suppositories.' (This was about sandwiches he had called 'in the shape of a suppository' and that he ate at the lycée for lunch.) 'They filled me up completely and it could not escape because I had too many of them. So I could not eat any more.'

It is rather extraordinary, the puberty that was about to happen and that provoked a flourishing of old infantile fantasies. There was a confusion of all the orifices with an image of the digestive tract as a 'thing' in which everything you absorb piles up. He had the idea of an obstacle through accumulation and he said:

---

11 Translator's note: in French, '*il faisait tout le temps des Laïus*' – an expression that means to be talkative, and a pun upon the name of Oedipus' father, Laïus. In the child's mind, Oedipus killed Laïus because he talked too much.

'You know, it's like when pipes are blocked, you have to unblock them,' and this is why he had unblocked his stomach with an opening of the abdomen with the kitchen knife. He had to kill the ghost to become real. In his case, anal castration had been given by the sister. That is to say that it is with his sister that he identified at the time of being able to acquire the mastery of his motor self and of the world around him, in a sort of fake twinning in which he believed himself to be like her. He knew about sexual differences but there were no behavioural differences until the day that other boys' desire became directed towards his sister. Then he was lost because he had been abandoned by his auxiliary ego. He had not had any real autonomy until then despite very good intellectual development and exceptional academic success. Anal castration had been given, but the masculine identification was impossible and Oedipus complex had been experienced with a blurred body image that was not that of a boy; it was a 'desiring-to-be-a-boy' that had an asexual or feminine body image that became subjectively asexualised because he realised that he was not feminine, but secondarily threatened (in his view) by feminisation when the boys' vote in class elected him prefect because they liked him in the way his sister was liked by boys.

One can see there that *anal castration has to be given by those who support, in the one to whom they give it, what we call identification with their sex*, the ego-ideal of the child – the envied model, the one with whom he wants to identify – and who forbid through gestures and words motor behaviours undesirable *according to the laws of the group: behaviours suggested by desire but which would be harmful either to himself or to others*. It follows on from this that if secretly, unbeknownst to the adults, the child, curious to experiment with his desire, disobeys verbal prohibitions that have been imposed on him, and not only does he not experience any harm but harvests only pleasure without damage to others or to himself, then he has discovered alone the means of satisfying his desire and through this has experienced a power of which the adults did not think him capable. It is the most important moment in the educational relationship between the adult and a child of between 2 and 4 years old. When this motor transgression is noticed by the tutelary agent, they should congratulate the child who has disobeyed rather than make him feel guilty for having disobeyed what was said, as the only goal of what was said was to protect him from a real danger and not at all to make him dependent upon an order forbidding motor functioning. This order has become obsolete as he does not need the prohibition to remain safe while taking risks according to his desire. *There is wherein lies all the difficulty in bringing up a child aged between 2 and 4 and in whom one wants to inculcate, because it is easier, that he or she should not disobey the prudent injunctions of the tutelary agent*: when he does transgress without any damage, one should say, 'Bravo. I forbade you this because I did not think you were big enough to do it without danger. But because you are, I congratulate you. From now on, you are allowed to do this; but do not do that other thing that you won't be able to do until the day where you will feel capable of it, because this or that problem could happen. Make sure that this younger child doesn't do it until he is able to.'

On the other hand, if in these transgressions or attempts at transgression the child has experienced his impotence through sustaining damage to himself or causing unintended accidental damage that was not part of his project, anal castration has to be given again in words at the same time as support should be given to his narcissism, as he has failed in a desire of transgression that was a desire promoting identification with the adult. We often see education being done quite differently. The child has suffered from his failure at the attempt at transgression and the adult, anxious that the child had risked an accident or had provoked an incident, attacks him and often verbally rejoices in a sadistic way, 'Serves you right, you disobeyed and you've been punished.'[12]

This way of giving anal castration is perfectly detrimental, inhumane. For the child, it seems as if the adult, whose magical words express his desire, is the agent of his misadventure. In the child's idea of omnipotence, it is the adult who wants to impose a motor impotence, an imposition that could later issue from the child himself, because of his desire to identify with the adult, and which will damage his success in reality. It is clearly necessary that the adult verbalises the real danger, the impotence of the child in the face of the action he wanted to accomplish. But the adult must also explain that the same impotence would be the lot of the adult if they attempted at their level acts such as that which the child tried to achieved and failed. In the first case, the adult gives the child a hope of identifying with him one day, in developing and in observing the modality of his actions; in the second case, the adult gives the child the proof that his impotence is not bigger than that of his parents if they had to deal with the elements at play in this dangerous activity within their own parameters. Anal castration keeps the child safe while supporting his freedom to desire and his hope of success.

The child, through experience, discovers that the prohibitions are safeguards as if he transgresses them, they bring real suffering. It is this experience that gives him trust in his parents and in what they say that limits his complete freedom. Nonetheless it is important to know that for a child every disappointment is a narcissistic wound, while at the same time the suffering he experiences from a disappointment caused by a desire that he has wilfully acted upon is in the order of castration. This is why it is important only to forbid temporarily anything that could be damaging to the child as such, but that an older child or an adult could do successfully and without danger when he has the wherewithal, according to the mode of the anal ethos. It is necessary always to affirm to the child that with time, patience, observation, a more developed competence and identification with the behaviour of trusted adults, his perseverance and efforts will be rewarded: he will one day access the same power he observes in his parents and maybe even a greater power than theirs. It follows from this that adults, parents or not, able to give the child anal castration with maximum symboligenic efficacy, as much for his playful, industrious, artistic and utilitarian power as for his social sense and

---

12 This can go as far as, 'God has punished you.'

respect for others, are those who do not in every situation project anxiety onto the actions of the children for whom they are responsible. It is those who are ready to respond to the questions asked by the child, without going further than what is asked, who are able judiciously to help him when he gets upset and discouraged by not managing to perform as well as he would like, because of a lack of adequate means.

It is also those who know how to say no to the desire of the child when this goes against the law against doing harm, either for example by taking possession – nicking, pilfering or stealing other people's personal objects in their owner's absence – or by really dangerous acts for their age. When I talk about a child having to learn to respect the goods of others in their absence, this is only possible if the child also possesses objects and the adult does not claim for himself the right to attack that property in the child's absence. For example, one sees mothers and fathers who regularly throw out certain of their children's toys under the pretext that they were broken. One also sees them confiscating toys or making the child entrust to them money they have been given as a present. They don't realise that in doing this they undermine the possibility of the child's respecting the goods of others. To begin with, the taking apart of his toys is part of the child's play and never should any possession of a small child be thrown out without him deciding this for himself. Also, no possession of a child should be confiscated as a punishment. If one removes an object from a child, it should only be because the object is precious in reality and to help the child himself, who risks damaging it and then regretting it later, the object's price or guarantee excluding the possibility of replacing it. But never: 'I'm confiscating your doll because you broke the vase.'

If one respects everything a child puts in his toy-box and holds dear, for personal reasons, the child will naturally respect the personal objects of others. *It is clear that anal castration can only be given if the parents are in reality respectful of the child and his goods, if they bring him up with trust in his intelligence and in the going-on-becoming of this little man or little woman, leaving a large margin for his own initiative,* reducing day by day the number of things forbidden to them according to their development and their acquired experiences – sometimes at the risky cost of transgressing parental prohibitions but that become successes if the child manages them without incident. When there are successful transgressions, when disobedience has benefited the child, then he is particularly on the look-out for what is said to him. Are you going to scold him for disobeying, or are you proud of his success? That an adult recognises that in continuing to forbid what the child is capable of, he has underestimated the abilities the child has developed, and the child gains even more trust that the adult is attentive to him for his own safety and not for the sake of keeping him dependent. If, when giving another prohibition, the adult makes reference to the child's past successful transgression in order to specify that in the present case, trying it would be too risky or even catastrophic for the child or himself, the child will listen and not disobey.

In many upbringings, the origin of character disturbances with regard to the family group or society lies in the period of anal castration – this being between

18 months and 5 years, when what comes into play is motor functioning, the value of conviviality in playing with other children, the value of mastering bodily functions, which is a source of pleasure and health. These disturbances are due to either inhibitions or the disrespect of all behavioural rules. The non-socialisation of children happens when their carers do not respect day to day his desires to take motor initiatives that in themselves entail no real danger but just because they are noisy or slightly mess up the tidiness of the room, or provoke in the parents fantasmatic anxieties that cause them to predict all kinds of evils and to threaten punishments, slaps or spankings – and this at the slightest transgression of absurd and sadistic prohibitions in relation to what is a healthy motor progression that rather honours the better judgement of the child.

This applies also to the prohibitions to getting dirty, to creating untidiness, making noise while playing, climbing on furniture (which can be fixed to the wall) or solid tree branches, to touching things that adults themselves touch, while observing closely how he manages in his turn to become skilful. The child wants to imitate adults – this is his duty, I dare say; he should be supported in this by an attentive solicitude. From the age of 22 to 24 months, children's hands and bodies can be as skilful with the external world as those of certain adults, even while they are not yet able to master their sphincters for absolute continence. At 4 or 5 years, when brought up in trust, the child is extremely skilful, if taught to use technology, and if he takes pleasure in helping the adult whenever he is allowed. Work and useful motor activity thus shared – games with parents, all activities where each takes pleasure in exchanging speech about what they are doing and what they know how to do – all this increases tenfold the pleasure of action in the child and prepares him for progressive and total autonomy by the day-to-day introjection of savoir-faire linked with speech and mutual liking between him and the adult, between him and other children, a liking he feels through shared activity.

I indicated above that *anal castration is so called because it has its origins in the voluntary functioning of the sphincters and the mastery of this*, even if the humanising power goes far beyond this one acquisition, which we call cleanliness, and concerns the child's autonomy over his needs, the maintenance of his body and unconscious continence during deep sleep. I would even say that this acquisition, when imposed too early, far from being educative, is mutilating. Then, it does not operate as a symboligenic castration that opens the child up to the pleasure of sublimation of the anal drive. Like all other mammals, the child is capable of spontaneously developing sphincter control: this happens whether or not it is asked for by the tutelary adult. Sphincter control is 'natural' as soon as neuro-physiological development permits. When adults put upon the child the demand to 'be clean' either too early or too late, it gives to basic needs a value that should only belong to the desire to communicate and have socialising exchanges.

This is how the behaviour of adults, which shows in itself the desire to control the needs of children, may come to pervert many of them, who then play with their retentive power either to please or to displease the demanding adult. This valuing attitude towards poo leads to the manipulation of the excrement while it is being ejected, the child acting like the adult who the child thinks takes pleasure in stealing it – to play with. A child who has never been asked for excrements does not play with them; they prefer to play with other objects – unless they have never had any toys or objects at their disposition. He takes this, because it is the first (mummy-ised) part object he can find in his space; but if he has toys, objects he is interested in manipulating, putting to his mouth etc., he will not occupy himself with his poo. If he is not induced to by mother's daily attitude of valuing the contents of his nappy or potty, the child will not make it an issue for himself. A healthily given anal castration – that is not focused on the wee or the poo but on the valuing of bodily and manual motor functioning – must allow the child to substitute (limited) excremental pleasures for the joy of doing, of manipulating objects in his world, as well as the pleasure in the promoting himself by identification with older siblings and parents. The hands are, in effect, the lieu of displacement of the oral erogenous zone after weaning. They act like the mouth in seizing objects: like teeth, like the clamping of jaws, the fingers sink into soft objects within their reach, they scratch, they break up, they palpate, in appreciating their shape. A baby likes to play at tearing with his hands with playful joy. This is the use of the 'hand-mouth.' Babies may experience overwhelming joy in ending up in reducing these objects into the elements of earth and water – the human joy of a first demolition that is for them a piece of work, transferred onto part objects pleasing to the hands from alimentary part objects pleasing to the mouth. Desire is never appeased by the tactile investigation of objects. The language of mother and father regarding their child explorer who 'is into everything' brings safety, if they are present at the first manifestations of pre-industrious observation and creation, even when to begin with, these investigations are apparently destructive and ravaging. It is only afterwards that manual activity, after a certain period of its apparently destructive exercise, becomes constructive, agglomerating, for example in piling up of cubes. And so, by the displacement of desires first oral and then anal, the child becomes skilful and intelligent, and observes physical laws according to sensory references acquired through experience, in particular the law of gravity that he learns to negotiate.

These real acquisitions of motor functioning and creation are obstructed when one gives stupid value to the 'problem' of wee and poo, to the early continence of the child. The child is always capable of that himself; the education consists, when continence is achieved, only of him putting the excrements in the place in which it is destined to be for everyone, children and adults – the toilet – and to manage proudly to do that on his own, as soon as it is neurologically possible. In effect, it seems to the child that the adults who go to the toilet and isolate themselves there are possessed of an extremely valuable symbolic key, all the more so because the child cannot accompany them. Doing wees and poos in the place reserved for adults and in a way that translates into continence – characteristic of the 'big ones' – confers on the child the right to attain a level of conduct that delivers, with the complete autonomy over bodily needs, the label of human dignity in society.

It is only among children who have been required to be continent too early that one sees a delay in the development of the body image with regard to that of the bodily schema. Because it is then for them the only way to stay a subject other than by opposing the pressing injunctions of the mother and depriving her of the pleasure she has – and that the child feels to be orally and anally incestuous – in occupying herself with his wee, poo and bottom, the region both shameful and sacred where needs and desire are at the origin of contradictory ethical values.[13] The child at the anal stage becomes policed in relieving himself and being continent in his sleep between 21 and 27 months at the latest, on the condition that there had been no educational training and that the motive of the tutelary agent in all other education has always been that of human promotion – mastery of motor functioning, sensorial mastery with its expression in verbal exchanges, extended knowledge of vocabulary, acceptance of the customs and regulations of society and the ability to be in the company of other children.

Natural continence is always spontaneous in a child raised in trust, in the respect of his human dignity in the midst of older children and adults with whom he has the right to identify as soon as he has the neurological possibility of doing this, without being rebuffed: 'Oh no, not you, you're too small!' It doesn't happen naturally in children who are not allowed satisfy their desire to act as and when they wish, in the way they see others acting, under the only pretext that they are small.

A child who has become spontaneously continent never bothers the adult unless they are intolerant of his questions, his demands, his attempts to do things, his initiatives in action. His requests, which sometimes tire his parents, are always intelligible; and the adults when they see him unable to realise a desire should rather encourage him to try again later rather than tell him: 'See? I told you!' Most children are kept for far too long in an unhealthy immobility, for example in public places and at table, for the convenience of the parents. And these same children at home are not helped in becoming skilful, which is what every child wishes. His clumsiness often comes from his inexperience, his lack of concentration, insufficient observation and mostly from the lack of explanatory speech coming from the adult whose activities he loves to observe. The child needs technological understanding and therefore verbalised help from the parents, explaining to him that if they had tried the same thing, they would have met the same impediment. But once again, it is only possible to reach that stage, this pleasure of 'doing' something technical with materials or objects, through the sublimation of the excremental pleasure, the pleasure of producing oneself the substantial part object, wee and poo, of which any other 'doing' is a displacement in its affective, ideational and language-linked investment.

It is true that since birth, the child's excrements are necessarily objects of interest for the parents as it is through their regular production and their satisfactory

13 There are exhibitionist and voyeuristic mothers who speak in public about their child's bottoms, stripping them naked to change them in any room and in front of anyone.

appearance that doctors and mothers judge the good health of the baby by way of his digestive functioning. In addition, for him, these interesting excremental objects have been relationally confounded by both the tactile and olfactive perceptions (the latter of which he experiences even when she is absent, if he has poo-ed in his nappy) with the co-natural link with the mother. It is she, who in taking them away in the course of cleaning him, in removing a tactile sensation at his bottom at the same time as he perceives the characteristic smell, adds facial expressions (language) that never go unnoticed by the child. It is she who initiates him into the role of manual mastery she has of this part object expelled because of need, and also to the role that the child, through his mastery, can himself have with regard to this object that also serves the desire as well as the pleasure that excreting can bring – a frequently solitary pleasure after having been shared with mother.

These are needs, as I said, but it is through all relationships with mother connected with need that the 'doing' initiates the child, after eating, into desire. With the development of his bodily schema, the child becomes naturally sensitised to what he can do through emission or retention, experiencing a local pleasure – or pleasure at a distance through the manipulation of the emotional climate of the adults towards him. The playful mastery of his excrement can at the discretion of educational demands become a valued exchange with others, the exchange of language and objects. We often talk (probably too much) about the 'poo-present' – this is very peculiar of certain, quite common ways of bringing up a baby.

From this comes the importance of the style of response the adult brings, in particular the mother. If she seems to give as much importance to the reception, the sight or the non-sight of the excremental part object, as to the whole child – chatting, smiling, manipulating objects and exchanging them with her – she gives a value of language to needs, the excrements as such, while it is something quite different for the child. The excrements as such cannot be a gift. They become this for the child if the mother rejoices in them more than she rejoices in his playful manual and vocal activities. The anus then becomes in some ways a substitute for the mouth as it is the anal signified that gains value because of her. This is how the poo can become – or remain – the 'poo-present.' Thus, we see mothers who rejoice and tell everyone about the wee-poo of their child! And the child, already 'pervertable,' tries even harder to please his mother in showing off, in exhibiting his talent. When there are visitors to the home, he brings his potty for everyone to see. This is the point where symbolic castration and not pure repression is welcome: 'Don't bring that, bring your toys instead, you have never seen your father or me bring our poo to everyone . . . bring cakes, show us the toys you like, come with us if you want but then behave as we do.' What the child wants, being sociable by nature, is to make himself interesting, to play a part in the group, be accepted by it, and this is how his mother can help him bring something to the social order.

This enormous value given to poo is something quite recent.[14] The importance of the excretory processes of babies and children did not exist before the use of nappies in the English way. It happened partly by way of the 'laziness' of the mother for washing swaddling clothes. The earlier the child became clean, the less work they had at a time where there were no washing machines and no wadding; it is true that it was an advantage for the child not to be as wet. When he wet himself, he was cold; when he was cold, he could have colic, and there was in this a whole anxiety-making situation in terms of both work for the mother and risk for the child. When I was a child, there were no rubberised pants, only woollen nappies, but the wet child could catch a cold and infantile mortality was the dread of mothers. Nevertheless, if the privileged means of exchange remain the substantial urethral and anal part objects, and still more because the production of these raw part objects is unconscious and necessary, the child comes to believe that his passive obedience to the desire to give his excrements at the moment the adult wants them represents a harmonious interhuman relationship. This perverts what would be the direction of creativity in the child. It is the germ of a compulsive warping that makes of this child a functioning 'thing' of an anxious mother when she does not have in the potty what she wishes to see.

It is a pity for the future humanisation of children if their mother believes that she needs to devote all her attention to 'training' them, under the pretext of education – that is, after the acceptance of food as imposed by mother, excretion at her will. Any 'training' is a perverse incitation to passivity, a prolonged parasiting of each other; through this the mother slows down the interest of the child in playful motor activity, access to walking and bodily and manual agility, all because of her demands and of the regularity she wants to impose on the rhythm of needs. These two activities demand muscular relaxation that is necessarily a source of 'accidents' in the pants. Before 21 and 28 months, the child is not yet able to control what he sees, hears, what his hands do in play and at work at the same time as controlling his sphincters, because of the insufficiency of his neurological and anatomical development. At that age, it is not possible for the child to focus on two things at once. Fortunately, mothers often get tired of not getting what they want and are interested also in all the other manifestations of the child's development, and delay this exhausting training, which is an uninterrupted source of quarrels with the little one if he has personality – which is a better omen for the future than if he obeys his mother in this.

For a child of 9 to 10 months at the earliest, the entry into the active anal stage of pleasure in the motor functioning of his whole body brings desire and pleasure to voluntary motor discoveries: first of the trunk and upper members, then the pelvis and lower members, which makes him capable of walking about, seated or on all fours, and of more and more manual dexterity, in an increasingly satisfactory

14 Some parenting books written by 'psychs' seem to suggest that admiration of the faecal gift is part of the panoply of behaviours of a 'good mother.'

and voluntary way. Finally, the child stands up and walks at around one year, sometimes later. Happy is the child who has discovered walking on his own and who has never been held standing up or made to walk, as is too often seen. It is a moment of extraordinary joy for the child when for the first time, he gets the revelation of his ability to move alone on his two feet, and it is certainly desirable that he discovers this without the close presence of an adult.

Anyway, it is through the desire to go towards his mother or towards something that attracts him that the child accomplishes his first steps. When he walks for the first time, he is completely surprised. If, when he is just starting to walk, an incident happens, he may not start again for one or two months, as he links the incident with that discovery.

In my experience as a mum, I was in the position of the mother who, in a discreet way, is present at the advent of verticality and discovers surprise in the face of her child. It is moving to witness the extraordinary joy shining from the little man or woman who invents afresh the standing position.

The child can now move in space. This motor displacement that happens first on all fours or on their bottom will be repeated on all fours even if he knows how to walk; and mothers must understand to what extent it is necessary for the development of the thorax, the muscles of the back, lower back and shoulders that children crawl on all fours for as long as possible, even when they know how to walk. Then, children like to use a stable support that they push in front of them, as this gives them enjoyment and mastery of their bodies at the same time as the pleasure of going towards or leaving mother by themselves; thus, the child measures at will his home and surroundings in his secure space, by the autonomy that mother grants him.

The autonomous displacement of external objects and his own displacement in space is for the child a linguistic metaphor – in the dimension of motor expression, thanks to the new abilities of his bones and muscles – for the digestive peristaltic movement that made the alimentary object move from the mouth to the anus.[15] This explains why a child who walks on his own for the first time, having dropped any support, returns on all fours to the place where he stood up and from which he left, and does this several times before discovering that he can walk further. Motor functioning must have been detached from its primary modality for it to be taken on as the rightful practice of a motor subject, and no longer dependent upon the conditions of the external space.[16] It is at the very beginning of walking that this can be observed. Let us repeat: the conditions that accompanied walking towards an object are the metaphor of peristaltic movement that went from the mouth to the anus, and the child therefore returns to the place where he discovered the possibility of standing upright and walking, to restart this experience. The child who discovers walking cannot immediately do the reverse experience, that

15 Maybe this explains the relative anorexia of some children when they discover how to walk.
16 Some children can walk at home and nowhere else.

is to say, he cannot return upright from the place he arrived at after a few steps at the end of this first daring try, when he fell back onto his bottom. He never turns around to go back when he walks. He always goes in a straight line, moving for a while in a space that is that of the oral schema (a metaphor of the trajectory from one hole of the body to the other).

The changing of levels – going up and going down – is a new discovery that can happen before walking and as soon as the child moves about on all fours. But the child who has climbed upstairs cannot descend them on his own. It is extraordinary to witness the first experience of climbing a stepladder with steps on each side of a little landing; in itself, it is as easy to go down but after having climbed one side, the child wants to go down the other head first, which makes him fall. In the same way that he does not believe it possible after a few steps to turn around and return walking, he can only come down backwards after a long apprenticeship. There is a direction in the order of things. The other direction would be, for him, disorderly. It is as if walking backwards during his first discovery of walking is to him unthinkable. It is a little later when he masters walking that a mutation in the behaviour of the little one operates, a mutation that makes him desire to act 'on his own' as the big ones do, while before he used the support of the big ones to 'play' at acting like them. From that moment on, he wants to 'be big' for real and not just pretend to be. The words 'big' and 'I can do it,' often mispronounced at a very early age,[17] become synonymous with promotion and narcissising goals. 'Look, Mum, look, Dad! I'm big! Do it on my own!' It is wonderful to see this phase – the pride of the child who wants to try on their own, to surpass themselves, to triumph in their identification with the older children. His attempt to imitate adults and older children makes the small child understand when he is unable to do something that his weakness is with regard to his pelvis and the lack of mastery of his legs. His hands have already been invested with an orality transferred from objects of dental aggression, taking to bits, throwing, displacing, putting together or separating. The feet now are invested with the aggression and tactility reserved until then for the hands. We know how much children like to explore their toes, heels and legs up to their root – their genitals, groin, anus and buttocks. They like to pinch themselves, this remaining the privilege of the hands and probably originating from the displacement of the pincer action of the mouth onto the hands that in addition open and close like a sphincter thanks to the opposition of the thumb and other fingers. The bottom remains the privilege of the hands of the tutelary adult as the child doesn't have arms long enough before around 30 months to reach all the parts of their body (it is at 6 years old that the right hand, the arm moving over the head, can reach the bottom of the left ear). But it is also because he doesn't know the tactile shape of the bottom crack and the anal region that he

17 Translator's note: the French '*grand*' is much harder to say for a small child than the English 'big.' She also adds, '*tou seu*' for '*tout seul*' or 'all alone' to suggest a young child saying he or she wants to do something by themselves. An English equivalent might be 'me do it!'

has to discover it. Also, instead of stopping the child touching himself, the mother should accompany his manipulations of his body with words that designate the different parts. From the earliest speech, when the child is only a few months old, provided that he manages to catch his genital region by chance – when his hands are only small pliers that squeeze everything they find and pull whatever can be pulled – the baby, if he does not then receive a slap on his hand by his mother, is able to find there sensations very different from those that he may have elsewhere and different also from those that his mother provokes through grooming.

When he has finally gained a generalised muscular mastery and the skills of the anal stage, the child discovers his whole body in a much more precise way than what he had known until then through the tactile contacts imposed by his mother. These are now his own discoveries and are at the centre of his interest. He needs words to specify all the sensitive regions he explores in his body and these words must let him understand that he is made like all other humans. He needs vocabulary to know the geography of his body and in particular the uro-genital region and the active excretory functioning, passive and retentive functioning with which he likes to engage without knowing yet how to put words to this pleasure.

His verbal expressions – 'wee' and 'poo' – are very interesting to him not only because they imply mastery of the words (orality) but also because they give value in reality as in saying this, he can control his seat. We have here a tuned-in mastery of words and function, while when the child says the word 'eat,' he cannot at the same time be eating. When he says 'wee,' he can do it or not. He cannot eat at the same time that he talks but he can poo while talking.

This is the whole difference between defecation and what happens in the mouth and it is also why the prohibition of talking about it leads the child to think that one wants to forbid him from experiencing what goes on in this well-innervated region and from experiencing the intelligent connection between on the one hand the mastery of the functioning of his body, just like adults and older siblings, and the pleasure that accompanies this functioning, and on the other hand, the sensual pleasures of its functioning in a way other than that of the behaviour that promotes him.

One cannot grasp how important are the stakes in anal castration, if one does not understand that it allows the obtaining of appropriate and humanised mastery of motor functioning, if only under the form, among others, of learning how to walk.

The decisive character of anal castration for the future of the child depends, in a word, on the narrow path that allows (or not) the sublimation of excretory manifestations into a form of creative and industrious 'doing.' At the same time, the relational phase of the child we are talking about is also that where he has to control his motor functioning, and where he has to take into account the behaviours he feels to be strange of other living creatures – animals, adults and children – that his autonomy in space make him encounter and are at first new to him, strange to his usual tutelary world. Until he could walk, he observed without risk from a cloud of familiar safety. This safety is now lacking and the child needs it in

imagination more than he did before, through words kept in his memory, supportive teaching about the new beings he will encounter – words that carry technical knowledge about the world to which he belongs and that he discovers day
after day, words that through their permanence in memory introduce him to the
manipulation of things, when the tutelary presence is missing. With these explanations that he can re-evoke, it is as if the tutelary presence introduced him to the
behaviour of beings and things yet unknown to him.

These teachings will allow him to consider unknown spaces to be discovered
every day, support him in exploring the familiar domain and every room of the
house without fantasmatic danger. He can conquer this thanks to the verbalised
knowledge that allows him to progress. Then he feels valued in his first narcissising trials when they are not stigmatised as silliness, and in his real success every
time he can act in the way he sees his elders acting.

In this intermediate stage between the very small person he is or the very big
person he would like to be, it is easy to introject failure and success as if they were
magical effects due to the malice of things – due to a wish to do harm of animal,
vegetable or even inert things that the child anthropomorphises in the image of
his all-powerful mother. At this stage, the child projects anthropomorphised intentions of devouring, rejecting or harming anything that resists him, and rightly or
wrongly, into anything that causes him anxiety, in his contacts with objects.

A 9-month-old child who crawled very fast on all fours and put his fingers in
an electric socket was told by his father not to do this; he was told that if he continued, it would be very painful and that it was completely forbidden by father.
Like any intelligent 9-month-old, this one tried to transgress the interdiction and
once, when nobody was watching, committed the forbidden act. He screamed and
people came. Fortunately, that day the damage was not too great, but the child
pointed at the electric socket and said with terror, 'Daddy, here!' Three days later
when his grandparents were visiting, he signalled to his grandfather to come with
him, crawled ahead, and pointed to the electric socket from afar, saying again,
'Daddy, there.' In short, the person who voiced the prohibition was for him present there, where having transgressed the prohibition, he received the unpleasant
electric shock.[18]

Narcissistic wounds push the child to withdraw into known and therefore non-
dangerous pleasures for his bodily schema. At this age, all the bodily pleasures are
focused on the cavum, the mouth, the anus and for the boy the penis and the girl
the vulva and clitoris; pleasure is produced by the use of their hands. Too many
prohibitions of touching objects external to his body oblige the child to consider
their hands as dangerous; and if he is forbidden to touch his own body, he may

18 This is what adults do when transgressing the laws inscribed in reality that they have not properly
    understood; we think, 'God or the gods are against this.' In the same way, when our neurotic
    processes lead us to failure or illness, we look for a persecutor to blame – an evil spell – in short,
    the 'enemy.'

come to believe that all or of parts of his body are objects in danger, breakable and devourable, and to believe his sex to be threatened by his own hands – which are themselves worrying for certain children to whom people are always saying, 'don't touch!'

His wish to break down, to take apart, to touch everything is a way of discovering that like adults, he has hands capable of dealing with things other than his mouth, bottom or sex. He develops manual dexterity, visual, auditory and tactile knowledge of objects; at the same time that he masters this, he tames the dangers the objects represent, experiments with their utilitarian or agreeable aspects – in short, he reconciles himself to the world by becoming familiar with and learning about it and himself.

A technical misadventure may provoke a reaction of mockery, crossness or anxiety in the adult, who sometimes adds to the experience phrases such as 'this child will kill me,' or 'he's going to kill himself,' 'this child only does naughty things,' or even 'serves you right, that will teach you to disobey.' When this happens, the child is suddenly thrown into a petrifying solitude in the middle of dangers that lurk under anything attractive, dangers that threaten him and with which the parents are complicit and therefore persecutors, and this has a destructuring dimension for the desire of the precocious child. Anything attractive causes the functional motor image to emerge in the body image. Cleverly used, desire pushes the child to seek a pleasure that if obtained will confer upon him greater autonomy.

Faced with failure, the child always needs words to explain the cause of the failure without blaming him and that thereby reconcile him with his intention, removing any magical aspect to the danger he was exposed to and that he believed had been intentionally put there by his parents. It is necessary to establish clearly with the child the technical aspects of his failure – technical aspects that the adult also has to take into account because they are to do with the laws of the reality of things.

Faced with his failures, the child feels humiliated in his own eyes and asks for comfort either by screaming or by going to his mother to complain in a plaintive and regressive voice. However, the child who comes to ask adults for help because he has been clumsy while pushing himself to do something new often receives the conclusion that his case has no merit or even aggressive words: 'Shut up and leave us alone!' Or else, the adult stupefies the child with his own anxiety by coddling him rather than putting him back in front of the obstacle and showing with his own hands or feet while explaining in words how he could have been successful in his experiment. Let us say that if the adults do for him what he has failed to do, it is as bad as if they didn't do anything because they suppress the desire for the experience by providing the immediate result. This leads to an increased dependence, whereas the child was trying to become independent of his mother.

As soon as the child likes to sit and manipulate small objects for his pleasure, then when he crawls on all fours or on his bottom, and even more when he walks and likes to explore everything, the way in which the adult present behaves determines the development of this child. The role of the adult presence is to ensure safety in the environment, so that the child feels free to act as he is tempted to do, as far as possible. Of course, there will be disorder created – the objects displaced and thrown on the floor, which should be left there. All this implies a tolerance that many adults do not have, especially in small homes. However! If the adult knew how much sensorial and mental intelligence is spoiled, as well as trust in oneself and in others, by not tolerating the noise and disorder of healthy babies and children up until the age of 3 and 4, I am sure they would abandon playpens and the 'don't touch!' style of upbringing; they would discover the precocious intelligence that is expressed in this continuous and apparently disorganised activity.

The presence of the adult, occupied with household chores or professional tasks while lightly supervising the child, who is sometimes perplexed and discontent because he doesn't manage to achieve his goals, allows the possibility for the child to learn through example and verbal explanation and learn how to do technical things; it is enough for the adult to put words to efficient operational gestures that the child wants to observe.

To this should be added the encouragement of friendly words without anxiety; and never to scare the child with regard to something he desires wishes to do (unless there is real and inevitable danger). One needs to allow the child to perceive his impotence and faced with it, promise that with growing up, he will be able to do this or that – but never do it for him in his place, nor lure him through a physical aid that makes him cheat the difficulty.

It is therefore very important to understand what the education at this age is about. Sphincter cleanliness, naturally, is part of it, and every child who does not acquire sphincter cleanliness when they are 4 or 5 years old becomes those whose motor education has not been delivered to them but has been faked through an attitude of excessive and infantilising help. This makes them dependent for life; they remain, except in their sleep or in moments of inattention, at a stage where they did not have full mastery of their sphincters. In fact, the education of the small child at the age of touching everything, which is walking age, is about making the hypothesis that the child is always asking: 'Explain how I can do this on my own as well as you do.'

The narcissism that pushes the child to identify with adults he admires expresses itself by the fact that he has become able to mother himself when he is hungry, to feed himself, to help himself to food, to dress himself and put his socks on, even if he cannot buckle his shoes or do up his laces. He can shelter himself from things unpleasant to his body exactly as his mother would have done – sheltered from tensions and needs when of course there is food available. He can also help a younger one, mimicking the role of father or mother in an appropriate way. Then, he behaves towards this human object to keep him away from danger and suffering (obviously when jealousy has been overcome and more readily so if it is a child from another family who has been entrusted to him for a while). In psychoanalysis, we say that this child has already elaborated a pre-superego with regard to anything linked to the body and its survival, his as well as that of others. Unless the child is in a state of emotional disturbance, he can no longer be injurious to another anymore than he can forget to feed himself or to go to the toilet. At most, he attributes to everyone the same desires as his own, which will give rise to some very useful incidents, precisely in what is in the line of anal castration.

In effect, *the difference between the imaginary of the 'doing-with-another' who is supposed to be similar to oneself and the reality, where the other does not want to behave as expected, instructs the child in this: his imaginary desire does not fit the imaginary desire of everyone.* If the other refuses to be his object or his collaborator, for example in playing with him, he feels disappointment. But if the tutelary agent explains that everyone has his own desires and that it is when these desires meet that there is pleasure for both, he will discover one of the keys of life in society. Alas, the adults often force an older child to play with a younger one when the children don't enjoy it and it is not at all necessary for the younger one. *It is never healthy to teach a child to have pleasure at the price of the displeasure of another*, to inculcate this in him in words or by example.

Other frequent situations: the child whose tutelary adult accepts to be used as a plaything, to be wound around his little finger and gives in to all his desires – this child is in danger and will be fragile later in the company of children his own age. Why? Because he is not castrated anally inasmuch as anal castration bears upon the making of a distinction between the imaginary experience of something being done to oneself or of doing something to another, and the reality of an encounter with another whose desires do not conform to his expectation instilled in him by his parents that he can manipulate others.

It is the same when older siblings receive the perverse advice to give in to their younger brother or sister under the pretext that they are small, or agree to let them invade their time and space, their activities and completely different interests. One sees that constantly in families – these injunctions as perverse for the older as for the younger ones, but it is for the younger ones who do not receive anal castration that the impact is the worse. This perverse ethic at the anal stage will follow the child in a neurotic way at the genital stage.

I mean by anal castration the prohibition to do whatever one likes for one's erotic pleasure. Limiting prohibitions should be imposed on 'doing' as soon as the 'doing' provokes displeasure in or danger to others, from the moment where the exercise of freedom actually hinders the freedom of others to act.

Anal castration must teach the child the difference between his possessions, with which he can be totally free, and those of others, his use of which must happen by way of his asking that the other lend him the things he wishes to use while accepting that the other may refuse him. Beside the urge to possess part objects, the respect paid by others to his personal ownership of an object triggers in the child the understanding of personal space that extends into the external world, and he also comes to respect that the space of another extends through his or her personal objects to which the child has no inherent claim but only that which is *negotiated in language*. The education of the drives from the anal stage must leave the child free to give or not, to another an object that belongs to him and that the other covets, or to barter – an activity often unfavourable to the naïve child who is trying to make friends or is tempted by an object because it belongs to someone else.

The exchanges of buckets and spades at the playground happens very early and would be very socialising if mothers did not stop them: 'That's your bucket, don't let anyone else take it!'

As the child grows up, one witnesses the gifts made thoughtlessly, the bad trade-offs, the excessive profit (according to the monetary value of the object received in exchange); on the condition that the objects really belong to the child partners in the exchange, it is clear that this should not be forbidden but explained. *There are no implicit rules for giving, there are for barter.* But if a little car has more value in the eyes of a child than the beautiful toy given for his birthday, that is his problem. It is hard to accept for certain parents, but for a child – and still for many adults – the value of things is more emotional than monetary. It is in talking about it with a child that the child learns, but not if the parents feel they still own what they have given to the child; nor should the parents judge the affective value the child does or does not give to a present they have received.

Anal sadism?

It is my opinion that when one talks in psychoanalytic writings of anal sadism, as if the pleasure in hurting is normally linked with the drives of this stage, one makes a serious mistake. What people are talking about is children who have been brought up in a perverse way without the respect due to their person. If the child receives limitations for real reasons of causing harm to himself or to others, in gradual accordance with his desire for motor functioning, while still being supported and consoled by a tutelary agent who reassures him that he will succeed in future, this child, supported to overcome his feeling of impotence by comforting words, will absolutely not develop a desire to hurt others, any more than he will understand there being pleasure in destruction. The child is never sadistic except at the very beginning, when cutting his teeth. Sadism is oral and not anal. The perversion of ethos at a particular stage due to castration being badly given or not at all (here, it is in weaning) can contaminate with perversion the following developmental stage. *Any coercive behaviour of the adult towards the child is an initiation into sadism and incites the child to identify with this model.*

One can therefore see that anal castration is (for oneself as for others) the prohibition of damage or theft of other people's objects and of all detriment to the bodies of human beings, and also of gratuitous harm to everyday objects needed for the activities of all within the family or society, to animals, to aesthetically pleasing or useful vegetation, just for the pleasure of the one who uses his strength and power: this is vandalism. The verbalisation of prohibitions by an adult who provides an example by conforming his acts to the prohibitions – this again is anal castration.

Anal castration, which has to be symboligenic in the psychoanalytic sense, is also not received by a child between 24 and 33 months, who is in full triumph of the anal age, that is of voluntary motor functioning, if everything is forbidden and if there is no time in his day and in the space in which he lives for the freedom to research in an intensive and auto-erotic way the pleasure of his movement, of his acrobatics, of his rearranging of objects that he can move around. He cannot sublimate his drive in a socialised way if he has no companion with whom to play. It is thanks to same-age companions, a bit older or younger, that in learning by experience, he manages to avoid unpleasant moments caused by the strength of older friends, and those he could cause to younger ones just in enjoying his power over them.

Anal castration is the prohibition to harm others, given day after day, from walking age, by tutelary attention that allows the child's muscular activity to have a useful and pleasant impact, by allowing him freedom of initiative, supervising him at a distance and helping in an educative way by gestures and words and at the same time by continuous example. This is the healthy attitude that needs to be given to a child with regard to the drives marked by anal castration. *It is desirable that any activity in which the child freely engages because he likes it is respected by adults when it does not inconvenience anyone, and when the child plays with interest, it is important that he is never disturbed by the adult, any more than he himself has the right to disturb the busy adult.* Here, example has even more impact than words.

The adult, male or female, parent, older sibling or someone *in loco parentis* – if he gives this castration judiciously over several months or even two to three years, and if his words regarding the actions of the child are not sadistic interventions intolerant of the desire of the child and aimed only at his own comfort – this adult, the only kind that is a healthy educator, does not appear anxious, tense or complaining when he forbids an act. He is on the contrary brief, affectionate and respectful of the child, and if the child asks a question in connection with the prohibition, he knows how to explain it without simply saying that whatever he has been deprived of is 'for his own good.' He tries to explain the reason for the prohibition, for example that the act could harm the child, but does not equivocate by quibbling nor use the blackmail of 'do this for me.' Nothing is more humiliating for a child in the real sense of the term than prohibitions given in the style of 'because I say so!' or 'because I'm in charge,' without the child feeling there is a reason justified by danger for him, that is to say without the child feeling that he is loved within his own development rather than as an animal commanded by others and who needs to be reduced to obedience. The educating adult avoids anything that could unnecessarily create anxiety in the child and therefore make him repress his drive. He also avoids anything likely to over-excite the child in sexual anticipation. An educator for early years is one who understands quickly the temperament of a child – the ones who need stimulation, and those whom one must, while supervising, avoid paying too much attention to the child that could trigger exhibitionist tendencies and for whom on the contrary it should be about developing a sense of authentic progress and not just for the eyes of spectators.

What is educative in the attitude and the words of the tutelary adults is everything that will develop the interweaving of the bodily schema, which is now complete, with the body image – far more than what will develop the dependence of the child on his visual and auditory drives and the flattery of his entourage. To judiciously look after children and truly deserve the title of educator, a title that parents bear but for which they rarely have the qualities with regard to their own children (but may have towards other children), one has to take seriously the socialising role that some older children may have in developing a younger one, whatever his temperament,[19] on the condition that this connivance between the children is not exploited by the parents to avoid their role. The socialising role of elders is important in the development of younger ones, as when a child asks to be looked at and performs something he considers an exploit, it is necessary that he knows the adults trust him and allow him these exploits.

This is why the exhibitionism of children lasts some time before they are able to renounce this feeling they seek of being admired. Any child needs to be looked at by their mother when they do something. This should not last, but exists always at the beginning. Otherwise, the child develops without social sense and only for himself. It is also necessary that the adult shares and ratifies what he does by saying, 'That's good, you will manage even better,' and when the child wants to take risks, it is important that the adult knows to say, 'Do it if you feel you can but I don't want to watch because it scares me. It is for you to judge if you can do it.'

This is when the child will or will not take responsibility for doing something he feels capable of without being seen. The important thing is that the educating agent supports him in accessing personal experiences, the fruit of which will allow him to acquire the means of being autonomous and valued in the company of children his own age. At the same time, the educator must answer any question the child asks and never say that it is not his business, as if the child shows an interest in something, this something is 'his business,' or more precisely it is his business that the child has observed it and wants an explanation about what he has seen. Supporting the curiosity of children rather than limiting or forbidding it, as the epistemological drive is one of the most fundamental,[20] is the key point to an education of oral and anal drives without sadism. The interdiction given to children to take interest in something is anti-educative and even toxic – taking interest in something is never harmful. In words, every time a child asks a question, one should answer truthfully what one thinks, knows, or one should confess one's real ignorance. It is in this way that the bases of sadism are neutralised. There may be sadism later, at the time of the urethral stage, but not at the time of the anal stage. Sadism is, then, a regression of the urethral or genital drives onto the anal stage;

19 Translator's note: Dolto has a footnote here specifying that she is talking about the younger child being a group with older children and being looked after by them (without being a nuisance), listening to them and observing them in their games.
20 The drive that pushes human beings to know, in short, curiosity.

but at the anal stage there is none when the child is supported in the realisation of their motor activity, and when this is not feasible, it is spoken about and a delayed permission is given to be used in future, 'When you are able to do this or that.'

Supporting and valuing the curiosity attached to observation is one of the very principles of a humanising education. If symboligenic castration supports that aim, it is because the person who limits the direct and known access of the child to his desire herself represents for him a more evolved human being, possessing a power and a knowledge he wishes to acquire – power and knowledge that she is happy to delegate and transmit to him in words by predicting an experience soon to be authorised. This is what it is all about: 'You will be able to, soon. It is not forbidden.'

The psychoanalytic treatment is precisely based on this permission to speak of one's desire. We also make children draw the thing that they confabulate, including, obviously, sadistic expressions. This means that we agree with the desire in itself, expressed here by fantasies of an exaggerated violence. From the moment the child realises this in and through dialogue in the situation of analytic transference, he has no more effective or real desire to harm in reality for pleasure. This is my experience.

The symbolised expression in language within a relationship in which the subject is recognised as valuable – therefore narcissised by someone who has no desire for the child but is at the service of his development, respects his person and those whom he loves – parents, educators – and does not aim at separating him from them – this is already a sublimation of desire. Symbolisation progressively moves the subject away from recourse to the pleasure of bodily contact, which eclipses the relationship of subject-to-subject. Any representation of drives outside the body itself of the desiring person is already a mediation on the way towards mastery of desire and the increase in his value as a human in agreement with the laws of social life. All human beings are naturally social on the condition that the social does not weaken desire in its search for satisfaction in pleasure.

Pleasure is increased in being shared with others – all the more as language allows us to communicate our experience, and from this arises the symboligenic value of the castrations that allow the drives to be expressed other than by the sole and immediate enjoyment of the body that made the tension of desire disappear, which suppresses the enriching questioning of the other aimed at communicating and sharing the emotions of the heart and the questions of intelligence.

The mirror

What allows the motor integration by the subject of his own body – an integration confirmed in relationship by anal castration – is the narcissistic moment that psychoanalytic experience has allowed us to pinpoint as the mirror stage.

Speaking of it as a stage is in itself misleading as it is more about the assumption of the subject in his own narcissism – an assumption that allows and covers the field of castration in the anal stage itself, and that makes the effects of this felt in the realisation of the difference of sexes (primary castration, as we shall see later).

I would add that we often emphasise the scopic dimension of what is called the specular experience – wrongly, if we fail to pay sufficient attention to the relational, symbolic aspect of these formative experiences. It is not enough that there is in reality a mirror. This is useless if the subject is in fact confronted by the *lack of a mirror of his being in another*, as this is what is important.

What is dramatic is that a child who lacks the presence of his mother, or of a living other, who is reflected along with him, comes to 'lose himself' in the mirror.

Such a child became schizophrenic at the age of 2 and a half, because she was put in a hotel room in which all the furniture surfaces were of glass and the walls were covered in mirrors. Until 2 and a half, she had lived in the United States – a perfectly healthy child who laughed, played, spoke; in France, after two months in this hotel with a person employed to look after her that she did not know at all, she became a schizophrenic child. She was lost, scattered in the space of this unfamiliar room with bits of bodies visible everywhere in the mirrors, in the glass doors and table legs, fragmented in space without a friendly presence. Her parents were busy visiting Paris and left her with someone as unknown to themselves as to her, who did not speak English.

Some children may also sink into autism through the contemplation of their images in the mirror – trapped by the illusion of relating to another child. I am not talking about those who fragment themselves in many mirrors but who have at their disposition a mirror. This image of themselves brings only the hardness and coldness of glass or the surface of stagnant water in which, attracted by the encounter with an other, like Narcissus, they encounter nobody, only an image. This is a moment when the child's feeling of existing is invalidated. The mirror stage, which can for the child be symbolic of their being in the world for another, inasmuch as he is an individual amongst others, can also be de-symboligenic for his body image if he doesn't recognise as himself the thing that is his own body, seen in the mirror.

Let us try to summarise what we mean by the individuation of the child subject in the mirror. What does this experience bring to bear on primary narcissism, from which emerges, after Oedipal castration, secondary narcissism?[21]

We have already said that the child can, by these images (anticipatory fantasies) provisionally supply the absence of a chosen other, who is indispensable for their survival. If this other is missing for too long, there is necessarily a regression, which is visible mostly in the exaggerated sleeping of the baby. If it is a traumatic regression, there is in the child's imagination a resurgence of drives dissociated from all fantasmatic images of functioning. The death instinct of the subject prevails. On the other hand, the pre-ego of the child originates in the dialectic of maternal presence and absence, in the safety-giving continuum of progressive

21 See pages 105, 110 (156, 164 in French version).

perceptions linked with the promised presence being expected and received, at the heart of the spatial and temporal media of his being in the world and by this being committed to memory in language. The child who can hear gets to know himself from those to speak to him; and day after day, these recurrent experiences personalise him, represent audibly who he is by the phonemes of his name spoken by that voice, by the perceptions he recognises and that make up the specificity of that person, the mother, who is repeatedly re-found. The return of the mother against a known backdrop is always a source of new discoveries. It is by way of the mother's language, both vocal and in facial expression, that accompanies the new perceptions that these take on human meaning.

The body image is therefore elaborated in language as a network of safety with the mother. This network personalises the experiences of the child, be they olfactive, in sight, hearing or ways of touching, according to the specific rhythms of familiar maternal ways. But this does not individualise the child's body – as the spatial limits set by what he can perceive by way of language are unclear – he is also his mother, his mother is also him. One can say that these closures, these separations (oral and anal castration) represented by weaning and autonomous motor functioning, have already brought about relative individuation, which has allowed the bodily schema of the child to become separate from that of the mother; and have also, by substitution, allowed the bodily schema, still in the process of elaboration, to be linked with the unconscious body image. This linkage between the subject and his body happens by way of the elaboration of a pre-ego narcissism that at the same time guarantees the existence of the subject in his continuing relationship with his body by way of an ethos that perpetuates a sense of safety after the anxiogenic trial of each castration.

But the notion of individuation belonging to the pre-ego narcissism that relates each to the tactile and visible limits of their skin and their cohesive reality leads to another experience – that of the mirror. This experience of the image he sees in the mirror, when he has the intuition that it is his, suddenly makes him grapple with the dominance of the scopic drive over all other drives – a dominance that is not obvious and is in conflict with the value of exchange and the narcissistic value of the other drives – smell, hearing and touch. Let us remember that *in the constitution of the body image, the visual drive has a very modest place – maybe even completely absent – with regard to the organisation of primary narcissism.* The mirror will bring this experience – the appearance of an unknown other, the image of a baby like one the subject might have seen elsewhere – and that he does not recognise as himself; this visual image must then be superimposed on the already known experience of the interweaving of his bodily schema and his unconscious body image. I mean that when faced with a mirror, he sees an image of which he learns he is the only cause, as he encounters only a cold surface and not another baby, and that if he moves, the image moves. The language of facial expressions and affects that the child has established with the world around him does not bring any answers regarding the image encountered in the mirror, in contrast to all the experiences he has had with others. This is why if the mother or a known person is not near him, in his space, there is a risk that because of the mirror, his body image disappears without the specular image gaining a meaning for him. The specular image only acquires the meaning of lived experience by the presence, beside the child, of a person whose body image the child can recognise by way of his own bodily schema: when he recognises this person in the flat surface of the specular image, he sees doubled in the mirror what he perceives of her near him, and can then endorse the specular image as his as it makes him see his image side by side with that of the other. He then discovers himself in the form of a baby, like others he has seen, while up until that moment his only mirror was the other with whom he was communicating – which could have made him believe that he was this other, but without knowing or genuinely knowing that this other had a specular image and he likewise.

It is only the experience of the mirror that gives the child the shock of realising that his body image is far less than what others know him to be. That it is not whole. This does not mean that the scopic image corresponds to him. For us all, this irreparable wound of narcissistic damage caused by the experience of the mirror can be called a symbolic hole from which follows the discrepancy between the body image and the bodily schema – which numerous symptoms will aim at repairing from here on. The repetition of the mirror experience vaccinates the child from this first stupefaction and proves to him by the scopic evidence that whatever happens, he is never fragmented since, for the others who are reflected along with him, the 'capturing' of their appearances does not damage the integrity of their whole being, as he continues to encounter them as before, in the warmth of their exchanges, in the opposition or agreement of their desires, which can be signified by language in the global sense of the word, as the visible aspect of the body cannot or can only be in a very limited way.

Because of this hole or gap, I wish to speak of a 'blank' – of a strange, discordant scopic relationship that serves as a living mask, always more or less treacherous to the subject's feelings. The subject discovers that in relation to the other, he is only authentic in his unconscious body image, which may or may not be linked with his bodily schema. This discrepancy between unconscious body image and the bodily schema evidenced in the mirror allows him to distinguish between fantasy and fact, and between a meeting with an other that may exist in his imagination or in reality, and who may be present or not. The mirror allows the child to observe himself as if he were an other whom he never meets. He sees 'himself,' but all his desire to communicate with another is frustrated.

Let us imagine a child blind from birth who encounters a mirror. It is for him just a particular type of wall, a cold space limited by a frame that is for him only a tactile reference. For a sighted child, the effect is totally different as he has, in this strange window, the lure of another whom he did not know, whom he will never know and who, rather than being a warm three-dimensional being, is a flat and cold plane surface. His image disappears from this surface when he is no longer in front of the mirror and appears when he puts himself back there. It becomes for him an experience concomitant with his presence but only a scopic experience, without response, without communication. His calls, his gestures are the same in mirror image. He may talk to this image but he hears only his own voice and no other voice replies to him. In this way, it is an alienating image if there is not in the space a person whom he knows and who shows him in the mirror that she too is subject to these same curious conditions of reflections on this cold plane surface.

There is here an experience of the lure of an encounter with the other that could bring him satisfaction, more or less as he derives satisfaction from a transitional object – trapping himself in it out of boredom in solitude, due to a lack of encounters with other people, the absence of toys, of distractions. For the child, the visual enjoyment could become a trap that removes value from intersubjective relationships, so that these lose the meaning of a shared pleasure. The trap could be a deadly fascination for the unconscious body image itself – the specular image becoming a conscious substitute for the unconscious body image, making the child oblivious of his true relationship with the other. He starts to consider only the appearance of the other and to give in his relationship with the other only the appearance of pleasure due to the encounter. His own image can be enough for his enjoyment: it is in memory of his own image that he pulls faces for the other as he does for himself – from this moment on, he no longer expresses himself truthfully. This is the trap that appearance creates. The trap is not a living being but a part appearance, a dummy, the mask of a living being. If the child can be fascinated by the repetitive appearance of living beings, it is because this has a reassuring effect with regard to phobic fantasies of living only with inanimate objects, but at the same time it is wholly a-dynamic.[22]

Every baby who sees himself in the mirror from afar, especially for the first time, is happily surprised, runs towards the mirror and, if he can speak, exclaims: 'Baby!' – while when talking about himself, he names himself by pronouncing the phonemes of his first name. So, this is proof that he doesn't recognise himself. He will be brought to discover his appearance and to play with it; up until then, while the body image existed in the relationship between the subject and desire, it was always unconscious and in intuitive reference to the desire of others.

This is where *people blind from birth can allow us to locate the difference in primary narcissism between themselves and sighted people: it is a difference due to the absence for them of a scopic experience in the mirror*. The facial expressions of such a blind person have an authenticity as moving as that of babies before the mirror experience. They never disguise what they feel and one reads on their faces everything they experience from their contacts with those they meet. But they don't know that we read them, so they don't know either how to hide their

---

22 A false response can stop the image-fascinated loner in his search for communication; this false response, a repetitive response that is only a frozen image of himself, a fetish of an other, is apparently less terrifying than solitude. He can be seen posing, playing at pulling faces, smiling at himself, pretending to cry – everything in which he can practice expressing feelings that are not experienced. It is pretending.

feelings; this shows how we sighted people hide from ourselves and from others what we feel because we were able to have the mirror experience. The sight of his image in the mirror reveals to the child that his body is a small mass at the side of many other masses of different dimensions and especially of the large masses of adults. He hadn't known that. There is also this that is new: the discovery of a face and a body thenceforth inseparable from each other. Therefore, from this specular experience shared with another, the child can no longer confuse in reality himself with the other, or with the other of the other, I should say – neither with the mother nor with the father nor with an older sibling, as he had willingly done before. No longer can he confuse in reality the narcissistic fantasies that brought him to imagine himself as he desired to be – as the child could easily imagine being a bus, a plane, a train, a horse, a bird; we see this in his play with onomatopoeia, translating into sound his supposed identity – sometimes he plays a person and believes himself to be them. From the mirror stage onwards, this will never be the same as before. He knows that he can never confuse a fantasmatic image with himself, that he can no longer play at being the other that he desires and is absent. In these imaginary games in which he likes to fantasise another identity, the conditional tense appears in his speech: 'If I were a plane, you would be . . .'

To better understand the complicated process of the mirror that requires to be dialecticised so as to go beyond the trauma, let's refer to this story – a document given to me by the mother of identical twins (that is to say, copies of each other in appearance but not in their nature or character, according to their mother). These twins, who had never been apart, nobody, not even those close to them, knew how to distinguish them from each other, with the exception of their mother and a baby born after them and who challenges them already with the help of distinct phonemes, discriminating between them without error. One day, when they were already in primary school, one of them had a cold and mother decided to keep him at home. She took the other to school and had returned to her routine, when she heard her son, who was playing in his room, begging. The begging tone increased in volume and became anxious, but the child was not calling for his mother. She approached the half-open door and saw the boy on his knees before the wardrobe mirror begging his own image to get on the wooden horse. His anxiety was increasing. The mother therefore entered and showed herself, calling to her son who threw himself into her arms and in a demanding and depressive voice said, 'X doesn't want to play with the horse!' Mother was disturbed to understand that the boy had mistaken his image in the mirror for his absent brother, whose image was his own. Holding him in her arms and taking the horse with them, she approached the mirror and spoke about the image it gave of them, that was theirs, but that was neither her nor the horse nor the absent brother. She reminded him that that morning he had been a little ill, but not his brother, that she had left him at home but had taken his brother to school and that she was going to be picking him up again. The child listened intently to her.

In this particular case of identical twins, the mirror, despite being on the door of the wardrobe in their room, had never posed the question of his appearance to the child. When he saw himself in it, it was probably having accepted that he saw his brother without being surprised that the brother could be in two places at the same time, and probably his brother had done the same (they were 3 years old). When the twin brother returned from school, the mother repeated the experiment with the two of them together, putting each child in turn in front of the mirror and making each see his image as his own, and the image of his brother as being his. She explained to them that they were very alike, being twins born on the same day. These explanations, attentively listened to, visibly and silently posed a serious problem for her sons.

Before the experience of the plane mirror, it was his relationship to the bodily schema of the mother, her body in reality, that gave meaning to the primary and fundamental narcissism of her child, and that sustained these. It is only after the mirror experience that the body image of the baby informs his own bodily schema, according to the language that constitutes the body image for the subject, in reference to the mother-subject. He discovers in it its apparent integrity – or not; its exhilarating character – or not; he experiences whether his narcissism is satisfied by the image in the mirror,[23] that everyone else can see.[24]

It is the moment of the clinical appearance of primary identification – the origin of primary narcissism, which follows the primordial narcissism that I also call fundamental.[25] Primary narcissism does not replace fundamental narcissism; it is grafted onto it. It joins onto it, extending the relational field of the child. The image of the heart of an onion enveloped by its leaves illustrates well the relation between fundamental and primary narcissism. The one is superimposed upon the other. There has first to be fundamental narcissism and only then primary narcissism, with the mental *reflection* about oneself, which refers to the experience of the image *reflected* by the mirror. Before this, the narcissism of the child was informed by and formed according to the unconscious of the mother, by the way in which she regards him. His being alive (his 'livingness') in the vegetative (passive) sense of the term, his 'vitality' in the animal (motor) sense, and his sex unconsciously agree with the feelings he has elicited and are felt by those who look after him, and who re-live the history of their own narcissism that the child causes them to remember. The narcissism of the child, this time as a subject, is

---

23 Imagine if, looking in the mirror, we did not see our reflection – what fear! But no fear at all if this happened before the first mirror experience. It is from this point that a reflective surface cannot be considered as a neutral surface.

24 The taste for dressing up and being made up originates here.

25 Translator's note: Dolto goes on to define in the following paragraphs what she means by 'primordial narcissism' as distinct from 'primary narcissism.' This could be a point of confusion for psychoanalytic readers as the term 'primary narcissism' is already well established in the literature, starting with Freud, who coined the term. Freud's use of 'primary narcissism' in reference to the newborn baby is very much what Dolto goes on to describe as 'primordial narcissism,' where what she calls 'primary narcissism' – starting at the mirror stage – is closer to what Freud and most other analysts would think of as secondary narcissism.

also constructed in his day-to-day relationship with the desires of the one chosen by his desire, and of those close to her; with his biological father, or any other adult of whichever sex who is the habitual companion of his mother, accorded the value of being his mother's partner.

Let us consider: up until now, the child has seen with his own eyes only the front side of his body – thorax, abdomen, upper and lower limbs. The volume of his body, its holes and projections, relief, face, neck, back, he has felt first through contact with his mother's hands, and then through contact with his own with the parts of his body he can reach, and by sensations of pleasure or pain. But up until now, he did not know his own face nor its expressivity. He could touch his head, knew how to point with his fingers to his ears, eyes, mouth, nose, forehead, cheeks and hair in the games mothers like to play with their children; but he didn't know that his face was visible to others as the faces of others are for him. This he learns especially by way of the mirror, as I have shown, in contrast with the blind person who knows but hasn't 'seen.'

However, children do feel themselves to be whole even before the mirror stage, thanks to visceral references – for example the subtle and continuous peristaltic sensations of his digestive tube, in which he feels the itinerary of the oral part object, showing his stomach when he finds what he has eaten to be good. Then, the perception of abdominal transit – he likes to touch and stroke his tummy. After this, it is the anal part object and its expulsion that relate him to specific sensations of touch and smell. All this constitutes a coherent continuum that is internal, within the limits of his skin, that tactile sensations have delimited during maternal care and carrying. One cannot overstate the importance of the mother or the nurse as the guarantor of fundamental narcissism, of narcissism up till the child walks, and further, when the child, having experienced relational difficulties with others in society, returns to find reparation with the mother. This is why the reunion with the mother, with its rhythm of specific references, is necessary for the durability of the narcissistic cohesion of the child. It is only after the specular experience, which the child repeats in experiments through his coming and going deliberately in front of the mirror, that he starts in some ways to own his own body and to trap in it his narcissism, which thus bears the name of primary. *The appearance takes on value that sometimes prevails over the feelings of the subject being.* In particular, one's face, revealed in the mirror, and which is now indissociable from identity, one with the body – thorax, trunk, limbs – convinces the child that he is similar to other human beings, one of them. The discovery of the relative size of his body in the frame of the mirror is not obvious. Is that not the reason why the absence of perspective and a non-proportional dimension of the human body in architectural frames prevailed in art for so many centuries?

In the same way that the child discovers through observation in the mirror the visible reality of his being in the world, facing it and almost immobile, the observation of the nudity of other children whom he knows to be similar to him and whom he sees from behind with at the top some hair without a face and lower down, buttocks, interests him far more after the mirror experience. Shortly after having accepted the fruits of the mirror experience, the child discovers that all children have at the top of their body a head, with in front a face and behind, some hair, if they have at the top of their legs, seen from behind, buttocks (if children seen from behind are all similar), but from the front, they are not all the same. Seen from the front, some have lower down a cleft,[26] as if they had 'little bottoms' there, while others have a protrusion. What about his own body? Has he seen this properly? The child then endures what we have called primary castration, the effect of the discovery of the difference between the sexes; and this is naturally linked with the face since the face is always visible from the front, as is the sex, with its openings – eyes, nose, mouth – and the mass of hair that forms the boundary between face and head. *This discovery of his own body in relation to those of other children cannot happen before the mirror stage. The repeated experience of this allows primary castration to be integrated into the conviction of being human*, and not experienced as a phenomenon of animality. To see himself naked, in conformity with the nudity of other children, allows him to know that naked as he is, he will become an adult man or woman and won't be a dog or any other creature that he may have believed himself to be before the specular experience. This is precisely the moment at which the child could identify himself with animals, without a human face, because the child identifies with everything he sees and finds interesting; but he identifies more strongly with his own image as soon as he has been able to recognise himself in the mirror, if this is given value by speech, and even if he is at first surprised, he is then promoted to being a human among other humans, going-on-becoming a man or a woman.

If the identification with an animal is not balanced by knowledge of oneself as a human child, it will make the perception experienced in his sex eroticised according to the way others speak to him about it, how others respond to his questions, and will make him link his sex with the narcissism of his specular image, positively or negatively. *There are cases where the child cannot integrate with pride the particularity of his or her sex.* 'Me, I . . .' doesn't feel valuable in being a boy or a girl, because of a reference to the phallus particular to his family, his place in kinship or the relative importance of the father or the mother in the family (if the parent of the same sex seems to be devalued by the other or in comparison with the other, in the words he hears or what he observes in their exchanges and behaviour). In these cases, the children feel themselves to be either with a face that fits what they are – boy or girl – but with an anatomical sex of which they deny the sensations (later, they will repress them), accepting only the pleasure of

26 Curiously, children only talk of the 'stripe' of the bottom, that dark line that separates the muscles when seen from behind. It is a word that talks about the visible and not the tactile, which would be the word 'cleft.' Children never used that word for the bottom. [Translator's note: Dolto is trying to make a distinction between two words, '*raie*' and '*fente*' – the second with and the first without tactile connotations. She suggests that French children use the one without tactile connotations for the bottom and the one with tactile connotations for the female genitalia. Unfortunately, we have not made the same observation of English-speaking children using different words for these things.]

linked with functional needs – constipation, encopresia, so-called urinary tract infections, or enuresis – or on the contrary with a sex that corresponds appropriately with their genitalia but that they don't show in their way of speaking and behaving. In society, they cannot make their face and their sex fit together.[27]

If a 'me, I' as animal is created or superimposed in the service of libidinal drives to which sex has contributed no value – in the service of the drives of a part erogenous zone linked with the genitalia before primary castration – there is a disparity experienced between the human face and their own corresponding sex. In these cases, the child experiences either a face or a sex – one or the other dominates, but they don't fit together. When the child experiences himself as sexuated, he experiences himself as animal; when he speaks, he experiences himself as human but of indeterminate sex. Between these two modes of expression, the subject is fragile and not cohesive. In the child whose structure with regard to their sex has been neutralised, academic success can, in giving him value among others, help him to keep face; but within these alternative images, psychosis or psychotic enclaves can fix themselves and remain in the background, to reveal themselves some time later, as, with this dissociated base, he can neither really engage in the Oedipus nor resolve it. It is particularly after puberty, in the crisis moments provoked by narcissistic trials, especially those that touch upon the failure of sublimations, that pre-genital castration anxiety is reawakened (the misfortune of the neglected).

It is without doubt in order to be rid of these pre-genital relics of desire that have not passed through humanising castration that de-humanising mimes, masks and dressing up are useful and spontaneously necessary to the games of all children, healthy or neurotic; but are ignored by psychotic children who, without masks, live non-humanised emotions. Probably, groups and social parties where faces are masked allow all to liberate repressed drives and not to sublimate all in accordance with the ethos of castrated desires. On certain set dates, they allow a guilt-free collective release, doubtless an adult enclave for certain sexual drives that date from a time these conflicted with their human face.

It is either a human face or the right to sex: this contradiction comes from what was not castrated and symbolised at the times of the different castrations and in particular primary castration at the mirror stage.

Primary castration deserves that we pay attention to it for a moment, inasmuch as it must be jointly found both in the experience of the mirror, which is initiatic for the imaginary, and in the taking on of the symbolic dimension by the subject, whose face corresponds with desire in accordance with his sex and with the intuition he has of the future. Primary castration happens after the conscious mental integration of the oral and anal ethical laws – the prohibition of cannibalism, vandalism and murder – which are linked with the narcissism of the child, the pride or shame of an act depending on whether it is ethical or non-ethical (human, indiscriminate of sex).

27 Pre-genital origin of the negation of the value of one's own sex.

To introduce the study of primary castration, let us say that it is a bridge between anal castration and Oedipal, genital castration, which follows it directly. Let us also say that it is since the experience of the mirror and the dialectic that leads to the taking on of the symbolic dimension by the subject that the child experiences a feeling of shame that incites modesty: do not show yourself naked to someone who could be dangerous, do not hide to see others naked, or look at the same time at the sex and the face of those who for him are his ego-ideal. For the child, there is a model person in reality who is the reference for his ego-ideal. The sex of that person will be revealed for the child at the Oedipal stage. The shame or the pride that shows itself after the discovery that the face and sex are connected is expressed by the way in which the head is held, whether the gaze is direct or not, the grace of the body in its poise and movements, or on the contrary in a gauche attitude, a sort of chronically inhabited mask of someone ashamed of his sex and of his non-castrated desires – desires that his face cannot assume without the risk of losing dignity. After the mirror stage and primary castration, pulling faces, masks and dressing up become the way of negotiating by camouflage feelings of impotence or of shame that the child experiences when he feels drives that could make him lose face, or deny the value of his genital sex.

When the mirror experience is integrated, whatever the mode of this integration, the representations of people are modified. The intuition that the child had of his truth and the primacy of his unconscious body image, invisible but represented in his drawings and modelling, gives way to the representation of visible and consciously valued images. The child draws characters as he would like the mirror to reflect of his body image, in an appearance in agreement with his narcissism. He gives human figures recognisable characteristics and masculine or feminine symbolic attributes if he is proud of his own sex.

If he is unhappy about belonging to his sex, his drawings translate through archaic references the oral and anal educational modes that he received with regard to the acceptance of his face, his body and his sex. In any case, after the mirror stage, drawings focus much more on the trappings of clothing and part objects – accessories linked with their characters, which aim at giving them value – than to the unconscious body images.

They project themselves into these characters and these attributes of power, of role, proving that sex in itself is always problematic; this will last for the whole pre-Oedipal period and then through the latency period, and in fact, this trait characterises children's drawings from primary castration onwards even when it is successful and followed by a successful genital castration.

The moments when we defend ourselves against the loss of illusions about our body, face, sex and power are the structural points of the ethos that from early childhood directs the narcissism that guarantees our cohesion and are always linked with castration anxiety. This raises important questions about the underlying identity in each of us, upon which are founded our feelings, speech and acts. Narcissism is necessary to defend the subject's cohesion in relation to his ego (his body) and through this the appearance he gives, which in certain relational situations has more or less to ignore his underlying desiring identity (unconscious body image) to avoid exposing himself to the risk of retaliation. During the Oedipus and also throughout life, we enjoy the conquest of successive identifications and the pursuit of the exaltation this brings. *These identifications come quite simply from the displacement of value attributed to the phallus; but none of these identifications can answer for our unknown desiring identity*, which since primary castration is without unconscious body image! This identity unknown to each of us, boys and girls, is perhaps moored to the introductory, luminous perception of the first face bent over ours. Did this gaze shine an expression of love when welcoming us, the new unknown host in the parental home? Was it the face of a professional technician of childbirth? Whatever, it is the gaze of this human face that is the first reference point of our value-identity.

Primary castration, sometimes called non-Oedipal genital castration

This is about the discovery of the sexual difference between boys and girls.

We have seen the child, after 30 months, arrive at a developmental level that permits motor functioning, locomotion, and shows him to be well or badly brought up, able or not to speak. Having hands and a larynx, he can show in his games and in his exchanges with others enough sublimations of drives from the oral phase (sense of smell, taste, vision, hearing, touch) to make observations and to have personal sensory experiences.

He has certainly encountered the mirror and observed all his bodily regions and their homologues in others, whether or not he has been given words for them.

In addition, the sight of other children's bottoms has revealed to him the visible shape of buttocks, while he has only seen the front aspect of his own body, except perhaps by means of rare games with the mirror. It is only by means of the tactile sensations of pleasure or unpleasure that he can feel the posterior region of his basal body, for example during toileting.[28]

A corollary of this is that in general, it is only after 30 months that the child notices the anterior face of the basal region, which serves in urination and as a sexual characteristic, in its difference in the masculine and feminine forms. (Similarly, while he may see adults within the family – parents, brothers and sisters – naked, he does not notice their patterns of body hair when he is very small.) In fact, it is not until he has known the back of other people's bodies that he takes interest in the front side of the pelvic region – as much his own in the mirror as that of others.

---

28 I am thinking here about children who receive spankings when they have done something naughty – it appears that mother or father locates the origin of their child's desire in this region. Why shouldn't the child in his innocence believe this, and play rebelliously at talking about wee and poo, or salaciously about poo sausages? After all, adults seem to believe this and to find such speech shocking! And they imagine themselves to be educating their children in so valuing their bottom!

On the other hand, the front of the body has already posed him a problem when, seated on the laps of adults, he compared the chests of women and of men. Looking at him- or herself in the mirror and palpating his or her chest, the child wonders why he or she hasn't got breasts? And why their father hasn't got them. Children verbalise all these questions when speaking freely about the body. And what is said to them about these bodily differences leads them to suppose, especially if they are boys, that the palpable protrusion of their sex and of that of men is of the same kind as that other protrusion, palpable on the thorax of women – breasts. It is not rare that children, and not only very small ones, have no other word for describing women's breasts than 'lolo' or 'pee' – names given by extension to their own sex. The word 'pee' when doubled, becomes 'pi-pi' in French, just as 'lolo' is a repetition of the phoneme of the vital element that like mother's milk appeases thirst – 'l'eau' or water. The word 'pee' onomatopoeic of successive jets that is given to children to describe the udders of cows, which can be milked by hand, is doubled to signify what is called the 'tap' of boys, I mean the penis, a word rarely given to children. It is when this interest in the breast and the penis – an interest translated by the words given to the child and that are at his disposition – that the child, girl or boy, asks himself the question about the difference of shape between the bodies of men and of women, between that of boys and of girls. How is it possible that boys have something 'down there,' dads too, mothers too (this is self-evident), and that mothers also have two 'up there,' while girls have nothing to show that is so beautiful or functional, neither 'down there' nor 'up there'?

Probably, the difference is already in the words, 'You are a little girl . . . you are a little boy,' but the difference has not yet been related to the body; at most, it has been to 'ways' fitting what is expected of a girl or a boy. It is through questions regarding the parents' different bodies that the child discovers the difference, but before that he has to notice that there is no difference in the back sides of the body between boys and girls. This is what triggers curiosity about the different fronts. When the parents have no words other than 'bottom' or 'bum-bum' to talk about both the front and back of the pelvic region they complicate everything, if even to discriminate the place through its functioning they add to 'bum-bum' or 'bottom' the adjectives 'big' and 'small.' For a boy, the first clear vision of the strangeness of the sex of a girl is a shock in the same way that the first clear observation for a girl of the sex of a boy is also a shock. There is no case where, if the children are free to talk, they don't strongly react to this first sighting. The boy thinks that girls have a penis but that it is hidden, momentarily withdrawn into the body; and girls immediately and unthinkingly want to grab it. How many of them, from the testimony of parents say: 'That's mine, you stole it from me.' They do not ask questions, they grab, sure of their right! When it comes to the boy, he is baffled by this interest or he laughs loudly and goes and tells whoever will listen. It is in connection with this experience of the discovery of sexual differences and the direct or indirect questions about it that truthful speech must be given to children of both sexes, confirming the accuracy of their observations and congratulating them for having noticed a difference that has always existed. *Truthful speech that links the appearance of one's genitalia to a future as a man or a woman is what gives the value of language and social value to his sex and to himself;* and this is what prepares a healthy future for his genitality, at an age when the genital drives are not yet prevalent. The child has heard since they were very small that they were a boy or a girl, but it was a purely verbal reference that had no connection with his observation of bodies. It is a word that contains relatively vague value judgements depending on families and, in addition, pleasant or unpleasant ideas for mothers and fathers who would have liked or not to have a child of another sex. In every-day conversation, girls are said to be pretty, boys are said to be rough; girls cry, boys must not cry; girls are softies, boy are dare-devils – children hear so much nonsense about sexual differences long before knowing how this is connected with genitalia, and how many are left without any explanation regarding these observations, which are fundamental to their general intelligence and affectivity, as this is the basis for all meaningful discriminations, supporting comparisons, differences, analogies, inferences and deductions and the vocabulary of kinship, citizenship and responsibility.

It is indispensable that children, when they express their curiosity, their doubts about their observations, or when sometimes out of prudence, they accuse another child of being interested in seeing or showing this region or when they make a false propos in order to arrive at the truth, receives at that very moment not an injunction to shut up or words that would make them ridiculous, but the right words and vocabulary to describe their observations, the physiological forms of their sex and that of others – forms that from birth cause a baby to be declared at the registry office as a boy or a girl – and that he will develop into a man like his dad or a woman like his mum.

True, fitting and simple speech – how difficult this turns out to be! Either it is a formal lecture accompanied by moralising and warnings, or more often, it is a refusal, 'It's not the right time . . . it's too important a question for me to answer you now' – as if it required a private conversation, which could be eroticised, and botanical or zoological words! In addition, people often suggest functional words that seem to confirm the illusion that its use is only, in order to cover the tracks of curiosity, about the pleasure that the child has already discovered and his questioning about it: what are these things for – erections, the observable genitalia of two kinds? And what is the use of what is experienced 'there' that is so interesting, so moving, in particular with regard to girls who do not have and can't talk about penile erections and have nothing that can be seen, where something can be felt.

As psychoanalysts who listen to adults on the couch know, and as doctors can also testify, many adults continue to have only childish words to designate their sex organs, in which the organ is named by its function or by soubriquets that verge on pejorative or jokey, or are slang. It is probably this that causes the impossibility for genitors to inform their offspring – father to son, mother to daughter – the impossibility of parents telling children what the child nevertheless has full expectation of learning from them. They mostly expect that desire or pleasure will not be silenced, as this is what is the most important for the child who has discovered it well before he realised the distinction between the pleasure that accompanies the evacuation of excrement and the one he experiences through the manipulation of that region or during certain emotional moments for which he has no explanation. *Around 30 months – at the end of the anal period or later – the epistemological drive of the child revolves around the 'what's it for' about everything*, looking for answers about the useful, the useless, the pleasant or the unpleasant, in the short or the long term; in short, answers to what has already provided the criteria for satisfaction or renouncement in the face of the dangers of the oral and anal drives. One of the banal dangers is to displease mother, and he notices this displeasure is about the pleasure that he takes in his excrements. The noticing of this displeasure is one of the means whereby the child can discriminate between what relates to sexuality and the excretory function while to begin with these are mixed up. They are mixed up mostly in the boy, as he cannot urinate without an erection up until the age of 28 or 30 months. It is only after this that erections independent of miction makes this organ and its independent and apparently functionless movement problematic. He cannot decode the meaning of this experience on his own. With regard to the girl, from very early on, the urinary function has no relation to the sensations of clitoral or vaginal pleasure, so girls are more precocious but maybe also they have more difficulties talking about it because their organs in erection, that is to say when they feel different, are not visible. These are intimate sensations with nothing visible that corresponds with what they could say about it.

For any child, it is the parents who are the keepers of all knowledge and what they say has authority, and what they say becomes law, after weaning, regarding everything connected with taking, acting and doing, for the child in their charge.

With neuro-muscular maturation, the displacement of interest from the digestive transit to locomotion in space makes the child register what he perceives as pleasant or unpleasant in what is said and done, both in his own body and in the harmony of his emotional relationship with his entourage. Castration delivered by the tutelary agent in words (and through example in the best cases), that is to say the prohibition that limits the freedom of the child, is about the good and bad for his body and that of others, for things and living creatures, plants and animals, in accord or contradiction with the pleasure experienced when acting on his desires or slowing them down in deference to the desire of others. The child is initiated by the tutelary adults into what is possible and impossible, allowed and forbidden, depending on the nature of things and sometimes upon a technical knowledge experienced according to their age, time, space and what the adult says, more than to the direct experience the child has of the possible or impossible. Sometimes, the answer he gets is, 'Later, when you are bigger.' The criteria for what is impossible, of which he has an intuition and that is taught to him (truly or not according to the anxiety of the tutelary agent) is the real danger, short or long term, and its corollary, the prohibition to harm himself or to knowingly harm someone else. Harming oneself, wounding oneself, making oneself ill, poisoning oneself, cutting oneself, mutilating oneself and maybe even dying – these are words he has heard and that pose him a problem apropos of everything that tempts him and is forbidden. The good and the bad relate to the body, but the ugly and the naughty relate to what is seen by the other. The good and the bad are complicated in their relationship with the moral good and bad, because the good can if you have too much of it become bad, and it is (morally) bad to disobey the tutelary agency in taking too much of what is good. It is (morally) good sometimes not to act when one is tempted to do so, because while it would be good (pleasant) to do it, it would be bad for another or if he was observed by the tutelary agent.

Since he was introduced to language, the intelligent child's work of mental discrimination makes him elaborate a value system – an ethos – regarding the imaginary and reality, while he is seeking pleasure, which is always the aim of desire, unconscious or conscious. There is the pleasure taken 'for a laugh' or 'just talking,' or that taken 'for real' – that which is taken in the realisation of desire. This underpins all the sublimations of the drives of children of both sexes. The structuring of the unconscious body image (let us remember that it is tripartite: basic, functional and erogenous) begins with the first umbilical castration, then weaning and then in motor independence, through the introjection of the words and the observed behaviours of the adult upon whom he is dependent for survival. The unconscious body image is structured by the informing of the bodily schema with parental discourse aimed at limiting the child's initiatives (pre-superego) because they might endanger the cohesion of the subject and his body, which mediates the relationship with his love object – mother, father, tutelary person. 'Mummy-Daddy' or 'Daddy-Mummy' – a two-headed agency as a familiar object to be manipulated and with whom he has a nuanced relationship, flattering each of them differently, but always inevitably building his own narcissism upon both of them.

Around the age of 3, the child, according to the verbal initiation and the example he received, already knows his name, his address, the family to which he belongs. He knows how to self-mother enough to not die of hunger or cold if there are things around to eat and to cover himself with; he knows how to take interest and derive pleasure from everything around him without excessive risk; and if he knows the space into which those close to him have introduced him, he also already knows how to behave – in short, to self-father. This child, girl or boy, grows up wishing to identify with tutelary adults, parents and older siblings. And so, his observations and desire for knowledge – fundamental drive of every human being – make him try to understand the purpose of everything, how it is made, how it works and why – and that makes him discover sexual differences more precisely, a surprising discovery immediately connected with the specific pleasure that this region of the body brings when it is excited. It is good, it is enjoyable – why? What's the purpose? And is this naughty? Why?

'Because you are too little,' he is told, with embarrassment. 'You will know when you are big.'

'And when I'm big, will I be like you?' says the boy to his mother, or the girl to her dad.
'Don't be silly,' is the answer. 'You will be like . . . you will be . . . I don't know, let's talk about something else.'

Thus, there is something mysteriously bad, something that makes asking questions forbidden. This is because parents, adults, have totally forgotten the thoughts and feelings of their early childhood (this is what Freud discovered and named repression) and feel put on the spot in the most intimate way; they are taken aback, almost embarrassed at the revelation that their child experiences a pleasure they thought reserved for adults in relation to feelings they imagined linked with a totally developed sex in a body with completely obvious secondary sexual characteristics. For an adult, desire and love before puberty are unthinkable and the possibility of a sexual orgasm even more. The interrogated adult therefore thinks that it is useless to answer questions that appear to him without foundation, but the child understands the embarrassment of the parents in a completely different way.

The child who sees that the sex of another is different from his has the fantasy that this is an anomaly or a mutilation submitted to(?) accepted(?) given by the parents(?). It is the very fantasy that sometimes awakens the child too precociously to his genitality. The parents have forgotten, but the embarrassment the child observes in the adult confirms to him that it is probably they who have done this to him or to the other, it is they who wanted it – and what for? From here, a completely unnecessary anxiety is added to the anxiety of the first awakening, which is inevitable and necessary, given the way the small child reason until then – either in his logic of forms (identical or different, big/small, more/less, good/bad, possible/impossible) or in his logic of the functioning of his body, always accompanied by the comments of tutelary people ('he is beautiful/ugly, he has eaten well/badly, he has been well/ill . . . and what a state you are in!').

The inconvenience of non-responses or inadequate responses to the questions of the child about sex confirms his hypothesis – it is his parents who have cut something or who have schemed to make it happen – opinions more credible for the child when he witnesses quarrels between parents no longer attuned in their sexual desire and love. There is a misunderstanding inherent to the respective ages of the questioner and the respondent; but there is also something that the adults cannot hear in certain questions of children because they touch their own deepest affective and psychic sufferings, that is to say, their own castration anxiety and their current trials and impotence.

In most cases – which will evolve healthily because of an educational entourage that allows the child the understanding of what he observes and loves the child as a future man or woman – the acceptance of primary castration entails for the child of both sexes the valuing of the penis as a beautiful and desirable form. This beautiful form of the penis inscribes itself in the continuity of the beautiful form of the breast. For the girl, it is secondarily and after reflection that she accepts that it is more valuable for her body not to have a penis to wee – as on the one hand she can (not standing up, obviously, but very well nonetheless), and on the other hand, in searching thoroughly in that region that maybe she had one or that it will grow, she discovers the clitoris that after all gives her many satisfactions; and because lastly, having learned that her mother and other women made like her are happy, she concludes that it is the condition of becoming a mummy, of having or making babies (conceiving is not yet thinkable) and of being pleasing to daddy. So, it's fine not having a penis! Let's accept this hole and this button (the vagina and clitoris) as they call it, and also there are these two other buttons on the chest. 'When will these become breasts for feeding my baby?' This is a girl's question, which bolsters the unconscious body image of the girl and consciously encourages the girl to accept her bodily schema. It is easier for her than for the boy to accept the uro-anal castration, that is to say the renunciation of the erotic pleasure with the excremental object. Sphincter continence is followed by the sublimation of tactile drives applied to manual dexterity, as seen by the child in the skilful women of the household. Similarly, the motor muscular pleasure is more quickly displaced in girls than in boys from the narcissism of the erogenous peristaltism and of the manipulation of the body in the area of the vulva onto the pleasure provided by the chores of pretend housework and home maintenance, looking after dolls and on the cleanliness of her own body, the styling of her hair, how well turned-out she is . . . in short, onto coquettishness, worries about dress, pleats, pockets, ribbons and bows . . .

Let us observe children of this age who negotiate this period well. Girls, happy in their chattiness, deny boys the value of their penis without fully believing in the denial, pleased to observe them weeing when they can, to contemplate them being 'strong' when they fight, but: 'It is us girls and not you who will be mums and have babies!' From this follows the playing with dolls, classically a girls' game, at least considered as such, while it is a girls' game indeed, but an erotic game with regard to a phallic-anal fetishistic child; as for boys, games with toy cars is displacement of the excremental part object onto an anal-urethral fetishistic object that he can drive and that he masters and cherishes. Similarly, games with weapons correspond to the fetishistic displacement of the penile part object, when the child has mastered his continence. As we can see, the little girl has displacement games with the anal part object where she trains herself towards maternity, and the little boy's displacement games of part-sexual objects, anal and urethral (internal and external – the penis) in which he expresses his developing virility.

In this sexual competition between boys (whose advantage lies in their obvious sexual organ) and girls (who feel they can trump the boys because they will have babies), the boy may be disappointed when faced with this information if he is not told at the same time that the woman can have a child only if a man gives her the possibility of conceiving by sexual union.

It is at that moment that it must be revealed in words that father and mother are each as much implicated as the other and responsible in fecundity, that is to say in the conception of the child. Any child of 3 years and above, when he asks the question 'what is the use of this?' (the genitalia) needs to hear this said clearly and to understand the responsibility of paternity and maternity in the union of the sexes. Parents who have problems finding the right answers may be helped by speaking with a psychoanalyst. When the child does not know his biological father or (more rarely) his biological mother, when he is raised by a single parent or by a parent with a different partner, it is more difficult for the parent to answer, while the answer remains indispensable.

Answering clearly and truthfully involves an allusion – implicit or better still explicit – to the sexual union of the biological parents during which the child was conceived and whether conception was deliberate or unknown to their conscious desire and enjoyment. Every child knows something of sexual pleasure and is sensitive to the way in which adults, when talking of his conception, refer without naming it to their reciprocal love and to their own pleasure or non-pleasure. The time that passes between conception and birth and that brings an emphasis to the maternal role also gives to the parents the possibility of delivering to the child his status as a subject. Once conceived, it is he who every day played his part in the foetal–maternal symbiosis. This clear response regarding conception leads to the truth spoken by the adult about sexual pleasure, which is not always in the service of procreation. If children are not told this truth, they innocently imagine the sexual act as strictly functional, animal, zoological. 'You did it twice' – if there are two children. And there it is, they have been inducted into total and growing incomprehension with regard to their romantic feelings and the desires experienced in their bodies when evoking or meeting those that they desire or love.

That the coming into the world of a child is a matter of reciprocal desire and pleasure of subjects who seek out each other, talk to each other and in a concerted encounter called unto themselves the being that they have knowingly or unknowingly conceived (in hoping for or wanting to avoid it); it is this that spoken in words the child perceives as truthful, reveals to him that genital sexuality is human, the language of life, and not only a functional process.

The genealogy and responsible parenthood of this child, on condition that he is told about it, gives fundamental meaning to his life as it is inaugurated – whether it was easy, difficult or impossible for his genitors to take responsibility for it. And this spoken truth humanises him for good with regard to what he has been able to see and know about coming into heat, mating and maternity in mammals and birds, and what there is in animals of parental pair-bonding. Generally, animal fecundation is not explained clearly to children. If nowadays one does not escape providing information on the technical aspects of fecundation and giving birth, most of the time it is with ambiguous words, for example, mating for the insemination of a domestic animal is called 'marriage,' the seasonal and instinctive heat of animals is verbalised in terms of desire and love as if they were humans.

The child cannot understand the vocabulary of kinship, in particular the relational vocabulary between familiar adults and himself, without a verbal explanation of parental responsibility in the conception and care of the newborn and the upbringing of the child by the biological father or a paternal replacement and the mother or mother substitute. *It is the knowledge of sexual union that makes him understand the symbolic meaning of words about the physical, emotional and social aspects of parenthood*, that is to say his nomination by a legal patronym declared at the registry office that the child will bear for life. The differentiation of these aspects of paternity and maternity – carnal, affective and legal – initiates the child into an understanding of symbolic relationships. People will say that a child between 3 and 4 years of age understands nothing of all this. This is not true at all; he intuits these meanings if the words reflect a reality experienced by him; words that the adult feel to be accurate and experienced as accurate by the child; this is what structures him as a human. He needs to know that like him, his father has been conceived by the sexual union of a man with his paternal grandmother and that the man who has given his name to his father is his paternal grandfather. His paternal uncles and aunts have also been conceived by the same man or in any case, it is the same man, the paternal grandfather, who gave them his name and showed himself before the law as responsible for them through their mother, his spouse, who is for the child the paternal grandmother. In the same way, he needs to know that his mother has been conceived by the maternal grandfather and maternal grandmother, that he knows or of whom mother speaks. His uncles and aunts are that because they are brothers and sisters of his mother, which means that they are born of the same mother as his mother or have the same father as his mother or of the sexual union of these same grandfather with the same grandmother. He then understands that his uncles and aunts are younger or older than his mother. He is their nephew or niece, their children are his cousins and it is the same on the paternal side. And if, for whatever reason, he does not have legal parentage on one or the other side, he should be given a true explanation why not. This explanation of the vocabulary of kinship has no meaning if the sexual union is not mentioned as the origin of his birth and kinship, the responsibility for which is assumed by the one who gave him his name and then raised him or not.

The enjoyment of the little boy of the penile erotic value of his body image, in the functional image of anal-urethral excretion, in masturbation partly sublimated in the mastery of playful and utilitarian objects, all of which invest his boyish narcissism, awakens him to consciousness not only of the pleasure he will later have as a lover in sexual union, but also of what will be his social value as a companion, maybe the husband, of the woman he will love; and most of all it awakens him to the procreative value of his father and his grandfather who until then were only perceived as pleasant or unpleasant satellites, companions, accomplices and allies of mother and grandmother. Every boy who does not know his father never ceases to want to know with whom his mother conceived him. I have seen many children of a single mother display numerous and varied behavioural disturbances following the non-response to an implicit or indirectly explicit question about their father: 'You don't need to have one, are we not happy?' or 'Don't you have grand-dad? Uncle? Your Nan?' This is what the child hears when he asks the only slightly indirect question, 'Why do other children have a dad?' In the example of this mixed-race child who had African hair and whose mother was blonde, as he was complaining about the questions his friends were asking about the colour of his skin, she answered: 'You're tanned because of your holidays in the mountains. That's all.' And to, 'Why do they call me a n****r?,' the mother's only answer was: 'They are badly brought up, rude.'

If these children are not too old, between 3 and a little more than 5, and their problem is that of their origin,[29] a true response from their mother can re-integrate them into the order of humanised behaviour. It is sometimes necessary for her to work with a psychoanalyst to understand what is at stake, to be able to tell this truth with the simplest words. This is what the child needs to know and be made to understand from the answers to his questioning. This is what gives him a healthy base for the finding of something I can only call 'his place.' But it is not indispensable to see a psychoanalyst for that – any mother could do it, if she knew how important it is to answer her child. In many of these cases, I only saw the mother. In some cases, it was useless to involve a third person – the psychoanalyst – in the humanising work of informing the child. The mother could do it herself as soon as she had understood her own resistances. But the truth about his origins could also be explained by the grandfather or any person who likes the child, knows his story and can therefore tell it to him with respect for the sexual union of which he is the issue, without blaming either one or the other of his genitors. It is necessary to tell the reality of the facts and if possible to bring details about the surname, the family of the biological father and the reasons why they were together and then split up. This human being, the child, is himself at the origin of his own life: it is his desire that caused his incarnation, that made him stay from day to day in the womb of this woman who was happy or troubled to bear him. All this was experienced by his body and therefore everything can be spoken of so that everything is humanised, nothing is left to a pseudo-animality and organicity *because nothing is only organic in human being; everything is also symbolic*. When children learn the truth of the sexual union of their parents, which is the origin of their lives, it is like the budding of their intelligence reinforced by the knowledge of their kinship and gives the foundation to the feelings they have for their mother, father and their dual lineage, if they are lucky enough to have this.

But in the mind of a child, it is a desire that is only verbally genital. What he cannot understand is his parents' responsibility in bringing him into the world, and whether they accept or avoid it; moreover, there is no moral discourse to be given about the true facts of his history. To be a mum or a dad is for the child a functional and probably erotic representation, but these are for him some functions of part erogenous zones of the body whose supposed pleasure is of the order of which he gives himself through masturbation with in addition some fantasies of happiness for two, the boy with his mother or a princess and the girl with her father or Prince Charming; but without the shadow of rivalry, it is not the Oedipus yet. That the

---

29 By this I mean both the physical power of procreation and the accepting of the responsibility of desire.

child does not understand the responsibility and the narcissistic mutations that maternity and paternity imply for his parents does not contradict for him what he believes is their happiness about his birth: they are happy to 'have him' and to play the parts of 'dad' and 'mum' for him. For him, moored to his own life, it is plain that love and joy go together with having a child; and having a child confers in his mind a 'discretionary power.' And for him this last (that they chose to have him) is quite compatible with the affection he has for them when he is young, whatever the behaviour of his parents.

But some might ask, if the emotional conditions of the birth of the child are unfortunate or even catastrophic, should he be told? Of course – as he has sur-vived them. As the child is here, after the trials of his mother, father, family or his own trials, it is that these trials have been compatible with his survival and therefore dynamically positive for him, and they are part of what has to be told in words while congratulating him for having overcome all that. The most precious good is life, and he is alive. Taking responsibility for oneself is achieved through the words of others who deliver the meaning and the strength of desire through the truth spoken about the difficulties he encountered. But quite a lot of parents would say that if children knew the so-called secret of their conception they will incessantly play with their genitals or tell anybody the truth about their kinship unknown to those around them. These are adult thoughts and not at all true; it is precisely the opposite. The child, appeased with regard to the questions he wondered about, enters into a period of understanding of triangular relationships and of life in general that conducts him towards the Oedipus complex. And this does not consist, as parents may think, of incessantly playing with their genitals. Other parents say, 'If I give this information to my child, he will repeat it to other children and what would others think of me?' It is always that question, asked by parents who think it is bad for a child to know the origin of their life in the love and desire of his parents! Because he exists, he represents a sexual union, and why should he not have the right to know this in words as it is this truth that made him the way he is. 'But he will talk about it at school . . .'

So, let's talk about school at 3 years of age and its role. At reception and then later in primary school,[30] the child could be taught elements of hygiene he needs to know in order to look after himself. He may also learn about sex and the role of accepted desire that conforms with social law: without neglecting the existence of desire expressed by children and which are not within the law, desires that some adults act upon and that cause them to fall foul of the law and end up in prison: forbidden desires of cannibalism, murder, theft, harm, exhibitionism, rape – pre-cisely the prohibitions that are the other side of the anal and oral castration these adults have transgressed. School should teach children to discriminate between

30 Translator's note: I have translated Dolto's 'grandes maternelles' and 'les classes primaires' as 'reception' and 'primary school' respectively in accordance with the British education system; this therefore concerns children aged 4 to 5 (in reception year) and older than 5 for primary school.

irrepressible needs and desire that can be mastered, and that it is this distinction that distinguishes human beings from animals.

The social life of humans implies the mastery of desire according to the law, identical for everyone; and from the age of 3 or 4 it could be said at school that one cannot marry his dad, mum, brother or sister, and while supported by the conscious knowledge of its prohibition in reality, children continue to live through and resolve the Oedipus complex in play and fantasies. *The only law common to the whole human species, which school never talks about, is the prohibition of incest, homosexual or heterosexual.* Children should be told that this rule applies as much to their desire for their parents as for their parents' desire of them, and also to the prohibition of sexual intercourse within their sibling group.

All other laws regarding genital sexuality, that is to say rules of validation and invalidation of marriage and those regarding the legal recognition of children born of a union outside of marriage, as well as what regards divorce, the custody of children, child maintenance – all these things that they hear spoken of or that concern them directly, follow different laws in different countries. Children should in school be made aware of this at the time where they have an interest in it, that is to say between 5 and 8 years old.

And then, in French schools there is now the problem posed by Mother's and Father's Days. What horrors these children have to endure on these occasions! Children have, for their mother and for their father, some intimate feelings that absolutely cannot coincide with the sentimentality of what they are told in class about it. The 'beloved mother' – God knows that these words are in some families completely out of order (because mother is ill, depressed, gone, has abandoned the home, is dead etc). What do these poor kids do with these Mother's Days that exacerbate the problem, when these occasions, if prepared, could be a celebration of the child himself, of his desire to be born of the sexual union of his parents, which had a meaning and which will always have one – the meaning of his desire to live, which connects him to his two lineages through those who conceived him. Some kids say in class, 'I have three dads' – 'It is true,' the teacher could answer, 'some have three dads but every one of us has only one birth father and one birth mother. One can have 36 dads, they are the partners of the mother; they can change, but every one of us has only one father, the one who gave the germ of life to our mother who carried us for months before our birth. We have all been conceived by our father and our mother when they had sex. Some parents love each other for a long time or all their life, others separate or divorce, but it does not change the fact they are the parents of their child.'

This is what the school should teach if it aims at educating. Truth can be told to all children. Nowadays, every child hears on television or radio about laws relating to abortion. They hear their mothers talk about the pill and contraception. Why can't they ask these questions? And why should their teacher not answer their questions quite naturally as should be done within the family? In this way, the vocabulary of kinship would start to make sense. What is a mother, a father? What is an uncle, an aunt, a grandfather, a grandmother? How can this be explained if the child is not informed of the laws of procreation and about the sexual unions by which means his ancestors became the parents of his grandparents, his grandparents of his parents, and he the focal meeting point of the encounter between two lineages that might continue through him.

It would be very interesting at school for everybody to work on a standard representation of a genogram with their father, mother and older siblings and grandparents, if they have any. In primary classes, children are given horrible stencils to draw and colour – why should they not be given the schema of a genogram? Those who are from different parts of the country or different countries would be very interested to hear their parents and teacher talk to them about the different customs of their grandparents and extended family, according to where they have come from. If they are of different ethnic groups, and there are more and more children like this in French schools because of immigration, they should be made aware of their family origins by looking at a geographical map and by talking about customs, habits and climate – moreover, their mother's and father's sides of the family may be different if the couple met in France. All this for me is work that should be done at school, since we know from psychoanalysis that *it is in this way that credible adults answer the questions that become explicit in the child's mind between the ages of 3 and 5 and that determine the opening (or not) of human intelligence, by which I mean intelligence linked with social law.* Before, the child's intelligence was by default employed in cunning, as they did not know any general laws.

When questions about his life, how he was made, have not been answered, the child no longer asks questions, at least not within his family. These questions should be raised again when he arrives at school to enlighten him, answer him and make of him not a nameless puppy of the human species but a subject to whom the responsibility of his history and desire is returned while his desire is recognised in its aim, its long-term masculine and feminine aim, 'when I am grown up,' within the laws of human society and in particular the one of which he is a part.

If I talk about the role of school in the information and education of children about procreation and sexuality, it is because children are entering earlier and earlier into social life, in playgroup and nursery and then in school, and there everything that has not been done in the family can be made up for. However, we see these poor little ones arriving at school without even knowing whose children they are – how, by whom and for whom their lives and their survival have a meaning, without knowing the meaning of the words they use: granddad, grandma, father, mother, uncle, auntie, brother, sister etc. It is the responsibility of school to give meaning to this vocabulary and *sexual education consists in the end of explaining the vocabulary of kinship.* Since Freud, we know that it is during the pre-genital stages, before the entry into primary castration, which is the discovery of the sexes, that the conditions for psychosis are established and that the response to questions about the sexuation of each child is one of the most important in making him able to love, care for and respect his body, to love the life that is his and to take charge of himself in the family that raises him, whether it is his own or not.

The child lives every stage of his life according to the words that elucidate the trials they will have to go through. In addition, each stage is experienced according to the way in which the previous stage was lived through, experienced and left behind. Children of today, especially in villages, receive so little upbringing from their parents that this role rests more and more with the teachers. In fact, has public instruction not become national education?[31]

Primary castration, that is to say the child's discovery of his sex and of the fact that he belongs only to this sex and what this means for the future, can fail completely to have symboligenic effects when the response of the adults is to tell them off, dismiss or otherwise provide no information to the questions raised by the child regarding what he has observed, heard spoken or experienced.

In school, all questions raised by children should be valid. Many schools have understood this and help children to observe and care for living beings: vegetal life, the growth of seeds, the care of small animals for which they take responsibility in class. All this is very well but is not an education about their own lives, sufficient for understanding and knowing them. What is extraordinary for a child when he discovers the sexual difference and when it is explained to him, is that it is the first time he encounters a law that does not depend upon his parents or any adults, a law that is a fact of nature and that for some shakes up their world. This has a symboligenic effect giving value to who they are, but could also have contradictory effects. In this case, it is important that school can help the child overcome the handicap that marks his sex according to the narrative or values inculcated by their families. Sometimes, this child, boy or girl, would like to be of the other sex for reasons of his own, could explain and usually has no trouble talking about if someone is willing to listen to him. The more I think about the question of the prevention of psychosis in children whose behaviour is still healthy at the age of 2, and of neurosis in those for whom some difficulties develop when they start school, the more I tell myself that it is the informative and educational roles of school with regard to questions about the body and sex of children that is not good enough, now that children enter society so early and have fewer extended families and less time to talk with their parents. In addition, everything they hear and see in the mass media, on television, adds to the confusion of what they experience: passionate feelings leading to murderous acts, or the exhibitionist amorous behaviours of couples. All this regarding the relationship of their parents and their own existence add images to the questions they ask themselves. School must change, must respond with a precise vocabulary to all the questions of children, in particular, notably 'why this child bears the maiden surname of his mother or the name

31 Translator's note: Dolto saw the change in the French school system from the title of *L'Instruction Publique* (Public Instruction, where Instruction suggests the teaching of primary skills such as numeracy and literacy) to *L'Education Nationale* (National Education, where Education implies a wider learning that includes life-skills that would in the past have formed part of what would have been the duties of parental upbringing).

of his biological father which is not the same as his mother's, or of one of his brothers, or that of a mother's lover who became her husband and recognised him but is not his father?' All this should be make explicit at school, as it is at school that all this is revealed to him. When the register is taken, how many children hear for the first time a name that they did not know but is nonetheless that on their birth certificate![32]

Oedipus complex and Oedipal genital castration (prohibition of incest)

The stage that follows the moment when children discover their belonging to a sex is the stage during which they enter what psychoanalysis calls the Oedipus complex.[33] As soon as the child has knowledge of their definitive belonging to one sex, his body image changes for him – it is no longer unconscious; it needs consciously to align itself with the reality of a body that will later be that of a woman or a man. With regard to the subject and to the desire he has about this future, it is the desire to identify with the being that he loves the most at that moment in his life. And as I hope I have demonstrated in detail, it is because of the function of the father as initiator to the law (successfully performed or not) that it is so important that an answer is given to the child regarding the role of his father in his conception and then his birth – his natural role in the sexual union, legal role in the recognition of the child at the registry office and emotional role in bringing up the child. The father has or has not given his name to the child, he has or has not helped the mother to bring him up. The child may or may not rely upon him to guide him, to help him become an adult man or woman.

In the absence of a biological father, another man who is partner to his mother can act as the tutelary father. From the entry into the Oedipus complex, the child develops an image of himself in the world where his imaginary life is dominated by his actual relationship with both parents as connected with the project he nurtures of his future as a seductive and successful adult according to his sex. The Oedipus complex can be either healthily conflictual or pathologically conflictual, which happens if there is a failure to belong to his or her own sex. This can happen

---

32 The desire to know more about one's origins by seeking a truthful verbal response from those currently responsible for his life (tutelary parents) is a sign of the child's intelligence. To violate this desire, to dodge a response, to prohibit this questioning as inappropriate or to deceive the child by responding in terms of the physiological functioning of pregnancy is to render stupid the man- or woman-to-be that is the child who asks questions about his life, to which in his eyes adults have the secrets. It is the desire for carnal alliance between a man and a woman, his genitors, who may or may not be prepared to take on the aftermath, the life of a new human conceived by their sexual union; this is what should be said to the child who questions mother, father or any adult about his origin. It is the triangular alliance of the desires of father, mother and child – girl or boy – that the words of the adult must signify, thus revealing to the child his own share of desire: to be conceived, then to be born and from then on to survive.

33 See the chapter on the Oedipus complex in 'Au Jeu du Desire.'

when the mother has not been able to or has not wanted to tell the truth about the child's parentage, girl or boy. But this can also happen if some ongoing dramas between the parents oblige the child to suffer the attitude of his father on behalf of his mother, or to misjudge his father – or the other way round. People will say: what can we change in the life of a child who has the misfortune to be born to a dysfunctional couple, or to be raised by a single parent or by divorced parents etc? A lot can be done by putting the right words to the existing situation and by helping the child to say what he feels guilty about hearing or of thinking, because a child always thinks positive things regarding his father and mother, even if he thinks negative things, even if he has visible evidence of their discord and suffers from the sometimes unbearable parenting style of some parents. These children always find an excuse for their parents. What is important, as long as the child is alive, is to support him and help him look after himself and to talk without shame about what is happening. It is neither easy nor pleasant. His parents are a problem for him, but to be able to continue to develop as their child, he must be supported in the effort he makes to keep some confidence in himself as their son or daughter. It is what I call in psychoanalysis 'supporting the narcissism of this child,' his primary narcissism (appetite for life) and his secondary narcissism (his interest in himself) in his going-on-becoming an adult of his own sex – either in modelling himself on people he knows or in knowing that even if his given models are not those he would like to imitate, he nonetheless desires and searches for a model upon which to become an adult of his sex.

Let us suppose that the child has parents who get on well enough for the child to continue developing. There is a difference between girls and boys at this point. The boy wants to identify with his father, as does the girl. Both want to be like both parents. But the boy, who has an intuition of his virility to come, takes the sexual initiative and decides that he wants to marry his mother. The girl too, when she enters the Oedipus complex, says she wants to marry her mother. This is because she still believes that the mother produces children through her digestive system and that if she makes herself loved by her mother, mother will give her whole or part of what her husband gave her – that is to say something with which to have children; because for her, in her fantasies, pregnancy and giving birth are exclusively feminine things and still have something magical about them. What do you need to make an anal baby? This is what she would like to receive from the loved adult, man or woman. Dad, if he is present in the home, would remain Daddy, her dad and her children's dad. The boy is far more directly implicated in the Oedipus complex. If he admires his father and feels that his mother admires his father, he is proud of him, wants to become like him and tries to identify totally with him and naturally, to have his father's prerogatives in intimacy with his mother. This is where *the father can and must give his son what we call in psychoanalysis castration*; tell him: 'It is forever impossible for a son to love his mother like another man loves her. This is not because you are small and I am big, it is because you are her son and that a son and his mother can never live in a sexual union and have children.'

The boy

What body image is in play for the child who enters the Oedipus complex? Let us talk about the boy. The active genital drives, which we have seen are rooted in the urethral, remain penile part drives that move centrifugally towards the object of desire. It is these drives that the child transposes onto part objects, which themselves represent part images of his body, the penis in particular, that he displaces onto all hitting instruments – weapons aimed at attacking, the penetrating aggression in ballistic games, in sadistic puncturing actions and in targeting girls by playing at killing them. Here the child projects quite literally either his desire to throw a murderous liquid (excrements are seen as bad in that they are rejected by the body), or his desire to throw something that would make a baby, since he knows that this is what will happen one day in his life; he knows this through what adults or older friends at school have said. These alternatives are in no way contradictory. Children who play at killing want absolutely their victim to get up again immediately afterwards. It is 'just talking' and 'for a laugh'; here the drives operate in fantasy and not 'for real.' Then, he hears of the birth of a baby: where does this come from? And what about death? It touches the child's entourage. Where do we go after death? Life and death are the most important questions for the child when he is in the full Oedipal stage. Then he will stop his aggressive penile games, or at least those that are not regulated in quasi-social games; and this, thanks to the prohibition of incest, which has to be spoken about as much in relation to brothers as to sisters, that is to say as much homosexual as heterosexual. Boys transpose unconscious or preconscious outwardly directed penile aggression onto manual or intellectual activity, and the activity of their whole body, playful and production. It is through the speech of the father and examples given by him of respect for women, for his wife and his daughters, that the boy grasps the difference between his urethral-anal desire to master the body of another, of hitting it aggressively to feel virile (something of the rutting of animals), and the fact of one day giving life to a child through a choice arising from love linked with desire; with an understanding of the responsibility that causes people to commit to each other as lovers, and then as parents, and then to bringing up that child until he reaches his majority. *When this is said by the father to his son, it is the initiation of the son to human life. This is the Oedipal castration. 'I forbid you your mother, because she is my wife and she brought you into this world. Both things are important. Your sisters are as sexually forbidden to you as your mother is.* I did not marry my mother, your paternal grandmother, or your aunts, who are my sisters; your mother did not marry her father, your maternal grandfather, or her brothers etc.'[34]

This is how the child hears what is going to introduce him into the order of genital humanisation. This is where school should also play its role, talking about

---

34 It is very important to say this again and again to a child of a single mother whose surname may look like that of her father, in comparison with those of other children.

the difference between the human genital drive, linked with love, and the procreative rutting of animals, which obeys a blind coupling instinct between male and female without love, without a sense of responsibility and commitment even if some animals observe a period of couple-formation to assist in the raising of the young until they are able to find food for themselves.

The deficiency of the father who is inadequate to giving castration

If the father does not deliver it, or if nobody delivers this education in the mastery of desire by the prohibition of incest, the boy can for all his life hold onto the idea of an exclusively narcissistic object choice, which may perhaps not be his mother or sister, but whose sole destiny will be to gratify his genital desires: an object that might be chosen because it can be held in dependency by intimidation and violence. It is the submission of the father to the law of respect and non-violence towards his partner, the child's mother, that awakens the child to the fact that adult relational life is not of the urethral-anal kind that he imagines, based upon his way of feeling and according to his infantile narcissism, but of a type other than that which he wishes for at his age. It is here that a violent father, or the complete absence of a father, plays a disturbing role. Those who are aggressive or drunk and odious to live with in a family, who come home to beat their partners, who are irresponsible and don't talk to their children – none of these help their children's emotional development. Equally, men who take no joy in their families, but who are seen by their sons to take violent possession of their wives, are pathogenic because their young sons still admire them. These males seem to them fantastically powerful and are for them more animal than human models. Such fathers, with the submissive complicity of their partners, give their children a model of irresponsible masculine behaviour. When the children are small, this 'virile' behaviour appears to them magical, we could say narcissistic, oral, anal and fascinating. It is what one finds in the ogres of fairy tales and the monsters of mythology. The behaviour of father towards mother exemplifies to boys, who have otherwise embarked on a normal developmental course between primary castration and the end of the Oedipal stage, the claim to domination that is also seen in the disdain of the boy for girls.[35]

If the father continues single-handedly to lay down the law in the household within the register of oral, anal and urethral drives, gratified by alcoholism or by paranoid behaviour, the fact that the child sees this man as the absolute master of a terrified woman, who from time to time has babies with him, confirms in the eyes of the child who bears his name that it is by means of urethral-anal drives that the man is a valued citizen of society. Great then is the sensitisation of such a boy to homosexuality – either a passive homosexuality in identification with the

---

35 Children of the other sex also boast of this domination and disdain, at least between brothers and sisters (a way of underlining the repression of incestuous drives that often are common).

sometimes depressive but otherwise valued mother, as she is the only protector of the children from their father, or as an active homosexual structured in relation to his father, whose example leads him to think that this is what it means to become a man in the real sense of the word. This is how men come to behave in a paranoid way and violate both women and laws as soon as their impulsive and irrepressible desires are challenged in the slightest degree. These are adults who in their childhoods never completely formulated an Oedipus complex or who never received castration from their fathers. They remain masculine individuals without ever becoming truly humanised, led by rather than in mastery of their drives – querulous, making up the law for themselves, often intelligent and logical and (as the child can witness down the pub) liked by their mates. In fact, these are in society models of homosexual affectivity and at home in their relationship with their women, animals in heat. Women who feel obliged to accept such a situation are obviously also born and bred in difficult family situations in their youth.

Here, the role of the adults around them, the adults at school and the doctors who know these children, is very important: not to separate them from their families but to allow them to understand the lack of upbringing that is at the origin of their father's difficulties. They may not love them any the less, but the fathers will be less harmful as identificatory models. In addition, such fathers are very often, early in life, slavishly in love with their women – as much as sons as lovers; these are men who have had serious Oedipal difficulties, and who re-live this in becoming jealous of the love and interest shown by their partners towards their children, especially their sons. A doctor who knows about psychoanalysis and who is familiar with this kind of family life can well deliver the prohibition of incest to the boy and tell him that he can no longer console his mother by cuddling her when he sees that she is unhappy with his father – that this is not age appropriate, that he would do better to work hard at school, to respect his father and mother and stop behaving like the exclusive friend of his mother. His father has not always been this way – what he sees at home – and in addition his mother can say this in front of the child to the doctor. The father has often entered into this situation because of depression, burn-out, or to the concrete difficulties of life. All this greatly helps a child to see in proportion the dramas he witnesses, and in another way, it helps both parents, through the child. When a boy has reached to an impossible Oedipal situation with a pathogenic father, the work consists in helping him understand that he will learn better in class, succeed better if he leaves the family home and asks for himself to board at school, if this is economically possible or with social assistance. But this request has to come from the child. It is not because the situation is difficult that we should separate the child from his family, barring exceptions. We should wait until the child asks for himself. It is within the family that the Oedipus complex must be resolved.

The girl

Let us now talk about the Oedipus complex of the girl, of whom I said that at the start is as much homosexual as heterosexual, as the little girl enters into her genital life with the aim of seducing someone who will make her a mother like her mother. For her, in reference to the phallus, it is clear that men have penises but women have babies. Her desire to identify with her mother leads the girl, if the parental couple get along, to want to have the prerogatives that father recognises and confers on mother. But the girl cannot enter into the Oedipus except on condition that she tries to transgress the prohibition of incest by making her father fall into her seductive trap. The girl has not got the centrifugal (outwardly directed) active penile drive of the boy. With regard to the phallus, her drives are centripetal (inwardly directed). She attracts to herself. She is on the look-out for an object who represents power and that she can have for herself. In fantasy, the transgression of the incest taboo by her father or brother gives value to her person and her kinship. To be taken and penetrated as mummy is by daddy, even to be forcibly subjected to this seductive power – this is what explains her dreams of pursuit, kidnapping and of rape by a man whose face is never seen but who has this or the other characteristic of her dad or one of her brothers. In reality, her desire is to attract.

This makes her develop feminine qualities useful to social success – learning at school, working conscientiously, behaving well, getting good marks and developing feminine qualities at home – cleaning, doing the washing up, all the activities she sees done by adults, as much by mother as by father and that she will do to please them both, and if possible to please father more so that he values her as much as his wife, and perhaps even more. From this arises the fact that the 'perverse' attitude of girls is more obvious and visible than those of boys in the Oedipus complex. They are 'perverse' in the sense of being seductive, in making the other evade the law, from the moment that this law has been expressed to them. This is why it is so important that this law is expressed to them. 'If he really likes me, if I am more valuable than Mummy, he will see that I am the one who understands him the best, that it is I who would be his best partner'; to which is added the fact that this expression of desire for the father often takes on a so obviously untruthful aspect, cunning and slanderous towards the mother. So, when father comes back home: 'Mummy's gone, you know, and I don't know where she is, or if she will be back for dinner.' Other little girls' fantasies go as far as mythomania, in which they have attracted men who have had sexual contact with them – fantasies they never verbalise to their mother – they are aimed at making father jealous, so that he will do with them as much or even more than these imaginary men they say they have managed to seduce. The perverse attitudes of girls are overall far more verbalised than the perverse attitudes of the boy, which are more often lived without being verbalised. It is known that girls are chatterboxes and use cunning to satisfy their aims (or cravings – always more or less oral in their genitality).

This comes from the fact that *girls have discovered that their seductive power depends on their acceptance of not having a penis and on their desire that another will give it to them – not to have it but to be the mistress of the one who has it and can therefore satisfy them.* What better target than their father or their mother's lover, the one who satisfies their mother? How to differentiate between these fantasies told by little girls and reality? We constantly read in the press stories of sexual seduction and we hear a lot of these stories in our sessions. How do we distinguish truth from falsehood? It is rather simple. There is a great difference between the way a girl who has been the object of seduction talks, with realistic details, and the ones who make it up. Alas, these fantasies that deceive adults have sometimes traumatising social consequences for everyone, and every psychoanalyst has had to treat women whose verbalised Oedipal fantasy destroys the credibility of their entourage, up-ending and ruining their lives. On the other hand, they also have to treat women who as children have exposed themselves through their careless seductions to the assault of men in the family or close to the family, and who were not able to talk about it at the time because they felt both guilty and proud to have attracted the attention of an adult. Here again, I think that *the role of school could be very important in teaching children that sexual relationships between adults and children is prohibited* so that the child can distinguish reality from his fantasies, and if the child is in reality exposed to a disturbing situation, he will know to tell an adult, 'But this is forbidden'; generally, children don't have the words to escape the advances of perverts because they have never been taught them before they undergo the experience that leaves them completely lost.

Speaking the incest taboo gets the boy out of the Oedipus complex, but on the contrary draws the girl into it, super-charging it in language and therefore in her sublimations into speech and actions of oral and anal drives, so providing the means of transgressing the taboo or rather of making an adult transgress it. Her coquettishness attracts gifts, which pleases her, small objects – rings, earrings, necklaces that sparkle to attract the attention of men to her appearance and that make her the envy of other girls. The father and boys continue to have for her a prevailing value, and she likes to attract them. She is also far more than boys attracted by mirrors in which she measures the seductiveness of her appearance. In fact, the narcissism of girls in how they show their femininity is lived far more on the surface than boys' narcissism, who live their Oedipus more deeply and in the emotions they feel for their mother, and in the rivalry they feel towards the father they love. The phallic activity of girls is enormous and is expressed through spectacular acts everywhere in society – at home, at school – and this is why girls are so easily successful in the Oedipal period and then during the latency period after the resolution of the Oedipus complex, especially if they keep the hope of pleasing both women and men through their phallic activities. The incest taboo provokes in girls sublimations of pre-genital drives, while in boys it provokes above all a reinforced awakening of epistemophilic drives. What is most in play for him is the question of knowledge – that he can understand and write 'seeing it.'[36] He wants to know how the world is made, how he can become its boss; he wants to know the laws that regulate rights between human beings, while for girls it is about 'being it' – appearing, attracting, winning whatever she can in order

36 Translator's note: In French, Dolto puns upon '*savoir*' (knowledge) and transforms it into '*ça voir*' – seeing it. This is to set up a contrast with the girl's investment of her drives later in the paragraph.

to impress authority figures. Backbiting and calumny are therefore her weapons against other girls in society.

Boy or girl, the child is fragilised at the time of the healthy resolution of the Oedipus complex as whatever they do, it is impossible for the boy to seduce his mother and the girl her father, these two adults having their desire taken up by sexual objects elsewhere, their partner or someone outside the home, Daddy's mistress, as is said by children who have heard their mother complaining to her friends. The child still needs the protection of his parents, or in any case the protection of supportive adults; he needs tutelary help for the difficulties that will arise in his path in society. The forbidding of his genital desires within the family catapults him into a desire to play within his peer group, towards auxiliary friendships, with human beings of his sex who have been marked by the same trial with regard to their parents. Among humans of the other sex, he aspires to conquer objects with whom he is in love and will be proud to obtain sensual and sexual privileges, and reciprocal love if possible; but then he encounters rivalry with others of his sex for the same object. It is this displacement of the Oedipus that colours the social life of children, particularly at school, although they are in the latency phase with regard to genital sexual preoccupation as such. Sexualised emotional preoccupations and the narcissistic search for partial pleasures never stop.

Numerous children have had poor Oedipal experiences or have come out of this phase without castration, I mean without having heard the prohibition of realising sexual desire within the family spoken, which would liberate desire to be realised outside the family milieu. Because parents may wish to keep their days off for themselves and so allow the child few opportunities to see other children, these children look to having pets, as much in order to love them as to have them as dependents. Cats, dogs, hamsters and even horses are loved by children because they are 'sweet.' This does not mean, by the way, that these children are not going to manage with time to resolve their Oedipus complex, but it will be later, as these animals are like the transitional objects of earlier times, which linked them in imagination with their breast-mother. These animals, which they love to cuddle and pet and whose love they gain, which they command and in which they may inspire fear, are for them transitional objects for their relationship of diffuse sensuality with their parents before the resolution of the Oedipus – before they realise for themselves that they have no hope with regard to genital desire or future procreation with their beloved parents. This attachment to animals may become the aim of sublimations that later in life continue in a vocation linked with the animal world. I do not mean that all good relations with animals are the sign of a body image that has not emerged from the Oedipal relationship, but it is the case where the masters' love for the animals isolates them from their fellows, because his narcissistic need is for a mute emotional confidante.

After the Oedipus, during the latency period, the role of adults (parents and educators), although radically different from that of friends and comrades, remains important for children during their failures, their narcissistic disappointments and their trials in friendship and love. The way adults react can support the child or make him feel guilty in his distress. He is sensitive to being attentively listened to by an adult whose presence is felt to be chaste, compassionate, non-reproachful and non-moralising. It is possible for a child whose parents are attentive, helpful and above all confident in themselves to develop confidence in himself, including by way of his failures. A father who says to his son, 'You will do well because you are my son and the son of your mother, and we are good people and you too are a good person, even if for the moment you are finding things difficult,' is not a father who preaches morality but who supports morale – and the child needs this as much as he needs congratulations for success. The same is true for the girl who castigates herself and complains to her mother: 'Boys don't like me, I am ugly, I will never find a husband,' – 'But you will,' replies the compassionate mother, 'You will find a good husband because you are a good girl. Your father is a good person and we have a good daughter. You are disappointed for now, but you will succeed next time. You too will be a good person.' And she should point out the assets the girl has in reality in the game of life. It is only through the parents' recognition of their own value and of the love and confidence they have in the child that the child feels valued and supported by a self-confidence linked with being the child of these two parents, and is thereby able to overcome his failures.

This confidence, this love and this chaste interest, one could say, of the parents for their child are irreplaceable after the Oedipus complex, because the love of his parents is necessary to the child at the very moment when, knowing that he is forever banned from sexual and sensual intimacy with them, he believes that he no longer has any value in their eyes, that he is no longer loved, or is even rejected. The moralising discourse, as much as the intimacy of a soothing tenderness, is harmful in the short or the long term because the child must continue to disengage from dependency upon parents. The adults' difficult role is to contribute to this liberating flight through their true love for him.

The contribution of Oedipal castration to narcissism in the freeing of the libido

After the Oedipus, what about narcissism, its ethos and how it affects the relationship of the subject to his body? What about the unconscious body image?

We designate as *secondary* narcissism the relationship reached by the subject with himself when he has taken the structural step of the last of the castrations, which is the obstructing of desire by the incest taboo, in other words the acceptance of genital castration. This last castration is an initiation into social life. It is delivered by parents when they can and know how to do it, supported as they are in this (as much a trial for them as for the child) by their parental ego-ideal and their chaste love for their children.

It is clear that parents who received the same Oedipal castration in their childhoods from their own parents find it much easier than others to take on this task in the child's upbringing. This is why the role in society of teachers and others *in loco parentis* is important as parental auxiliaries in supporting the child in going beyond his pre-Oedipal and Oedipal modes of reasoning and affectivity. It is especially important in initiating and supporting the child whose parents are themselves badly Oedipally castrated and experience ambiguity in their love relationship with their child – a relationship that may be philic or phobic (in caresses or blows) and is felt by the child to be incestuous because of the interest his parents have in his body and the feelings that this brings him. Let us review the evolution of narcissism since early infancy:

1   Primordial narcissism is linked with the taking on of the fact of umbilical castration by the newborn – the fact that he survived birth and discovered his respiratory and cardio-vascular autonomy, olfactive sense and the peristaltic movements of his digestive tube.
2   Primary narcissism results from the experience of the mirror that reveals the infant's face to him. This mirror experience is concomitant or joins on to the knowledge of his body as having a masculine or feminine sex and creates a distinction between the possible and impossible that does not depend on the will of the parents.
3   What is added by the incest taboo, the source of a different kind of narcissism, named secondary, is the prevention of sexual impulses remaining in society without a humanising law – remaining animal, so to speak, and instinctually driven (the 'I didn't do it on purpose!' of the child). From here on, the child has to learn to master his desires and to tell the difference between thinking and doing something. He learns to act in his own name, which constitutes the identity of this subject within the social group. He is responsible for his behaviours. It is then to himself that he feels obliged, and risks losing face in his own eyes if he is not the master of his desire and if he responds to impulses to which he must submit without understanding their motivations.

From the moment of Oedipal castration, the child must know consciously that his genital desire – like that of all human beings, adults and children, regardless of age and race – and the pleasures of bodily sexual intimacy and procreation with his parents and close family, are definitively and forever banned. He has to renounce his first heterosexual and homosexual objects – father, mother, grandparents, brothers and sisters – as incestuous objects, as they too must renounce the realisation of their sensual fantasies towards him. However, it must be recognised – and all children feel this – that *it is only the incestuous goal that has sustained him throughout his humanising promotions*, as since birth, his desires and motivations have been focused by his mother, father and close relatives. This is what leads to anxieties about kidnap, eviscerating rape, castration and murder, according to the child's sex and whether active or passive drives dominate, according also to his fundamental fantasy and the sensual pleasures expected of receptivity or emissivity; in order to survive, he has to renounce the pleasures of his violent drives and the incestuous eroticism and ethos of his primary narcissism. In effect, what until then characterised the dynamic of desire of children who mixed fantasy and reality was that unbeknownst to them it depended upon their incestuous desire, which leads unconsciously towards the exclusivity of genital desire for the parent of the opposite sex, without however renouncing either the subjects' fundamental narcissism or their future fecundity as individuals.

Unbeknownst to the parents, the child may obtain satisfaction for his burning erotic drives in bodily contact that he preserves by engineering caresses or sleeping in their bed, a situation as erotically disturbing as the corporal punishment that he forces his parents to give him. When this happens, the child risks regressing and failing to maintain the cohesion between an age-appropriate body image and bodily schema, a cohesion that allows him both to remain the subject of his history and to win his fully human status. This human status is won by the human young in the image of their parents; but they don't understand that the only humanising semblance is in the acceptance of the laws that govern the exercise of the drives in acts between humans. They believe that the humanising semblance consists in imitating and mimicking the ways of adults, as if the adults were playing a part that they themselves have to take on. Might this come from the traps of spoken language in that it is stereotyped, including all roles and civil behaviours?

The words uttered by adults are the same as those children use but have different meanings that depend on the different lived experience of each. It is through the body image that underpins what the child says (and that he reveals to us through drawings during sessions and mostly in his commentaries upon these) that one can understand the ambiguities and misunderstandings between children and adults.[37] There are thousands of examples. To cite one: 'to love' for a child at the oral stage is putting in his mouth, the way one does with food; then, after weaning, 'to love' is not signified by cannibalism or biting but by its mimicry in the kiss. When a child is well brought up, the kiss must become silent and be used ritualistically within the family. With regard to kisses said to be 'the kisses of the nurse' – noisily applied to the cheeks or bottom of the baby – might we dare to think that for them, as for the baby, this is an allusion to cannibalistic enjoyment and at the same time an allusion to farting, a prelude to defaecation? Another example: I remember a formal social gathering when as the children talked to each other after having greeted the guests, two of them shared their thoughts: 'I say, that lady called Mrs General – she is so wet when she kisses!' This lady had given everyone a rather wet kiss because of her dentures. One of the parents reacted in a horrified way: 'Be quiet! You don't know what you're saying!' – the maliciousness of words![38]

37 An 8-year-old boy, upon being enlightened by his mother about how babies are born, reacted with horror: 'But it isn't polite to be born! You see them naked!'
38 Translator's note: In French, the child had said: '*Dit donc, la dame qu'on appelle La Generale, qu'est qu'elle mouille en baisant!*' *Baiser* means to kiss but could also mean to have sexual intercourse, so the child's words were heard by his mother rather differently to how they were meant.

It is in his fight to preserve in his own way his semblance with adults, to win a human status, that the *neurotic subject represses the non-castrated drives of different stages without being able either to act upon them or fantasise about them, until they are crushed, together with desire itself. This is what causes both the subject's suffering and his dignity. It is also the difference with psychotic subjects whose narcissism no longer suffers from the loss of a human semblance that would be threatened by the pleasure of acting on his drives. There is no longer any distinction for him between fantasising and thinking or acting in reality.* If, out of narcissism, the child renounces during various castrations the enjoyment of the primary means of satisfying his drives, it is also because human adults are for him, when he is small, an image of himself with added value; before primary castration, I mean adults of both sexes and afterwards, the adult model of a particular sex. During Oedipal castration, he no longer has just to resemble the image of what he believed he had to become to confirm his identity, but he has totally to identify with the parent of his own sex, taking his place, power and prerogatives.

He realises that until then, he had been mistaken. *It is with the parent's submission to the law that he must identify, and not with the image of his parent, nor with his parent's affectively determined self-representation.*

It is from another subject, like him castrated with regard to his incestuous desire, that the child subject must receive the anticipatory recognition of his erotic value – which in his eyes is momentarily eclipsed – of his body, sex, person, dignity of man- or woman-in-becoming: because whatever he does, he cannot gratify his desire, until then incestuous and impossible for him to separate from the fact of loving his parents or of being loved by them. He can no longer see what is pleasurable in loving or in being loved.

However, Oedipal castration happens in the life of children at the time of the loss of milk teeth. When they see themselves in the mirror, they judge themselves to be pathetic, and very often they are told: 'Oh, you look frightful like this!'[39]

Losing teeth in adults' dreams is a frequent image of castration anxiety. The loss of teeth – mediators of the active and sadistic oral drives – ratifies the Oedipal acceptance and the mutation of primary narcissism into secondary narcissism in the bodily schema. The unconscious libidinal economy before the Oedipus

---

39 Someone outside the family must reassure the child that his face and his person remain capable of eliciting love and desire. Not to be like her mother for a girl, or like his father for a boy, not to become similar to them in their appearance, confers upon the child his status as a subject and guarantees that he will become the man or woman that his birth foretold. It is important to explain this well to him (once again, this should be the role of school); until this time, children live in the illusory hope of becoming an exact copy of their model, and this hope is moored to their child's face or their behaviours, always validated by the pleasure or non-pleasure they gave their parents. It is at this point that the sometimes contradictory meaning in honouring his parents and loving them or being loved by them could be revealed to them, at a time when to love had only the meaning of 'to please' the beloved. Without the integration of the taboo of incest, to please is ambiguous and can be perverse.

complex could be described as a homeostasis, guarded by a pre-superego, between the id, the ego and the ideal-ego. This economy is modified because the ego no longer has an ideal-ego; an ego-ideal, unrepresented by an existing person, has taken its place as the goal that supports conscious and unconscious motives of desire. If his persona continues to exist and grow, it is no longer a pre-superego that was always affiliated with the tutelary entity who watched over him to control his acts and upon whom he was dependent. Now, it is a superego linked with the fantasies that he himself created when faced with his impossible desire for the incestuous object, the castrating or murderous fantasy for the boy ('your purse or your life!'[40]), the fantasy of kidnap or of mutilating rape for the girl, rape of which a woman can be the executor in complicity with a man. This superego, the unconscious heir of both the pre-superego and the fantasies triggered by the taboo of incest, has the energising effect of pushing the child to leave the narrow family circle to win licit objects in social reality, or more precisely those not forbidden to his sensual and amorous genital desires. That this desire is not only not forbidden but is licit and valid as long as it does not apply to the pursuit of incestuous objects is what must be verbalised to children.

It is in this conquest, which gives them value with regard to boys and girls of their own age, that the latency years will be used in children who have received castration. Adolescence, with the physiological push that puberty represents, rekindles desire in its genital manifestations and the love affects for desirable objects. This confirms and reinforces secondary narcissism, which incites the young man or young woman to promote him/herself in society – both to reinforce his own image and to conquer the right of a bodily encounter with the love object, in triumph over rivals. This fantasy of success in any non-incestuous amorous or sexual relationship supports the secondary narcissism of the subject from the latency phase onwards and even more after puberty.

It is therefore the barrier, put firmly in place by father or mother against the incestuous desire of their son/daughter, that frees the libidinal energy of the child for his life outside the family. This taboo, to which they themselves are subject as much as the child, suddenly ennobles the child and puts him on the same level as all citizens. It allows him the free play of his drives in society from the moment where he expresses these within the rules. It is from this time that games, with their rules, are so important; and also the acceptance that the game be recognised as much more fun if one doesn't cheat, even if it can be a terrible trial not to win when he finds that either chance or skill are on the side of the other. There is another manifestation of this. Pleasure gets directed towards effort, work, the learning of everything that helps him to understand the world, others, the laws of nature, of commerce between humans, and everything that gives the child value within his age group, which has become much more important for him than mummy, daddy, brothers and sisters. Then it is important that mummy-daddy bear

---

40 Translator's note: In French, '*la bourse ou la vie!*' where bourse means both purse and testicles.

the loss of much of their importance for their child. If they want to teach their child the respect owed to them, it is only through giving him the example of their respect for his person. The child in any case does not 'owe' them anything. It is to his children that he/she will owe, having become father/mother, what his parents did for him/her.

If, on the contrary, the parents claim a debt of love and of recognition during latency and even more during adolescence, this will be damaging to the child and through the long-term effects of their guilt damaging for their grandchildren. Certain perverting parents talk incessantly of the sacrifice they made for their children; these 'sacrifices' are in fact inherent in their responsibility as parents and do not entail any debt from their children towards them.

The latency period covers first a physiological latency: the volume of the genitals – in the newborn disproportionately large in comparison with the rest of the body, as is the head – remains the same in the body of a girl or a boy of 8 or 9. It is the pubertal growth-spurt accompanied by the rapid development of the genitals and of secondary sexual characters that brings back into the imaginary the representations of desire known at the time of the Oedipal castration. It is as if the adolescent had to re-live in a few days or weeks the significant steps of their evolution from childhood to the Oedipus complex.

The technical and cultural aptitudes acquired during latency for narcissistic pleasure or sometimes to win over a rival are reshuffled and re-orientated towards what we would call a vocation. This is the long-term desire to play a role in society by the devotion of one's strength and the acquisition of arms. 'Going out' is the magic word of adolescence.

They would like to be able to assume responsibility for their needs and to live elsewhere than in the family home, not only to be available and free to see friends of their own and the other sex without being supervised, but also to be able to take their part in social and civic life. The value of work continues to be gauged according to the pleasure one takes in it, whatever the effort needed, but the earning of money by tasks and even unpleasant efforts with the immediate aim of being free of parental control also becomes important. It is, as one says, earning your daily bread. This is why the current economic difficulties in countries with a high unemployment rate are a drama for youth, and a lot of them regress to a pre-genital narcissism. The impossibility of licitly escaping parents by earning money through one's work undermines the meaning of life inherent to the genital drives and contradicts the anal drives of action that would give value to the adolescent in his age group if he could find a job. This explains in large measure the small acts of juvenile delinquency that seem to be increasing and are the expression of the difficulties faced by our young people. How does one have money, live under one's own roof, be able to have the object of one's desire and live together as a couple, if it is not possible to work? How does one take the pleasure necessary to preserve one's narcissism if only passive desires – of patient waiting – are authorised when there is no work? Passive desire does no honour to a young man who wants to win a young lady, and tends in young women to favour only attractiveness of appearance. Passive desire linked with pre-genital drives, for example olfactive eroticism, leads to solvent abuse (glue, ether) and more expensively, cocaine; the oral eroticism leads to drinking and drugs; anal eroticism to false and empty imaginative creations; and a lot of young people sink into these passive regressions.

There is, fortunately, the possibility of using some socialised and active drives: music, dance, love and discovery of nature, sport; but this also costs money and from this arises the current great difficulty for young people – even those who have been through the perilous pass of the castrations and who have been humanised by education – who end up during adolescence without any cultural or educational interest. They become young adults in social difficulty, unable to assume responsibility for their own subsistence or sexual development that would be given meaning by couple-formation, even transitory. However, regression to active anal drives when coupled with the anxiety of hopelessness leads to violence.

Chapter 3

Pathology of body images and analytic practice

Early dangers of the alteration of body images

We can start from what can be considered to be a sort of general law. Even with no neuro-muscular or neuro-vegetative defects, a human being can find himself unable to construct his first body image or even to sustain his fundamental narcissism; it suffices that he suffers damaging ruptures in his early bond with his mother, be it during his symbiotic foetal life or his life as a nursling, in the period where the equilibrium of the mother–baby dyad is essential to his going-on-becoming[1] a human.

During pregnancy

It may be surprising that there could be such ruptures during a pregnancy otherwise physiologically sound and medically supervised, but this is what we sometimes find in the archaic structural premises of paranoid children and adults. It could happen, for instance, to a baby in gestation whose mother suddenly loses a loved one and who forgets for a few days that she is pregnant; it is highly possible that one may later find a trace of this forgetting, of which only she has a memory, in the paranoid reactions of the child. This observation can only be possible in the course of an analysis, and no doubt we cannot generalise. It must be understood that what attacks the vital symbolic link of which I am speaking is not any conscious hostility of the mother towards the foetus, either because she does not want him, or feels him to be parasitising her. Nor is it shown in the classic irrepressible vomiting during pregnancy, an attitude of an uneasy body or an uneasy affective conscience, as these displays and affects, however negative they may appear to us,[2] are nonetheless proof not only that

---

1 Translator's note: One of Dolto's most often emphasised ideas is that of *allons-devenant* – translated as 'going-on-becoming.' Based on the Winnicottian concept of 'going-on-being,' Dolto's expression highlights constant development as a fundamental quality of being human.
2 Translator's note: Dolto had in her practice a woman who complained of vomiting during her early pregnancy, and her response to the patient was that this was not a bad thing, as it showed that

DOI: 10.4324/9781003312499-4

the libidinal symbolic link between mother and foetus is still present in mother's consciousness but that it is maintained in her unconscious and can mobilise feelings towards the child in her conscious affectivity.[3]

It is the continuity of this unconscious bond of desire between the foetus and his mother and vice versa that allows the child to live a healthy foetal life. It is not the same if, as I have suggested, the mother forgets that she is pregnant. In fact, this forgetting is impossible to any pregnant woman, even during sleep; for all women, such forgetting seems to go against nature. Such forgetting arises from a powerful psychological trauma in the gestating mother, which shakes the very meaning of her life; and to have an effect on the foetus such as we have seen, perhaps causes her even to forget her own existence and that of her husband or lover. These psychological traumas of pregnant mothers, who may completely forget them and then bring into the world babies psychotic from birth, can only be discovered through psychoanalytic work. These are very rare cases, or at least it is rare that the foetus does not die through abortion or premature birth with all its complications.

At birth

Something similar happens to babies whose mother suffers heavy post-natal haemorrhaging. It is a danger to babies who are born with placenta praevia and without a caesarean section, and who survive. For them, it is like an interruption in their symbolic link with their mother, and hers with them, broken for the hours during which she is in danger of dying, and the child is in intensive care. The rupture in the bond is experienced in an *après coup*. If later, their psychosocial difficulties bring them into psychoanalytic treatment, one discovers that these children live as if they had died at birth. It is the *cohesion of subject–body image–bodily schema* that could not be constituted, because going towards life was for them risking death. Something was also broken in the symbolic link between the mother and her newborn, arising from the replacement of joy at the moment of birth with anxiety about imminent death. In addition to the 'relational blankness' of the mother towards her baby, which may go as far as her not learning its sex before falling into a coma, there may be murderous fantasies on the part of the mother's lover, the genitor of the child, towards the newborn who is causing her mortal danger.

If the mother finally dies of complications of this dramatic birth, after a period of intimacy with the baby, this could have the effect of preventing the child from structuring himself in a cohesive primordial narcissism. The two shocks to the baby, one after another, of being born at the risk of dying followed by the death

the baby was very much in her unconscious mind, and that they were somehow learning to live together. Source: verbal report from Anne Marie Canu.

3 Let us not forget that negative or positive, affects in the libidinal sense are alive and therefore operational – dynamic.

of the mother, break the first humanising link, which will take a long time to be displaced and then reconstituted with others in the family, especially if it is one of them who takes over from the deceased mother. Very often in these cases, the family bereavement confers upon the child the guilt for having killed his mother. Of course, this is never actually said to the child, but the family's way of being with him, or looking at him, of thinking about him, and the saddened discourse around his cradle all create a depressive atmosphere that is felt by the newborn, who is always extremely sensitive to affects that concern him. He is like a murderer and incestuous at the same time – having unconsciously violated the two great taboos of humanity, which all children have to construct after weaning and after anal castration (which is, remember, the stage of autonomous mobility).

For the nursling whose mother dies prematurely by accident, while she is nursing and caring for him, what happens is that the mother takes away with her the breast to which, in the child's understanding, he is still attached: this mouth-breast is gone with her. And if she disappears without having verbalised to the child that he is to be cared for by someone else, then unbeknownst to all, she takes with her not only the breast but also the relating and language-orientated mouth of the baby, something of his nose, lips, bronchioles, tongue, hearing and sense of smell, which are in imagination attached to the vanished breast of the mother – her voice, her smell and her vital touch. The early death of a mother who has been totally caring for her baby removes the place of the bond in the body of the child, which mediated between the child and language and the human existence procured for him by this unique adult. He continues to exist as a mammal, but he has lost what animated him in a uniquely human way – his mother. What in him continues to eat is 'it';[4] but suckling no longer means the re-finding of the known and rediscovered pleasure of him-her, her-him. The narcissism of this nursling, girl or boy, is deeply wounded by this, cracked we may say, and very much weakened for the future. There are two levels of wounding:

1   The wound to the relationship between the subject and his body in itself, due to the fact of the amputation in the body image of the erogenous zone that is gone with the mother, and that was the sense of smell and the swallowing reflex. This body image can be returned to him if one can bring him either materially or subtly the odour of his mother that remains in her clothes. What then regains life is his body. It is his basal image, the body itself; it is the functional image, the possibility of suckling; while without the smell of his mother, he no longer knew, for example, how to suckle or swallow.

2   The other wound, the deepest trauma, is the loss of the relationship that already existed, sometimes very strongly, between the mind of the mother

---

4 Translator's note: The French translation of Freud's 'es' is closer to the German original: ça; this has been translated in English as the 'id' and this sentence could be translated as *what in him continues to eat is 'id.'*

and that of the nursling. This wound cannot be repaired or gotten over except by someone known to the child to be close his mother and father speaking true words to him about the ordeal that both he and his mother have undergone. Analytic work with babies precociously separated from their mother for whatever reason – death, illness or abandonment – show that over and above the hiatus of the erogenous body image there is a hiatus in the intersubjective relationship. Only speech can re-establish internal cohesion in the child, in a symbolic way; but if we want to help the child get over this trial, we cannot help him 'economise' his pain. It is astonishing and we don't know how, but children, babies and even nurslings understand words when they are spoken to communicate to them a truth that concerns them – words that recount what we know of the facts without value judgements.

When the baby survives the imminent symbolic death that threatened his erogenous zones to the depths of his existential desire to communicate, the most minimal residual consequence of these mutilating and traumatic events is speech delay and difficulties – the sticking to the palate of the tongue that renders the pronunciation of some or all phonemes impossible. There are cries that are just a continuous expulsion of sound or, on the contrary, a total absence of sonorisation by the symbolic death of the larynx as a place of pleasure taken in the active modulations of communication.[5]

The oral stage before the child walks and talks weaning and its failures

A generalisation that can be drawn from studying such early trauma is that the toxic aftermath always lies in the fact that weaning did not happen. *There has been no weaning*, that is to say a loss of the skin-to-skin contact that until then had been a constant feature of every feed – a separation experienced as painful for both sides and put into words, followed by the return of the mother who cuddles and talks about the weaning, but no longer offers the breast. The 'work' of weaning has not happened; there has been an abrupt and unexplained separation. Moreover, it is always relational difficulties with the mother, difficulties negotiated with her around the acquisition of walking and autonomy, that help the child develop his individual narcissism. Some traumas can happen during this stage

---

5 This partial symbolic death, which could probably be classified as precocious hysterical symptoms, should not be mixed up with the death drive of the individual as the nursling is not yet individualised and the subject – present from conception – cannot therefore invest his body with unified desire. His body is the constituent part of a mother–child dyad. In this particular case, what looks like the death drive of a desiring subject is that in losing the use of the larynx, the nursling saves the future individuation of the baby. This place of communication in sound with his mother is gone with her. Is it a displacement of the afterbirth onto the larynx, another aspect of what is left behind at birth, the placenta – a first step towards individuation?

(called anal castration), when for example the mother engages in strict sphincter training without allowing the displacement of excremental pleasure onto the pleasure of manipulating all the non-dangerous objects within reach of the child. Castrations have to be mediated – birth and the umbilical severance; weaning and being fed in another way than through bodily contact with mother; autonomy and the autonomous satisfaction of needs when the child acquires mobility; speech, minor incidents, complicity, joys and hurts – all these should happen slowly and not abruptly and not without any conflict or without words. It is the occurrences *without* conflict or speech that cause serious disorders of non-structuration of the child's personality.

In the extreme case where weaning results from the abandonment or death of the nursing mother and is what I would call a 'wild weaning' rather than a humanising weaning, what is left in the nursling as a desiring subject manifests itself in a behavioural regression due to the recurrence of pre-trauma fantasies. The archaic origins of what made up the prehensile image of the mouth and tongue involved in the communication of desires as much as needs may also reappear in a way that reverses the developmental possibilities of the bodily schema when linked with an unconscious body image in communication with the mother. The larynx and cavum can lose the vocalising abilities that the baby had previously acquired.

What happens then is a psychogenic mutism not caused by any damage to hearing, but we can also observe an apparent loss in recognition of familiar voices of those in the child's entourage; these children become not only mute but also psychogenically non-hearing. They no longer hear voices and speech, but they do hear the noises of life. He annuls what is said to him and removes from his attention the humans around him, while still able to receive whatever he needs to survive. The most archaic body image, the respiratory image, with which is linked cardio-vascular rhythms and the peace of sleep, can be altered by the emotional suffering born of the painful weakening of the mother–baby bond. We can explain the everyday respiratory illnesses of blocked windpipes and dripping noses as signs that the child needs to try to return to the prenatal image of a foetal body in which this region – cavum and respiratory tract – were as yet non-eroticised and bathed in amniotic fluid. Children said to be psychotic, mute, volatile, walled up by incommunicability or mental suffering rarely have any functional physical alteration. The subject that was at the origin of their incarnation from the moment of conception, and that survived birth, appears absent. But where is he? In any case, it does not, by the mediation of the body image, assume a bodily schema that lives on its own, an anonymous specimen of the species. When the subject disassociates from his body, it is this that I call the death instinct of the subject. This should not be confused with the desire to kill the body of another, or even oneself. It is only a sort of withdrawal of desire of the subject, who tends in reality to rest from the work of living with his body; it is as if he is reduced to a single focal point where the rhythms of organic life are maintained, preserving for a while the continuity of the subject who is 'on holiday' from his libido. We see this in children who sniff everything but who never do anything with the object they smell – they pick it up and simply drop again. They sniff the body, the feet of the people who approach them. We could say they are obsessively seeking an odour – maybe that of the genital tract of their mother, the archaic mother; perhaps that of their birth, in which they re-find themselves as subjects of desire, of inter-psychic communication. Sometimes, when one puts into words the hypothesis that they have elaborated about the meaning of their search, one can see – in an intense gaze that is addressed to the depths of your own eyes – that something true about their distress has awakened them for a moment to a human relationship that has no future.

Such abrupt and lasting *dissociations of the body image from the subject, without any possibility of repair, are frequently encountered in the aftermath of early hospital admissions and of successive changes of maternal objects before the age at which children can sit or start to be mobile*, that is to say before four months and again between four and nine or ten months. The child regresses to a state where his vital needs are satisfied by people around him with whom he no longer has subtle exchanges based on language, facial expression or motor responses. He becomes autistic. These drives, directed by desire, remain without issue and are symbolised pathologically in hallucinations of dangerous jaws somewhere in space. Is it his own mouth that he feels he has lost, and could it be his own cries that appear under the shape of terrifying hallucinated vocalisations – his own cries sent into space and that remain there as timeless hallucinations? The whole thing leads to a picture of major phobic symptomatology in the mute and psychotic child. The fantasy or the memory of his body held in the arms of his vanished mother manifests as a demand, an attempt at communication from mouth to breast, not linked with a cohesive unconscious image, a demand at first unrecognisable by the observer. This unconscious subject may still be linked with a pre-ego cut away from the mother, his 'you' seems to be reduced to something of the functional and erogenous image of a biting jaw, as may be his perpetual, silent and pleasureless rocking. Sometimes he self-harms, targeting in this case his arms, forearms or hands, which have remained the fetish of the maternal breast in his body, the only memories of the breastfeeding relationship linked with the mother's breast and the mothering arms that signified love. This self-devouring is seen in clinical work with psychotic children every time they experience an increase in the distress that gnaws at them (but where?), the distress of impossible lost communication and of the terrifying loneliness of those ill in the realm of language.

All phobias correspond to archaic part images that use drives that the subject does not now recognise as his own and that are projected into the external world. This defensive and extremely early phobic symptomatology gradually invades all the libido of the child, while using, translating and fixing in place the child's anxiety; and while phobic anxiety, if shared and understood by adults, can be a way of getting reassurance from the adults, the same anxiety when so precociously experienced cannot gain expression and be shared in a humanising way with another in the external world. Then the autism becomes worse day after day; it aims to curb the phobias and to prevent desire from attaching to objects but fails in this, because being alive is constantly accompanied by symbolic functioning in human beings and remaining with only his lonely images of intentionless part objects becomes increasingly terrifying.[6] The phobia becomes persecutory and the child falls into a serious psychotic state. The traumatic autism that we have just described can appear without it being possible to connect it clearly with an incident that happened in reality. It could be an early and sudden separation from the mother. It is nonetheless always the consequence of a symbolic trauma, added to a trial in reality or accompanying it. What the nursling suffers are trials associated with castrations that have remained non-symboligenic. The trials of the child are often concomitant with trials experienced by the nursing mother, who because of this pays little attention to her baby outside of urgent physical care – feeding, changing – but without words or cuddles, or fine attention to what is happening in the baby and that at some other time she would notice. Is it in fact an absence of structuration that provokes these partial mutilations of the body image? In cases of an early psychosis that is just beginning, the work of the psychoanalyst is to accept the death instincts into her person, by way of the transference, and to decode from them the perverted human ethos, compared with the first human ethos, which is the desire to communicate. In such cases, it is about having a careful, preventative attitude towards desire in the face of the anguish of all relationships in reality, as if the child subject rationalises by saying, 'If I go "no, no, no" to all present' (avoiding the possible danger of communication and therefore a second painful separation), 'I am not present, I won't be targeted, and I therefore risk nothing.' I say this, of course, to explain the child's apparent non-transfer onto its therapist. But as soon as the therapist understands the sharp intelligence of a psychotic child and his defensive strategy against suffering, he or she is able to talk to him about it without blaming him for the mask he wears – that of indifference, mutism and animal behaviours. This is how we help him to re-find himself as a human and the subject of his desire, and to accept afresh his wounded humanity into his bodily schema and to reconstruct through transference a body image that fits with this, as if breaking a spell.

The psychotic child is afflicted by a veritable tumour of symbolisation, we could say an imaginary tumour constructed by *a symbolising function that worked in a vacuum without any possibility of a relationship with another human being*, because the human targeted by the drives of the child was absent, or if physically present, was psychically out of reach for the child who was therefore all alone.

These phenomena are more or less what we see in what is called, following Spitz, hospitalism. This arises in children who experience many changes either of nurses or of institutions in the first 18 months of their lives, but especially in the first 6 months, which seem decisive. We can also speak of 'bourgeois hospitalism,' where the nursling is left by his parents in the charge of a string of mercenary women, themselves often frustrated in their own sexual lives, and who raise him like an animal or a plant, without speaking to him other than about what relates to

---

6 Desire obliges the subject to disguise his needs – as if they were the desire of an invisible other.

his needs, and without respect and liking for his parents and sometimes even with some hostility towards them, which he inherits.

For all these children who have suffered early chronic or cumulative trauma, the passive oral and anal drives are satisfied in a solitary way that must be described as invisible, imaginary and masturbatory – in a non-observable form that could be olfactory, optical (e.g. squinting), involving the lips, swallowing, the tongue or the rectum or urethra, the bodily parts eroticised during these early stages. This eroticism makes them use their own body-thing to evoke and elaborate fantasies of bodily contact with the absent mother in the solitude of the cot. Thumb-sucking, banal in most cases, can become an inveterate passion in some babies and is here certainly one of the least serious manifestations because it is compatible with later development towards a banal neurosis. Here, the imagination of the baby, supported by all the normal desires of his age, has as its only stable references the moments where the adult brings food or takes away his excrements, toilets him and manipulates his body as an object. This way of raising a child without shared joy and without words, which happens with some mothers, turns the child into an object and does not allow the subject of desire (and mostly his pre-ego of verbal language) to be constructed through an exchange of perceptions in a dialectic with the other. If this child develops solitarily until discovering the ability to grab, his necessary masturbatory activity, linked with thumb-sucking, fixes itself to an unnameable object that he keeps under his nose, sucking it, breathing it, his being in the world being totally absorbed by the sensations that this gives him.[7]

This unnameable object constitutes an archaic fetish of his relationship with his nursing mother who had been indispensable to his security, and for this child this fetish is a metaphor for 'him-his-mother,' promised to each other as interminable bodily contact in suckling. The child is thrust into the greatest anxiety by the occasional absence of this fetish, which is the only symbol of the subject in a relationship of continuity with his known environment and relates to the tutelary relationships of the mothering space. We know this anxiety of children who, when they go to bed, don't have their transitional object; but if the mother is present and comforts them, she allows them to regress with her and the more she talks of this object with them, the quicker they will get out of the regression that is a reaction to loss. What puts children in serious danger when they lose their fetish is when this object is the only remnant of their past: they have nothing else onto which the relationship with their mother can be transposed – no varied games, no songs, no words. While they had their fetish, they had some relationship with the world; once they lose it, they progressively enter into a secondary autism that

---

7 Winnicott has named this object the transitional object and has studied its security-giving function in the raising of children. It can be compared with jokers in a pack of cards, which are used to replace all the missing cards in a particular relation to the trump (here, the mother is the trump card for the baby). Translator's note: Dolto plays on the word *atout*, which means trump and adds in brackets, *ici la mere, 'la Tout'* ('the everything'), *pour son bébé*.

looks like a form of sleepwalking, without anybody realising it. The archaic oral drives cannot be transformed into anal and pre-genital drives in their relationship with their nurse or other people. The subject loses some component of his body image that connected desire with his body and reaches the point where he presents somatic disorders (mostly insomnia and digestive disorders) accompanied by distress. This state provokes in the parents fantasies that the childminder provided bad care that caused the child to fall ill. This child is admitted to hospital for observation, and you can see the chain reaction of children traumatised by the loss of the object that was there to replace the mother – the loss operates as if it was an early separation from the mother herself, as I described earlier. All these early disturbances of communication always cause sequalae, even if the child manages to overcome the ordeal. They always leave some abnormalities of language in the widest sense of the term. The bodily schema of his age has not been interwoven with the mediation needed for the elaboration of the corresponding body image, resulting in a psychomotor and language delay.

Then, what are the symbolic mediations needed? We have mentioned them: they are the auditory, tactile and visual data that comes from the mother in response to her baby, as she pays attention to the enjoyment and suffering of the baby and talks to him. Apart from the indispensable physical care – feeding and changing – that causes the mother to handle the baby's body, apart from the mother's bodily holding of the child, symbolic mediation consists of her words, her songs, her rocking, her cuddling, her telling off – all the language of the emotional intelligence of mothers, when neurosis has not blocked off the avenues of maternal intuition through the anxiety of being a woman.

From birth, every baby takes the woman he has turned into a mother back to the familiar source that springs from her own forgotten relationship with her own mother and father, from the depths of her early childhood, and that will now feed this new mother–child relationship, the old one overlaid by her current relationship as a lover to the man who may or may not be the genitor of the child. This baby, boy or girl, elicits in this mother, his nursing mother, speech that is from her heart, which awakens the smile and the heart of the child and awakens his mind to listening – in the same way that in deserting the womb of this woman's body he elicits the coming in of the milk, his milk, suited to him for the continuation of his development. This dialectic of body–heart–mind of the foetus, and then the nursling, with the mother is rooted in his physiology; but as everything is symbolic with human beings, he elaborates for himself an inter-relational psychic component of which this is a metaphor. Thus it is that the relationship of every human being with his mother – the source of his existence – appears enrooted in what for lack of other words we may call the sacred. This is about the evidence felt by every human being of an aesthetic and ethical experience of contact with nature and its beauty. This sacredness is for the child haloed by the light of the face leaning over him in the first hours of his life, in the first days of his trials.

Every mother is the model of pacifying mediation of needs and also, because of the link between desire and need, the source of confusion between the two. The child's reactional sensibility develops according to the emotional peculiarities of the mother's first sorrows and joys, intuitively grasped by the child in the forgotten first upsets and joys of his life that were centred on her; and this sensibility is umbilically joined with the dream of existing, of finding oneself and continuing, that was first induced by the mother, and that now becomes reality day after day, night after night.

People often say, 'this woman is not a good mother.' This is an absurd statement. No mother can be said to be good or bad. She is the mother, therefore it is in her that this human being effectively rooted himself, as he is not dead and has survived this so-called bad mother. That he suffered from it is another matter, but once again there is neither a good nor a bad mother; there are mothers who support more or less the child's narcissism in the overcoming of castrations that are for everyone the trials necessary for the construction of one's identity.

Even if we suffered and it was difficult, it is the first perceptions of our mother as we experienced her, and that for us she was life itself, that fed umbilically our dream of existing. This long dream of our early childhood is progressively reprised and reconsidered by reason throughout our development and is moored to flashes of technicolour memories of gaze, hearing, speech and events linked with the idea of a mother. This taste of 'sacredness' linked with the idea of mother is for everybody an agency that is both masculine and feminine. This could seem surprising as every mother is a woman. However, you just need to think of the constructions in which human beings honour Providence to see that they are crowned by shapes with phallic references, domes and cupulas referring to the breast, towers and spires referring to the penis. These are body shapes, sacred part objects of the bodies of our parents, perceived as giants. Our own active and passive drives are projected into the shapes of the procreative, magical adults – shapes that recall for us the living source of our being, one could say recall us to the coitus in which we were conceived, which links the permanency of self-consciousness with the living fruit of a sacred marriage – a permanent and fertile union between the sublimated active and passive sexual drives, from the most archaic to the most current. To say it in another way, every one of us is as a baby totally dependent upon the adult and can survive only if his thirst and hunger are appeased and we are protected from the dangers of the external world. These two conditions are met by the mother with her breast and by the father with his protective vigilance. As to the baby, he is alert for the vital breast and the protective force. The baby is in a totally passive libidinal position towards these two parental agencies that he experiences as active with regard to him. While he is necessarily passive in his body, in his heart, he lives an ardent, active love for these parental agents, with their double protective aspect in his eyes. These all-powerful masters of the space, these two phallic bodies, mobile like animated steles – he perceives them as endowed with palpating and stroking extensions that magically rule over a space in which he is totally impotent, subject to their goodwill and discretionary power. His fragile mind is moored safely to their faces, brightened by the shining stars of their eyes and the timbre of their voices talking to him – loving and helpful presences without which he would be lost, without bearings in time and space, to the indifference of the natural world and the elements that constitute his body. It is not surprising that having become adults, still impotent before the Creation, human beings build their houses of prayer with the shapes of phallic masculine and feminine beauty.

The mother is also the first credible source of information regarding dangers and the messenger of a love that once given by her cannot be taken back by her. Furthermore, she is the one who can give death. Man is not the representative of death in the unconscious; woman is, because she is the source of enjoyments that make the subject forget his body and the child his being. When he was starving, she appeased his hunger; when anxious, she comforted him, and he felt himself becoming her; but it is she the child has to renounce – girls as well as boys. She does not take back what she has given, but the child has to divest himself of her solicitude at a certain point in his development and refuse to give her the pleasure she wants from a certain point, which is, at the latest, that of the Oedipus complex. This is why I think that mothers can be the symbol of death as much as of life.

Maybe this is why psychotic children are afraid of their mother when they are reunited with her – because the one they re-find is not the archaic mother they were looking for, and their experience of her is not what they expected on reunification. Between the moment they were separated and the moment they are reunited, she is not the same. We have seen how a long, early separation from their mothers of certain children between the ages of 5 and 9 months can cause some of them to enter into an autistic state. They fear the renewal of their relationship with her as if she were the incarnation of death for them. For the subject, the continuation of the search for a lost archaic enjoyment makes of him a human being maladapted to his age, without language, without the complicity of the gaze, without a re-engagement in motor games from before the trauma.

On the contrary, sometimes the child moves ceaselessly and aimlessly – hyperactive, as people say. Sometimes the child is totally immobile, frozen, stupefied. He can only be distracted from his stereotyped behaviours by the tension of his excretory needs or the need to eat – anything. Playing with his faeces would be the only distraction that seems to have a certain meaning for him. In fact, he survives like the non-weaned child of a ghostly mother – death – who threatens him and whom he staves off by forgetting himself and by mimicking, as if he were becoming 'other,' the mother who when he was small appeased him. There is, in everybody, one of these archaic stages that have more or less stagnated for a long time, a leftover of the way of relating to the world and to the mother from before the narcissistic level of the Me–You and of spoken language, then of the Me–I.[8]

Some speech delays are in fact language delays due to the invalidation of the desire to communicate that unfortunately is only recognised from walking age onwards. I am asked: from what age can we talk about a speech delay? Well, from the beginning of life every child is in a speaking state; although himself unable

---

8 Is it not the consciousness of this in every one of us that is called a psychotic kernel?

to verbalise, he hears speech and is constantly in search of communication with the other, except when asleep. And he needs constantly to be surrounded by communication, proof that he is participating in the world; and even when he is asleep, speech does not bother him. The non-structuring or the destructuring of the oral and anal body images appear clinically in a way that is unmistakeable only when the child reaches the age where he can move as an individual; it is then that the social entourage alerts the parents, who had not noticed anything in a child whose habits had become that of a domestic animal who would no longer communicate even with his masters. Yet, it would have been easy to remedy his distress if the mother, the entourage or the paediatrician whom some worried mothers alert in vain ('you are worrying too much about him,' 'that will sort itself out once he goes to school') had been able to understand and detect the indifference that provides the first indication of the child's difficulties. The absence in the child of the smile, the gaze, of babbling, of calling out, of his seeking out mother and of constant communication with her, the silence of a 'well-behaved' child or on the contrary his stereotyped continuous crying – these are things an attentive observer can read as signs that the child is not in collaborative, flexible and truly relational communication with his mother.

This indifferent, passive baby that is sometimes called 'good' and placid, but who doesn't react to his mother and other familiar people, is without expression, doesn't grab playfully, who is apparently always satisfied, sleeping when mother puts him to sleep, eating whatever he is fed – this baby is nonetheless worrying, although not to many doctors so long as he gains weight, has normal stools and cuts his teeth . . . 'What more do you want?' they say to the mother. 'He is doing fine.' And this is how, quietly, psychosis or early neuroses are prepared in children who could very well have been helped if someone had noticed in time their suffering, their loss of communication and the lack of expression of their suffering. At the developmental age where the bodily schema should become the mediator for the body image between self and others, the dominant drives are only actively engaged in the satisfaction of the natural needs of these children. These drives give rise to desires that are non-verbalised and express themselves in the guise of an insatiable need to drink or to eat. He puts everything in his mouth – little objects, stones, excrements – everything with which he is presented. If anything, the only recognisable signs of a disturbance are those of sleep and of the digestive tube. 'He eats all kinds of rubbish,' it is said. There is vomiting and constipation but rarely diarrhoea. He is doing everything he can to preserve in himself a little of his secure space, acquired at little cost. But his dehumanised space that he engulfs and sometimes vomits doesn't speak and nourishes him neither psychically nor emotionally. Growing up, this pre-psychotic child acts out his desires in a compulsive way, going sometimes to extremes: for example in mad flights from home, losing himself or almost drowning himself in water – he cannot discriminate what is dangerous. He commits acts that are damaging and destructive, is dangerous to himself and to others. He attacks plants, flowers and small animals; in every case he makes his own acceptance within a group of children impossible

– which is what the mother had hoped would help him out of his difficulties. Alas, this is what is often noticed as a mark of 'maladaptation' that in the mind of the parents and of many doctors leads to a placement, that is to say, his segregation in an environment 'for children like this' – so-called specialised education that tries to at best adapt this Martian to the behaviour of earthlings of his time and apparent age, but it cannot promote this subject. To achieve this, he should remain with his family for the time needed for the parents to engage in psychoanalytic work that prepares the whole family to hand his education on to another holding environment. It is in a triangular situation – the psychoanalyst, the daddy-mummy (or alternatively one and then the other) and the child, if the child accepts it – that psychoanalytic psychotherapy can be established. The psychoanalytic psychotherapy of a psychotic child on his own, while the family exists, is useless. In cases where a child in a foster family is helped by psychotherapy to regain consciousness of himself, if the trauma of the separation from the parents is not spoken about in a piece of work between the child and his parents supported by the psychoanalyst, it will prevent the child from re-finding his subject self from before the trauma, and there will be an irremediable hole. This is why I insist a lot that no work with a psychotic child should start with him alone, a piece of work with the parents is needed first, and then with the child and his parents before thinking of any educational solution.

This is not about educating or even re-educating the child but about retrieving authenticity and distinguishing it from the mother's imaginary world that concerns the foetus and baby, and the father's imaginary world with regard to the child, and then of the child's imaginings vis-à-vis his parents, according to the events related by the adults and that the three of them have lived together. What is at stake for the mother is the residue of her own daughterhood, as I have shown in every case for mothering, and similarly for father, the residue of being a son to his mother or his father, depending on whether the psychotic child is a girl or a boy. Psychoanalytic work with a psychotic child means the rebooting of a communication circuit between the three characters – father, mother, child – of his primal scene. The parents are helped by the transference of the psychoanalyst onto their child; his way of working, his search for the interlocutor locked in the prison built by the child for himself, sometimes changes the stereotyped behaviours of the child before their own eyes. Seeing their child questioned by this other person, the psychoanalyst, who is truly interested in his life and personal story, the parents can see that a different kind of relationship is being established between the child and this adult. This rehabilitates in themselves the hope of a human relationship with their child – a hope that they lost day after day when faced with the seriousness of a state about which until then nobody understood a thing. It does not mean that today psychoanalysts understand more, and this is not what is important. What is important is that the child makes sense of it. In the psychoanalytic work, the parents, in thinking about what they themselves have suffered in life, can understand how this interferes in their relationship with the child and in the ordeal he constitutes, and the ordeal this is for other family members, especially siblings if he has any, which they had not realised up till now. At the very least, one of the advantages and fruits of the psychotherapy of a psychotic child – even if one does not manage to return to him his *joie de vivre* as a free, autonomous citizen – is that the other family members, his brothers and sisters, will not be marked for life by the trauma of the suffering endured by them because of this child.

For the psychotic child himself, the treatment begins to bear fruit around the rediscovery of the first relationship, that of a very small nursling with his parents. Difficulties arise from the panicky terror of living differently that the child has to experience in order to escape the anguish that is, in general, patched over. At the start of a psychoanalytic treatment, particularly when the treatment starts to take effect, what occurs are periods of aggression and dysregulation in the child's behaviour and in their visceral functions, which very often cause the treatment to be suspended because these disturbances are taken to be counter-indications to psychological treatment or for an organic illness. Hospital examinations ensue and the adults' cycle of anxiety starts again. Once again, the child is isolated instead of continuing the treatment despite the occasional perturbations of bodily functions, which the psychoanalyst should seek to understand with the child as being a language in reaction to his anxiety about getting better – an anxiety he communicates to his parents, his mother and his GP.

On the contrary, this dysregulation in somatic functioning with regard to the frozen stereotyped behaviours of the child's 'good health' before the psychoanalytic treatment is a sign favourable to the continuation of the treatment. It proves that the subject in this psychotic child is seeking to retrieve communication, but that before being able to express himself in affects, words, representations, drawings, models, acting and games, he begins by reacting with the language of the functional body, the unconscious pre-ego. It would be desirable therefore that lots of doctors be versed in psychoanalysis and that psychoanalysts also be child psychiatrists. What is needed are GPs and paediatricians who will take on the somatic medical treatment of these children while encouraging the parents and the child himself to continue the psychoanalysis despite the various dysfunctions by which he expresses his suffering. It cannot be the one who takes care of the child's body who does the psychotherapy, but it is possible that the one can support the other so that the child can continue this work, which is difficult but worthwhile, especially since psychotic children are generally intelligent, precocious and sensitive human beings behind their depersonalised mask.

At present, many children present this problematic of early maladaptation for which the diagnosis fluctuates between psychosis and neurosis. We could say that infantile psychosis occurs in families in which both parents suffered an unconscious traumatic episode in infancy due to their relationship with their own parents before the Oedipal stage. This episode, repressed in their minds, is expressed in their child in a way that cannot be noticed except by psychoanalysis. However, we can also see children described as psychotic according to their symptoms, whose state is only explained by very early disturbances in their own personal history, that have no resonance with the infantile trauma history of their parents.

Oral, anal and subsequent phases
before primary castration

Before I continue with some clinical examples and so that these have their fullest meaning as illustrations of my thesis, which is the link at every point between the body image and the bodily schema, it is necessary to summarise the main points about the regressive process or the minute steps in the destructuring of the body images, which is the inverse of their structuration. Let's not forget that the process whereby the body images develop depends upon an emotional relationship while the bodily schema can develop even in conditions of emotional distress.

Please excuse the abstract aridness of some of these clinical vignettes; they provide the necessary reference grid by which human pathology can be understood. Beware of coming too quickly to deterministic or even quasi-biological conclusions: it is in the language relation between the child subject and his entourage that the process of linkage between the body images and the bodily schema is revealed to be the defensive, narcissistic personalisation of the subject. Whether this is reversible or not depends on the transference of both patient and analyst over the course of a psychotherapy treatment. So, here are some generalities for a clinical understanding of pathology by way of body images.

Let's remember that the body image is tripartite – a basal image, a functional image and an image of erogenous zones – all of which are subject to fantasmatic sensorial representations that are communicable between subjects. Children reveal the existence of a dynamic image, either linked with this tripartite image, representable in drawings or models or dissociated from it, without representation except as a rough spiral or at best a dotted line: a dynamic image riveted to desire, which absorbs the potentiality for representation. This dynamic image, integrated with the subject when awake or in a light sleep reduces to a dot in deep sleep, leaving the bodily schema to enjoy, under the influence of the death drives and in the absence of all collaboration with the subject, the vegetative peace of the organs without representation or feelings of lack.

Nicholas

I remember Nicholas, a child said to be psychotic, who was nearly 6 years old when I saw him. He was three days old when Paris was evacuated. He remained without milk, without the possibility of being changed for more than two days, but fortunately, with his mother. Both were alone without food or water in a carriage deserted by everyone.

Nicholas was the last in a family of five children; the four older ones, girls and boys, had been lost for several weeks, separated from their mother, evacuated during the bombardment of the train that was taking them to meet their father, who had already been evacuated with the administration to the south of France. The mother and nursling should have been taken to hospital but found themselves unexpectedly taken to another town. On top of this, the train was very soon immobilised in the middle of the countryside, stopped by a bombardment of the line that prevented it from reaching its destination. There was nobody, and no cows or water, in the neighbouring farms – everyone had been evacuated and all pipelines blown up. This woman, separated from her four older children and anxious about them, remained there with her nursling but without milk, which despite having come in normally had stopped because of anxiety. She survived 48 dreadful hours completely exhausted and impotent, witnessing the death by starvation and thirst of her baby, whom she could not change. At last, things improved and she and her baby were saved. Nicholas had escaped death by dehydration and grew – this is what she was able to tell me about the child. When I saw him, he was more than 5 years old and psychotic, but he could be helped out of this condition by psychoanalysis. I cannot recount the unfolding of the treatment here, but when I think back on the history of the case, there was nothing pathological in either the mother or father's relationships with their own parents during their childhoods; the war caused no important bereavements or separations to the families; the four older children survived the trauma of evacuation and were quite well. For the duration of the war, the children and Nicholas in particular remained in the free zone in the countryside and suffered no deprivations. But he remained in appearance a wild child – indifferent but not avoiding the gaze. What was immediately noticeable about him – and I mention this as a clinical sign – was his mop of unruly hair. He had a raucous voice, he was anxious, moved aimlessly in all directions (like his hair) coming and going with elbows and knees bent, speechless, not nasty or ill intentioned but unpredictable. He did not really play, he 'did stuff' – moving objects here and there. He had to be watched constantly in case of accident or incident.

This was in 1946, when I had little experience. The only sign Nicholas gave that his appointments with me at the clinic mattered to him was that on those mornings, he was up at six o'clock, trying to dress himself and waiting for his mother near the door. One of the most curious things was to see, before anything else, the evolution of the child's hair. Among all his anomalies and behavioural oddities, his mother never thought to talk to me about this one, which had such immediate visual impact. The effects of treatment commenced by making his hair soft and tameable – to the surprise of his mother who then told me that at the same time, the child have developed a normal sleep rhythm that he had never had before; little by little he developed diurnal continence, then nocturnal, a vertical gait, pleasure in playing, the expression of affectionate feelings for his mother and finally speech – at first grammatically poor but appropriate to what was happening.

Any invalidation of a functional image, whatever the reason and nature, when the subject is animated by a desire, first of all stimulates the intensity of this desire. On the other hand, this invalidation, if not resolved, provokes the resurgence of a past body image, of a past where enjoyment linked with the satisfaction of tensions was known and in which narcissism remains invested. The subject can live on a fantasmatic archaic satisfaction for a certain time, during which the real functioning of his bodily schema in this way drains him of vitality.

The representation of real death, a representation of the body becoming an inanimate thing – archaic, like a poo object or a thing – stimulates all the current drives to focus on the re-finding of the functional image and of the erogenous image in search of an object that is always linked with the first lost object in sensorial reality, but not in the imaginary.[9] In the case of non-satisfaction, of the unsuitability to desire of any object, where the person as total object and also any part object linked with him is absent, the dynamic image after having vainly attempted an unsuccessful over-activation at the place of the current erogenous zone displaces itself onto an erogenous zone that corresponds with an earlier erogenous or functional body image. And where this regressive zone has itself lost all relation with its archaic object, or if it involves a functional image, which does not procure any pleasure, the dynamic image sets up a tension with the basal image that by definition is without an erogenous zone. Without an object of desire and without a representation in the body of the tension for this object, the subject is lost. As neither emotion nor consciousness can get hold of it, the malaise appears to be somatic – sleep disturbances such as narcolepsy, epileptic or absence seizures.

When the basal image is dissociated from functional or erogenous images, which cannot happen without some initial panic, we have the schema that Freud found in neuroses, to do with secondary narcissism, and which he explained in

---

9   This is well illustrated by the ending of Nicholas' treatment: after a few months of weekly sessions, the healing of his psychotic state announced itself in several sessions during which he appeared to act out his death. He would throw himself face down on the floor with more or less violence, stay there for a while and then do it again. I remember maybe at the last or one of the last sessions, the most elaborated of these fantasies: he would show on his own body, before falling, his thorax-abdomen around the navel, as if it contained a mass. Me: 'What is there?' Him: 'Stone.' Then, as if this weight made him lose his balance, he fell forward face down, stayed down for a moment, then crawled on all fours, then stood up again and repeated the process. 'Draw?' Hastily, Nicholas drew: 'House, window, a man' (he shows himself), an enormous black stain on the body. He drew a line indicating a movement: the body fallen from the window onto the ground. There, it became no longer head, trunk and arms, but a vague, small rectangle with three extensions – 'legs' – looking vaguely like a dog without head or tail on the ground surrounded by scribbles that more or less form closed shapes – 'leaves.' These leaves – 'What are they?' He showed me his face and hands, fragmented into 'leaves' around his 'defenestrated body.' 'Who is this?' Nicholas pointed to himself and said: '*Vis eux mord lo pas la, va las, fi, ni, ma l'a pu*' (untranslatable gibberish) – which could be written of the fallen, '*Vieux, mort, l'eau pas la, pas la, fini, moi y'a plus*' ('old, dead, no water there, not there, finished, me no longer'). Was this his initial trauma? This scene was not for me but I witnessed it. It was a sort of mime with sounds emitted with sustained passion, a kind of medieval Mystery play. The drawing executed at my request was not presented to me; it formed part of the trance-like performance of this child. As a young psychoanalyst, I was there, accepting but not understanding much. He would not say hello or goodbye. He would enter, impatient, tense, and would leave more and more happy to be back with his mother. 'It' healed. Nicholas' gait straightened; his head became free on his torso where at the start of treatment he would charge into the room like a wild boar. Very quickly, his sleep and his appetite improved, and then he gained diurnal and then nocturnal continence. He spoke better, with words linked grammatically. Nicholas had started to kiss his mother and father tenderly and to act in a coherent way. He began to be able to put subject, verb and complement in the right order.

Inhibitions, Symptoms and Anxiety. In the situations he described, he showed how symptoms of the genital phase come from pre-genital drives that can only be expressed by way of pre-genital body images. For example, the male subject, instead of being able to have sex, has diarrhoea; the woman, instead of having orgasms, has uterine cramps or nausea. The symptom becomes anal or oral, with either a tightening, like a sphincter contracting in vaginismus, or with vomiting, as with the rejection of a phallic part object, that becomes oral – food. Libido, refusing the genital body image, is displaced onto oral and anal body images that divert desire but fail even to give the pleasures of these regressive drives. What happens is linked with the genital zones of partners, but produces oral and anal phobic images. Let us note that all of this is easily interpretable in terms of the unconscious body image but is only valid for individuals who have, at least in principle, achieved the integration of their genitality into a relational image of their bodies, that is to say the mirror stage of which I spoke earlier.

However, when this applies to a child before primary castration, which is to say before he has the intelligence of a 3 year old or knows his or her sex, and still more if it applies to a child who cannot yet walk and whose bodily schema is still neurologically incomplete, if he has not at least the saving grace of sucking his thumb, then only the bodily places that link him with his mother can be the sites of the anxiety created by the frustrations of the appeasement of tensions; and this notably results in symptoms of dysregulation that could be called autonomous – of the digestive tube or the openings of the cavum, encopresia, enuresis, naso-pharyngitis and otitis. While the erogenous zones of the face, mouth, anus and buttocks – the homes of oral and anal drives – are no longer integrated by pleasure, neither in a language relation with the nursing mother (even when she is not there) nor with functional images (the functional oral image being the normal peristaltic movement from the mouth to the anus), nor of the corresponding basal image (the abdomen, stomach and intestines when at peace), there is a regression of the subject towards some disturbed cardio-respiratory and peristaltic images. There can be a call for an impossible return to the foetal mother in cases where the child cannot recognise his own odour, or a call in vain to a tactile and vocal mother, which provokes some asthmatic crises, cyanotic breath-holding spells or croup. Sometimes these anxieties and the events that trigger them pass unnoticed by the mother or on the contrary cause her to panic. Either because she is not attentive or because she is too anxious, she cannot nestle him, reassure him or cradle him – that is to say return him to the rhythms of foetal, then aerial and oral life of the first days by holding him in her arms, rocking him and talking to him reassuringly about what is happening. The child suffers and no longer has the security of the relationship of subject with the total object that is the mother by way of a part object specific to her such as her voice or smell. And so, the body image of this child lacks being signified, as the expressions of his sick body are not verbalised and he suffers in not eliciting compassionate speech and acts from his mother. The image becomes mute for him and he is reduced to a bodily schema battling against the death drives. This is what happens when the child stays in a hospital cubicle without frequent visits from mother to feed and change him, and if the hospital stay is prolonged, hospitalism may ensue – the hospitalism to which I have already alluded and that we will see shortly in the case of Sebastien. In children who escape dissociation between subject and body image, there are always serious disturbances of temperament that take a long time to disappear and to which there are always regressions.

Beyond these anxieties, reinforced by the silence of the mother or carer if she doesn't speak to the child of the traumatic events he has experienced or experiences, these early psychological traumas permanently or definitively alter the development of the body image, especially if the secondary reactive symptoms remain along with the non-recognition of the meaning of the somatic language taken by the mental distress. The prolongation of the child's stay in hospital may consummate the rupture of the mother–infant dyad that the latter tried to reconstitute fantasmatically through regressive symptoms. This is the origin of most cases in which children become psychotic through early traumas of their body image, in particular those who are traumatised in their basal image at the foetal or oral phase, and less seriously in the basal image of the anal phase (the basal image of the anal phase being cohesion of the head, torso and limbs).

This general picture is of capital importance for the understanding of what plays out in paediatrics, at nursery and in hospital. We remember mostly that the basal image is always linked, at the origin of the subject, with the foetal image before the first umbilical castration that follows birth, and that it returns us to the primal scene in which the child is conceived and to the original desire of this human being that his parents should want him as theirs, not only that they want his conception in the moment of their reciprocal desire as lovers but that they want his survival and accept his or her sex.

Sebastien, who became autistic at five months

To clarify the early effects of the difficulties regarding the body image that cause psychosis, let us bring in here the example of a 5-month-old nursling, Sebastien, whose parents had to move three times in one week. The parents, a young couple of whom he was then the only child, were waiting for permanent accommodation that was not ready. The child had been breastfed until four months and in the interval between four and five months, the mother weaned him. It went well and she planned to return to work to pay for the furnishing of their new home. She had looked for a nanny who would look after the child in their home. As she had to change accommodation twice in a few days and as their current accommodation had been loaned to them and was therefore temporary, she had to change the childminder as the flats were in neighbourhoods distant to each other. In a few days, the child had two different homes and two different carers. To spare the child a third change of scene, mother decided to find a childminder who could look after the baby at her own place until they were able to move to their permanent home. Neither mother, child nor father knew the new childminder until the day the child was dropped at her house in the morning as mother had restarted her job. When mother came to pick up her baby in the evening, the nanny told her, 'Your child is at the hospital, he had green diarrhoea at eleven. I had a baby who died of this before, so I took him immediately to the hospital.' Naturally, the hospital admitted the baby as an emergency; however, when the mother arrived, she was told, 'We have not seen any diarrhoea but do leave him here for observation.'

This is how I received the maternal testimony about the beginning of the mother–child separation. I came to know this case when Sebastien was already 7 or 8 years old and was a mute schizophrenic. He would never sit down, as if that caused him suffering. He lived standing up or lying down. Mother told me about what she called his constipation, which went back to what the doctor at the first hospital had said when Sebastien was discharged. She referred often to the word 'constipation' but, she said, the various doctors involved with Sebastien had not been interested in this. Give him suppositories, one of them said; give him some other medication, said another. In fact, this child was terrified of having to defecate. Around every fortnight, howling with pain, he would expel an enormous stool that according to his mother did not to appear to relieve him. The doctor to whom I advised the mother to take the child diagnosed an anal fissure that he treated, and having gauged how dangerous a hospital admission would be for this child undertook at his office under general anaesthetic, with the mother present, the extraction of a faecaloma the size of the head of a baby. He had to cancel all his patients that day as the smell of putrefaction in the clinic was unbearable. This child had borne this faecal putrefaction, this faecal foreign body, for more than four years. From time to time, he had an enormous 'big poo,' screaming of pain. The mother was telling doctors, 'He's constipated, that's all.' Sebastien refused any food likely to cause constipation, such as the chocolate that his mother and grandmother thought was good for him (why?). The chocolate that Sebastien refused was a cause for conflict between these two women. From the moment that his peristaltic movements were re-established, first by the medical intervention and then by the treatment with me, who was verbalising what happened in the presence of his mother, Sebastien became able to sit and to enjoy eating a varied diet. This doesn't mean, unfortunately, that he was cured of his psychosis, but already his life was more pleasant and he was less anxious.

Let's go back to the development of the psychosis. At 5 months of age, the alert baby was without explanation put in the care of a childminder he didn't know, and felt himself to be rejected and placed with three different unknown women successively in one week; it is without doubt secondarily to this that Sebastien became dysregulated in his digestive peristaltic image. The third of the childminders had once before taken care of a baby who died of toxicosis that began with diarrhoea in her home. On her first day with Sebastien, she took charge of him at eight o'clock in the morning and by eleven was horrified that he had diarrhoea. She took him to hospital and left him under observation in a cubicle. This is where the mother, shocked by the childminder's report, found him that evening, without being allowed to enter his cubicle or speak to him. In a few days, Sebastien regressed profoundly and also contracted bronchial pneumonia in hospital. The paediatrician said to mother, 'I have not seen any diarrhoea, he seems more constipated. He is fine but we'll keep him in for a few days as a precautionary measure.' This suited the mother, as they had not yet been given the promised accommodation. It was of course a trial for her to be separated from her 5-month-old child, but she had her work and was told that the baby would be as well in hospital as with an unknown childminder. And also, she had no idea what was happening to the child; it was only when speaking of this period that she remembered the distress of the baby in the cubicle. Behind the glass, he became unrecognisable in a few days. Then he had had bronchial pneumonia. Where did that come from? From a respiratory image that lacked the odour and the presence of the mother. He looked for her, and at the start when he saw her behind the glass window of the cubicle, he screamed; but after three or four days, he became indifferent. His pulmonary respiratory image was deprived of the smell of his mother, who had deserted his olfactory erogenous zone. His eyes and ears no longer perceived his mother, and abandoned by the desiring subject, the functional respiratory image became prey to the death drives. There are always microbes in the environment that, being living creatures, ask for nothing more than to swarm over a body whose circulatory functioning is not excellent. The bodily schema is badly ventilated when the child's oral and olfactory body image suffers from not being able to re-find the smell of the beloved mother. In terms of the peristaltic image, as this is about constipation, the functional image of the digestive tube regulates the pathway of the alimentary contents according to the bodily schema of the digestive tube; this functional image became frozen, as the doctor said, 'about this diarrhoea – your baby is showing constipation, but that's okay. Give him suppositories and then take him home, he is getting fed up' – this is what was said as soon as the bronchial pneumonia was better. But no, he wasn't taken home as the apartment wasn't yet ready. And this is how this 5-month-old baby, superb on arrival, came to stay in hospital for six weeks. The precociously laughing baby, able to recognise his mother, father and grandparents, became a sad, apathetic and lost child, no longer gazing at or playing with anything. When the mother, having begun to settle into her new apartment, came to pick him up thinking that everything would be fine afterwards, Sebastien did not get better and shortly afterwards showed increasing signs of autism. How could he re-find himself, in a new apartment in which his parents had prepared for him a child's bed, which they thought very fine, but which was not his cot (the part object linked with the 'him-mother' he had known before five months)? The mother who had temporarily stopped working as much in order to set up her home as to look after him expected nothing of him and he, nothing of her. She was very busy and he was, as she said, very good. If we wish to generalise from such a dramatic but alas not exceptional example, we could say that the symbolic functioning of the child who was not spoken to in such a way that he could recognise himself as a subject was disturbed – a disturbance that worked a mortifying and de-creative effect upon the body images, progressing from the current to the earliest that were embodied by their interweaving with the bodily schema, and so created physiological disorders.

Alas, all physiological disorders appear to adults as illness exclusively in the domain of the body, causing anxiety, not wrongly, to the parents and doctor. The dialectic of the tripartite body images closes in on the child's narcissism, and being a subject who expresses his feelings and his love for his mother in pre-verbal language that is neither understood nor recognised, he regresses. The desire for subtle subject-to-subject communication is repressed on the side of the child and then becomes impossible because of some functional disturbance that is not recognised as a language. The adult's anxiety focuses on the somatic disturbance of the child, who thus becomes represented only as a body-object. Thenceforth, all that the child's entourage seems to recognise of him is anxiety and his body, and recognised as such, the subject no longer exists in what he tries to say. People speak of his symptoms, but alas no longer to him.

In the new apartment, Sebastien's mother no longer spoke to him, as she recalls. She spoke to him a lot during the first four months when she was breastfeeding him and also during the month she weaned him, when they were still together and she was anxious about returning to work. Then she became preoccupied by various difficulties, then he became ill and she could see him only through glass in his cubicle. He became inert and indifferent and she no longer spoke to him or of him. She spoke of Sebastien to others as 'the little one' but he no longer was 'Sebastien.' She looked at him with sad, anxious eyes. After those catastrophic days of successive changes of accommodation, childminders and finally his isolation in a cubicle, a hospital admission for observation deemed by the doctors to be a temporary convenience for the struggling parents, was completely mortifying for the parent–child relationship and therefore for Sebastien himself – quite unknown to everyone. Sebastien was 5 months old, just weaned and at the most fragile age for the beginning of autism, when separated from his mother and, in this case, not just from his mother but also from the safe space he had known with both his parents. This change in the lifestyle of a baby who up until then had been completely grafted onto one person, at the very moment where weaning has been accomplished, requires enormous care and mediation. Every change in location and habit must be explained and spoken about to the child. He understands; he suffers, but it doesn't drive him mad. We know now that it is important to tell him; maybe among those who read this observation will be paediatricians who will remember and be able to warn of potential disturbances, while telling the baby that things are going to change for him, explaining the reasons why his parents are anxious and that they have to leave him temporarily with other people.

The symptom as equivalent to language aimed at parents

The symptom becomes a means of expression by anxiogenic dysfunction aimed at the parents, and this is also what happens in cases of regurgitation where the baby vomits onto mother the milk he has swallowed without having digested it.

In every case I have been able to see, the mother–baby relationship is disturbed because she leaves him the moment she has given him the bottle or even while she is feeding him, while the precocious, intelligent child desires a face-to-face conversational exchange. He wants a collaborative, emotional, animated interpersonal relationship after having dined. This is usually seen in girls, rarely in boys. The early vomitings of nursling boys, characteristically projectile, we know to be due to the slight malformation of the pyloric sphincter, which is easily treatable. But it is not merycism, by which I mean vomiting with no biological cause. In cases of merycism, one usually finds a precociously intelligent girl whose mother seems less bright, shall we say, than her child, and generally depressed after the birth. She doesn't speak to the baby and is concerned mostly about timings and doses, about weight and duration of sleep; she is not attentive to the displays of this little human and does not establish a cheerful relationship of partnership with her baby. Every time the baby calls out, she interprets it as being for food or a change. But when she changes her, the baby doesn't see her face in the same way as she does when she gives her her feed, so that the nursling understands that the only inter-psychic relationship occurs by way of feeding. And so she brings the feed back up so that at least the exchange lasts longer and she remains present thanks to this subterfuge. What begins as a mistake in channelling, a kind of points failure, becomes established in a chronic fashion. Instead of the sounds that come from the functional pulmonary image with air passing through the larynx, the nursling mistakes the functioning of the larynx in a sound bodily schema for the neighbouring pharynx, which should only function in one direction; and even more as her mother neither sings nor speaks to her. The milk that has arrived in the stomach serves therefore as a part object of a need to bring it back up the pharynx, while in reality what is desired is the prolongation of the soft and caressing sounds and reassuring presence of the mother. It is to be held in her arms that is needed at this moment and throwing up the milk is a clumsy way of trying to convey this.

Instead of eliciting the cajoling and speech of the mother, this constant regurgitation causes the mother and then the doctor anxiety. She no longer dares to pick up or move her child, and is advised to put her in hospital for observation. She feels guilty about the separation, which only aggravates the disturbance of the child's relationship with the mother. There is an over-valuation of the vomiting mouth that becomes a crying one, because of the buccal functioning when there is no longer anything to swallow or bring up. It is a subject making claims in vain for the face, now definitively lost, of the mother who welcomed her at birth. The child now both vomits and screams. To the enormous square opening of the gaping mouth, noisy (at the age of 3) but unspeaking, all part objects are good – poo, soil, every unnameable thing associated with the mother who calls her nothing but 'the little one.' Soon, everything that can be stuffed down and vomited begins to replace the mother–child relationship, which has nothing more to teach her. The mother is repetitive and stereotyped in her narcissism as an exasperated martyr. 'The little one' eats any old rubbish, putting everything in her mouth. The mother laments and shouts after her. These merycisms sometimes last two or three years, where the child eats and vomits everything, and yet gains weight and grows; but these are in fact serious neuroses, we could say experimental neuroses, caused by the fact that a request by the subject of her subject mother has not been recognised, a request for speech, for psychic and emotional communication. This request is therefore expressed by the only language the child has to hand, which is the vomiting of undigested milk as soon as the feed is finished, so that the perfusing relationship of mother and baby continues; perhaps as the displacement of the perfusion of the umbilical cord.

Every time there is merycism between a baby and her mother, as in the anorexia of nurslings, the treatment should be the care of the mother not by a psychologist but a psychoanalyst with the baby present in the mother's arms and recognised as a participant as much as the mother. Instead of this, a doctor, worried by the mother's anxiety, becomes embroiled in an infernal cycle of biological treatments, observations, tranquilisers and in the negation of the subject (the child and her desire), so that she is only cared for as a body-object. The body becomes the only thing spoken about, for lack of knowing how to speak to the infant, addressing her by her first name where necessary, and for lack of knowing that a nursling is already a subject, some more precocious than others in showing this, but always receptive of true speech addressed to them about their personal history and their search to be understood. One also has to listen sensitively enough to children and babies, as the following example shows.

What talking about one's pain can mean

Pierre

Pierre is a 3-year-old boy brought to me after quite a journey through the neurology department, because he complained about headaches in the months that followed his admission to nursery. At our first appointment, I met a completely stupid child with a sad face and eyes half drowned under their lids, and who repeated monotonously, 'I have a headache,' without touching it. In general, a 3-year-old child says while touching it, 'My head hurts,' rather than 'I have a headache.'

Wondering about his way of speaking, I asked in turn, 'Where does your head ache? Show me where it hurts.' Pierre pointed to his groin, near his crotch or his pubis, maybe his penis, saying, 'There.'

> **Me:** 'It hurts you there? In whose head?'
> **Him:** 'Mum's head.'

All this in front of stupefied parents. I then asked the mother, 'Do you sometimes have headaches, Madam?'

> **Mum:** 'Oh yes, I have catamenial migraines. This happens every time
> I have my period, ever since I was young. I have to stay at home for two

days. I have been a secretary in a company that took me on seven years before Pierre's birth so they let me stop work for two days a month as they know I can catch up later.'

Me: 'When did your son's headaches begin?'

Mum: 'He had just started going to nursery, he was very happy about it and one morning his father took him to nursery as I was not feeling well and my son was brought home by a nursery assistant with a note from the teacher saying, your son is ill, he says his head hurts. Fortunately, I was at home because of my period and my headache.'

Thanks to her headache, the mother was not at work. He knew that her return to the work that she had stopped at his birth was because he was now going to nursery. Work for mum, school for him, this was something they had agreed a long time ago and Pierre was a very clever boy. But that day, he understood. After three years together, he knew her well. It was the day of her period; she smelled like it. She would not go to work. So why should he go to school? He wanted to be with her as she was staying at home. He said these words, rather these phonemes, which for him had a magical effect, that of making mum stay at home. Why not him as well? 'I have a headache.' There you have it – these phonemes, this form of words had been taken for the expression of a pain in his head. He had been taken to hospital, kept for observation, and as nothing organic was found after all possible somatic examinations, he had been sent to a psychoanalyst. The head, where? There, at his genitals. Whose head? Mum's head. Which head is there? Doubtless the cut head, as there was blood there, which this clever child could not fail to observe when near his mother in bed for the two days of her period.

This little story shows us that *listening to a child is important but on the condition that one understands what talking means at the age he is at*. This depends on the body image, which is a language that only becomes one in the name of the child after the acquisition of complete autonomy and mostly after Oedipal castration. At this point, for the child who has negotiated the trial, 'his' word represents what 'he' experiences. He cannot always find the right words, but he is now putting his own words to his feelings, rather than those that worked like passwords or had some magical effect on others.

The cohesion of the three components of the body image, linked together by the dynamic image, is synonymous of security. On the contrary, their dissociation can allow the death drives to preponderate over the life drives. It is the red alert for the narcissistic integrity of the ego or pre-ego.[10]

---

10 Let us remember that the pre-ego designates the consciousness of the subject in his bodily schema and in his body image before primary castration (the not yet consciously sexuated but already erogenous body image because of local erectability; the bodily schema perceived as erogenous in connection with desired objects – erectile penis for the little boy, erectile clitoris and vagina for the little girl).

There is a risk of organic pathology when the dissociation is such that there is no reference to the history of the subject; then, the death drives start to prevail – something that at least supports the autonomous life of the body. When a child's bodily needs are well looked after but do not relate to his acts, his desires and pleasures, his relationship with his parents, his sex, his future and his history, it is as if his only value is in his body. When the body of a child and his needs are well looked after but his particular desires, pleasures, actions and sex are not considered in the context of his relationship with his father and mother, his future and his history since birth, it is as if his only value was organic. If it is only because of his body and its needs that he is looked after, he is induced to 'pretend,' to play the role he has been given, to be only an object. For example, he is seized by imperious needs or something concrete is missing or he needs to suffer in order to be looked after or to be given anything. What he says is stereotyped, always about sweets, a toy, a wee or a poo. In certain mother–child relationships, it is earache, tummy pain or any other pathology that brings attention. Then, only the bodily schema supports the child in a form of narcissism of metabolic exchanges. In his emotional isolation, if a real pain occurs, it can return to him the illusion that he exists as a subject, make him pay attention to this different perception, which is the only one he perceives. His primordial narcissism dissociates itself from the state of sensorial ease and becomes linked with a pathological state; this pain becomes company for lack of any person close to him. *The physiological malaise can thus become the specific signifier of the imaginary relational status of the subject with any other,*[11] *for lack of real others.* Through his imagination, a part of his body is like another person and they look after each other, him looking after his malaise and his malaise looking after him, wedding him to this part of his body.[12] This is the way one should understand the symbolic foundation of hypochondria, which is a neurosis bordering on narcissistic psychosis, quite different from hysteria – the hysteric has no other aim than to manipulate another person, while the hypochondriac manipulates oneself. When he has money and sees many doctors, he renders them impotent in healing him but does not even enjoy this. They are the witnesses of his interminable colloquium with the illness in his body, which is impossible to heal, for good reason. They have some similarity with certain neurotic and psychosomatic patients for whom healing should not take place completely – they need only some relief; healing would symbolise a narcissistic loss that threatens like death. They are excessively alone. This chronic feebleness, not very serious from a medical point of view and that does not threaten the life of the patient, spoils their existence and relationships but is necessary to them. It is a

11 Any others? Voices? Smells? Anthropomorphised tactile images that cause phobias in babies without the babies being able to speak of them? Also, gods and demons. In a 'reasonable' adult, one can spot the existence of this unresolved period of primordial narcissism supported by a psychosomatic chronic pain: 'It is again my liver playing up.' The liver is the 'other' to oneself.
12 See the case of Tony, p. 236.

way of loving themselves where they are at once mother and child (isn't that the theme of the song 'the pleasure of love lasts only a moment, suffering from love lasts a lifetime'?). It is a love that keeps you busy.

To say that *the body image is the symbolic incarnation of the subject* signifies that only symbolised emotions are inscribed in it, that is to say those that have the meaning of a language of interhuman communication, in any case those who have acquired this meaning for the subject. The symbolisation in question here is in fact pre-symbolisation. Symbolisation as such does not happen except with Oedipal castration and the accession to the symbolic order of the law, the same for everyone without prerogatives and exemptions for certain subjects over others. Indeed, it is only after Oedipal castration that the subject can say 'I' in his own name – 'I, son or daughter of X' – the name that signifies their kinship and justifies the interdiction of incest. He knows himself as an individual, born of his parents but different from the father and mother of whom he is the issue and connected by them to two families of origin. He accesses social responsibility for himself under the name given to him by his parents and his surname received from them but also regulating their parenthood according to the law of the country of which they are citizens. *As to the foreclosure of the name-of-the-father*,[13] a Lacanian concept, I think this develops very early in the child, much before Oedipal castration, at the beginning of primary castration, but I have not specifically studied the elaboration of this pathogenic absence of pre-symbolisation for the psychic economy. The foreclosure of the name-of-the-father produces a psychotic enclave, but this enclave is the guarantor of the narcissistic conservation of the subject and mostly of an oral ethos, itself guaranteeing the conservation and cohesion of the first body images, respiratory and digestive.

Pathology of the body image when only weaning has failed

Weaning has failed if it does not lead the child to a communicative relationship with his mother that is richer than the one he had at the breast; and not only with the mother who is present but also with an imaginary mother when she is absent – a mother with whom he is in constant conversation by way of his babblings during play, and in his attempts to put phonemes to all his observations and tactile sensations, as if he were in permanent conference with her.

Let's say it again: the effects of a badly symbolised weaning can cause the child terrors of being devoured, traces of which are found in many children. In the dark, they imagine wolves or crocodiles that could devour them, as if the oral erogenous zone that has not been adequately symbolised can roam in space and seize them – them as objects of their desire. This pathology of weaning develops because of

---

13 In my opinion, this foreclosure is correlated with a non-formulated absence, a negation or dereliction of the filial link with one's own biological father, which coexists with the narcissism of at least one parent of the psychotic subject.

maternal mistakes in the course of weaning, because of the lack of words spoken by the mother to the child to explain the reason for weaning; perhaps also because of the mother's suffering in depriving herself of the pleasure of being suckled by her baby. Another weaning situation that does not allow the symbolisation of forbidden drives, those of cannibalism towards the mother after weaning, occurs when there is a sudden movement of the breastfed child to a different space that separates him from mother for the duration of several feeds and changes, with mother being replaced by another carer. This may happen when a mother withdraws the child from the breast and puts him in a crèche or with a nanny the very same day, and the baby is not able to preserve the acquired body image in its integrity. He experiences the acquired body image as having been amputated, at least in part from his image of his erogenous zone, together with some of the functional image of the cavum (the images of smell, hearing, taste and oral tactility), which have disappeared along with mother. For the oral erogenous zone to remain alive beyond this bereavement of the breast part object, the child has to retain a sensory relationship with his mother, so that the total object of mother remains present, returning at sufficiently frequent intervals, and so that the breast from which he has been weaned remains in his memory. For this to happen, the mother must look after the baby at least as much as she did before weaning. Instead of by suckling and touching the breast, the child must continue to build the oral zone of his body image by discovering all kinds of other tactile sensations, tastes and smells of alimentary functioning in the known environment of his relationship with his mother, who comes and goes, talks to him and cajoles him, and he must be awakened to all the new alimentary perceptions along a familiar continuum of smells, voice, gaze and rhythms of manipulations that are specifically hers.

Moving to another person, another voice, at the same time as the loss of the breast and toileting care by the mother, even more so if this happens in a different space to the one in which the child has lived for months with his mother, may be enough to cause trauma – a rupture in the body image – that primes the start of psychosis in a sensitive and intelligent child.[14] As an effect of a failed weaning, there may also be a long-term discontinuity in the body image with regard to the relationship between the mouth (tongue and palate) and of the larynx and pharynx; the larynx becomes the heir, by contiguity of the bodily schema, of the deprivation of the pharynx of the swallowing of breast milk and of the breathing of its scent. Because of the absence of an image of pleasure, the larynx may disinvest pleasure in the sounding of phonemes – the child still cries but no longer babbles when alone in his cradle or in his mother's arms. Later, this provokes disturbances such as stammering, language delay or inaptitude in learning to speak, caused by the suspension of the images of the region at the same time functional and erogenous – a suspension that went unnoticed for the weeks after the badly achieved weaning, meaning sudden and non-mediated by loving speech that came in the place of the

---

14 See the case of Sebastien, p. 157.

body-to-body contact and above all, let's repeat, when the weaning happens at the same time that mother and the familiar space become absent. I take this as an opportunity to make a suggestion about stammering, which I think comes from the sudden destructuration of a taboo dating back to the oral phase, after a weaning without apparent problems in which sublimation consists in the appetite for all other nourishment than that coming from the maternal breast, and the elaboration of a new unconscious ethos built on the taboo of cannibalism. This taboo is connected to phallic drives; stuttering as a symptom expresses the disarray of the child weakened in his phallic pride by an image or a real experience, which collides with the impossibility of regressing to an active image of oral devouring not only of the breast but of the total object of the mother-subject, a living physical substratum.

To explain this better, I will cite the case of a young man whom I saw when he was 18 years old; let's call him Joel. His stammer began when he was 3 years old. He was in a tearoom with his mother and aunt – his father's sister. The women met there every week with him present. That day, the two of them were making fun of the faults of the boy's father – their husband and brother – as apparently they always did. Suddenly, Joel disappeared under the table, having slipped off his chair. He had lost muscle tone in his bodily schema, by an undermining of his phallic body image. From sitting on his chair while eating, he moved under the table without anybody understanding why. He was picked up, put back on his chair and, obviously, told off. He apparently looked puzzled. All this was recalled later, by his mother, when in his analysis, Joel remembered that scene in the tearoom and talked about it to her – she confirmed that his memory was correct. This was the first occasion on which he stammered, a stammer that never ceased afterwards, linked with the chocolate cake that Joel was eating while the two women were doubled up laughing at his father. This was a screen memory representing both the devaluation of the father and the stammering of the son. One can say that Joel had over-invested the phallus as the engine of verticality in the body image to the point that he could not keep his sitting posture and he lost the mastery of phonation, the sublimation of oral phallism as compatible with a future as a boy. It must be said that chocolate is by analogy of colour an image of excrement. There was a nullification of the possibility of urethral and anal-phallic transference onto the speech he had acquired and on the rhythm of his air column. Joel displayed a particular kind of stammer: instead of emitting sounds, he spoke as much on inhaling as on exhaling. He inhaled the air column at the moment where he wanted to pronounce phonemes, and he inflated so greatly his thorax with air that he could no longer sustain breathing. The air he had thus inhaled on stammering came out as disconnected from the rhythm of the speech that he tried to link with an exhalation that was at the same time windy and sonorous. Since childhood, no re-education could help him and God knows he tried many (he neither stammered when reading in a very low voice nor when reciting poetry by heart). The psychoanalytic treatment, in retracing his libidinal history, completely relieved him of his disturbance in phonation, after freeing his pre-3-year-old body image.

Besides the various languages disorders, the phobic neuroses also originate in the failures of castration of the oral stage, which include the new ethos of the taboo of cannibalism (the repression of biting), as I have already suggested at length. A common palliative of this phobic neurosis is found by many children in a transitional object, a true tactile and odorous fetish, associated with the sucking of one or two fingers. This fetish is meant to support passive drives as much as active ones, the satisfaction of which have been interrupted by losses due to the absence of the mother without enough of the mediating effects of speech on her part. This loss, for many, comes to affect the vocal, auditory or emotional interest in verbal language, which has been insufficiently invested as the replacement of bodily contact, a replacement that plays in the relationship of the child with his mother and then father. After weaning, the father, especially with boys, is the prototype of the total object that supports the development of the unconscious body image, and for girls as much as for boys, narcissism is supported by the relationship with father as much as with mother; sometimes, the image that serves as the ego-ideal involves a superimposition, a two-headed entity – the mummy-daddy or the daddy-mummy.[15]

Once cathected, the transitional object cannot leave the child without him experiencing an anxious panic. It expresses the child's desire to retain a tactile sensation of the breast at his mouth. Unfortunately, it is a breast deserted by speech and meaningful language. If he loses this object, it is as if he loses definitively not only his mouth and his tongue but also a part of his ego-ideal, which for him is linked with the fully complete body image. Thus, he also loses his cohesive certainty of being linked with the basal image of the unconscious body image (at the time of weaning – five to seven months – it is the abdomen and the respiratory and cardiovascular thorax), an autonomously assured certainty of being alive.

Pathology of body images that remained healthy after weaning at the anal stage and the child's individuation through mobility: pathology of anal castration

The period of learning to walk and of acquiring physical autonomy in space could be at the origin of the destruction of a body image that was healthy until then. The difficulty of structuration occurs in the context of a good relationship between the breastfed child and the mother, the child having in every way evolved without difficulties until 18 months. By 'healthy body image' I mean a body image that allows interhuman communication, the playful and utilitarian manipulation of objects linked with a certain intentionality, which creates a partnership in all things between the child and people in the family that is creative and fecund with regard to the child's developmental stage. A body image that allows the child to develop 'going-on-becoming within the potential of his sex,' with a well-established narcissism, in his own community.

---

15 See 'Mots et fantasmes' in Au jeu du desir, op. cit.

The destructuration in question happens in a child whose experiences, discoveries and wish for more active experiences, while appropriate for his stage of mobility, are not marked out by supporting words that advise caution and explain how to do new things so as to avoid major accidents. Before being able to walk, the child because of his auditory and visual attention was already taking part through a fantasmatic identification in what he was watching, in all the activities of adults and older children he saw moving around. It could be said that he was having experiences by proxy. It was an anticipating of his near future. As soon as he walks, he is obliged to reduce the body image that he had fantasised as the omnipotent image of grownups to the size of what is achievable for his little person, which has just managed to stay vertical and to become autonomous through walking, and this is accomplished through difficulties, failures and sometimes accidents causing physical pain. He needs to reduce this image to the reality of the experiences possible for his bodily schema as a child still not fully in control of his pelvic girdle and lower limbs, because of the late completion of the development of the spinal cord in human beings (at 28 to 30 months) – a time frame responsible for the lack of motor coordination of the human young and for their excremental incontinence.

The experience of reality

The child discovers through experience, sometimes painful, the limits of the safe space that surrounds him – a space defined by the fact that he can move in it without too many risks – and the determinants of a temporality that is not only punctuated by the appearance and disappearances of his mother. Now, because of his ability to move himself and objects, he can himself modify the appearance of his surroundings and seek or escape the presence of his mother. The acquisition of this new power, which leads to autonomy, is a difficult time for the child and also for mothers, especially if they are anxious, and for many fathers who are sometimes even more anxious than mothers. From the time he stands and learns to walk (from between 12 and 15 until 30 months), his future life as a human being will be influenced by the style of upbringing he receives – what is said or not said to him about his activities, the compliments or reproaches he receives from mother about the initiatives upon which he acts, the attention she does or does not give in accepting his sometimes clumsy attempts to help her, the encouragements or anxious warnings he receives from his tutelary agent, whether he is supervised only by her gaze and with decreasing amounts of help as necessary, or on the contrary if his freedom is limited by being kept in a playpen or in a reduced and unvarying space. The period around 18 months could be called the 'grab everything phase' – very demanding for mothers. The following four to six months are the most important for the child's education if they are used for the enrichment of language in association with free motor experiences within a relationship of trust with the adult. Verbalising whatever interests the child – that he looks at, tries to reach, touches and manipulates – creates richness of vocabulary, not immediately but eight to ten months later. Carried by this informational, even initiatic, language, delivered by the mother, that helps him understand the world around him, the child can renounce being carried. He has become too heavy and can progressively give up the physical assistance of his mother for his needs. On reaching 22 months, if since learning to walk (12 to 15 months) he has been allowed to practice doing everything like an adult, the child is quite able to eat cleanly on his own, to take skilfully what he needs, use implements at the table, help himself from a dish, like adults if he wants to have his meals with them. If day after day he is given the freedom to use the toilet for his excretory needs, he becomes proud to be able to do this, to wipe his bottom on his own (obviously if he has been taught how to do it and has been helped with it for long enough), and progressively to wash, and to get dressed or undressed on his own. He can also go to bed on his own when he is sleepy and let others sleep when he isn't. He can play with everything he encounters, listen to songs and stories, constantly ask questions confident that they will be answered and thus becomes very quickly confident in himself and his autonomy.

Autonomy of the child

The autonomy of the child with regard to the tutelary agent and in a safe space is the winning of a feeling of freedom, a feeling inseparable from that of being human. For every child, this depends essentially on the mother or main carer's tolerance of this autonomy, despite their own possessive narcissism. It also depends on the introjection of this tolerance by the child. It is certain that a child who is always penned up at home, carried or in a pushchair outside, who cannot try to explore the space around him at his own pace although he has for several months attained the muscular development that would allow this, is in grave danger: because his only experiences are visual, imaginary and 'by proxy,' by identification with others, without any real experiencing by his own little body, which becomes a part object in space when he is separated from his mother, who has been moving him either directly by carrying or in a car. It is obvious that a child brought up imprisoned in this way will be at risk of an accident as soon as he escapes, either outdoors or in the home but out of his playpen – he has no experience either of his body or of space, making the mother, who was already intolerant of his liberty, more anxious and inclined to put him in his pen 'for peace and quiet': thus, a vicious circle is set up. The child is heading towards a completely inexperienced bodily schema while at the same time developing a fantasmatically omnipotent body image based on oral narcissism and without motor experience; he will become more and more clumsy and inexperienced and will be in danger when the day comes that he no longer has the external impediments that for his mother represent safety but for him, a pathogenic prison. In this prison, where his anal drives have no outlet and are repressed without words and therefore not symbolised, they are reinforced by the imaginary oral register (in two dimensions) and used in fantasising omnipotence in an unknown bodily schema, not infirm but always experienced as without any relationship with the functional body image – an image that the child has built not through experience but in identifying with others, in watching them in action and in the mastery of their space. In imagination, he lends his immobilised body image to the images of the others that move around autonomously, whom he observes and memorises. He does not become Me–I, he is You, Me–You. Besides, many of these children when talking about their desires put them in the second person: 'you want this, you want that,' as if they are talking about themselves while being the other. These children are very inhibited in their motor functioning. After a satisfactory weaning, while the child was in a good relationship with the mother and could tolerate what she imposed on him, it is anal castration that he lacked. We could say that the imaginary umbilical cord that still links the mother and child limits the child for longer or shorter durations according to what the mother can tolerate. There are those who can tolerate no freedom for their child and others who know how to remove every chance of a serious accident around their child and, in this space of freedom, let him take initiatives and experiment with things. The behavioural, emotional and verbal language of the tutelary agent is interwoven with the playful and practical experiences that the child enjoys and that allow the child to memorise everything that mother explains to him about the objects to hand and the techniques appropriate for their successful manipulation – so that it happens without accident or failure. This is what contributes to the acquisition of autonomy. For the child, this is the way a pre-ego is built – limited by a cautious pre-superego that supports and encourages desire. This pre-superego is the internalised voice of the mother or the father, the You that is the reference of the child in his going-on-becoming ego. This voice, if it does not tolerate his initiatives, inhibits the relationship of the body image with the bodily schema. If on the contrary it tolerates his initiatives and verbalises the various aspects of his success or the causes of a failure, the subject can risk using his bodily schema in ways motivated by a desire that responds to the incitements of the external world. This introjected voice is memorised in him as if it was saying, faced with new actions: 'go on, you can do it, Mummy/Daddy would allow it if she/he was there'; or on the contrary: 'no, you can't, it's dangerous, Mummy/Daddy would say that, she/he said it.' This also explains why what can be a transgression to this child will not be for the other. Each child develops his autonomy according to the words – the phonemes, their tone, the timbre of the mother's voice – tense or amused, worried or happy – that accompanied his first initiatives. 'Mummy was here, she saw it, she said yes, or she said nothing, therefore next time I can go further.' 'Mum saw me, she was cross so I should not do that again.' It is this internal hearing that makes the child feel secure or insecure, according to whether he has been monitored with or without anxiety, loved or rejected in his daily motor experiences; it depends on the mother's words of interdiction and their style of delivery – yelling, threatening physical chastisement or the intervention of the father or the police or the bogeyman etc., and whether they were in fact connected with the reality of a danger the child was or could have been exposed to. In effect, if one day by chance, or because of a violent impulse, the child transgresses this interdiction and the artificial walls that had been erected around him and succeeds without encountering any of the misfortunes prophesied, he loses any superego, therefore any criteria for safety and as a consequence, any caution. As Mummy was wrong or misled him, there is no more Mummy in the sense of a tutelary agent to refer to. It is then an incident, a person outside the family or more damagingly an accident that conveys either the verbal interdiction or the boundary of the law to this child, who no longer accepts control and who through a healthy desire of living but without trust in his parents doesn't know when he is in danger. One can see that the nuances of a child's behaviour, ranging from inhibited to cautious to uncontrolled, are the translations of a body image that come from the way the child was raised and educated by his parents.

Symbolisation of reality

Reality is symbolised in relations between child and mother according to two great dimensions – space and time. The safe space is that in which he is left to be free and which the mother has invested with speech. This remembered speech helps him both in knowing what is permissible and in feeling accompanied in all he can find to do in this space during her absence. On the other hand, if what is said about touching, actions and motor functioning reduces the safe space and limits his freedom in living, the child feels that his desires and initiatives cause his mother anxiety. The *duration of separation from the mother* or all tutelary persons is also a reference of his safety. This duration may or may not be compatible with the rhythm needed in order for there to be euphoric reunions after times of absence – it depends on the child and also on the frustration felt by the mother during the separation and that he can perceive. In the best case, this separation is the sign of the freedom of the child with regard to his mother: it is not abandonment if she has warned him about it and if he is safe with known people. The reunion is joyful if at least the mother is not absent for too long, and if this does not cause the child to suffer anxiety that will inhibit his wish for freedom. Autonomy cannot be won except by safety linked with the loving attention of the tutelary agent. All the knowledge of the child – some of it acquired by the desire to transgress what was formerly unknown, some acquired in the confident ambiance of the tutelary agent, all of it experienced as play – brings him new sensations both pleasant and unpleasant. And it is this perception that organises his *body image interwoven with the time and space of his bodily schema*, like the warp and weft of a fabric. This is the fabric of the relationship between his desire and the world around him, that he does or does not come to master, that structures what I call his *primary narcissism*. All this happens in the period when his neurological and spinal cord development is coming to completion. This brings sensory-motor capacity with which the child experiments with pleasure – fine sensations in the soles of his feet, of the perineum and the whole uro-anal-genital region and therefore the sensory references of sphincter control performed for his own pleasure. This is the period when the child plays with retaining his excrements or expelling them voluntarily, even if he is relatively clean already, as mothers say, which means he is continent because of the attention paid by the mother to his excretory functioning and the pleasurable safety felt by the inexperienced and neurologically immature baby in being dependent on her.

The education of the anal phase

Sphincter control comes spontaneously for all human children, just because they are higher mammals. All mammals are by nature continent as soon as they are neurologically complete. Continence in itself therefore has no cultural value. But cultural value comes secondarily when the child discovers that continence can be pleasurable when he plays at its mastery and also that it allows him to satisfy or manipulate his mother, who reacts strongly to what she calls accidents in his pants and that are no longer that, from 30 months onwards, but proofs of the gross pleasure taken by the child with his anal impulses. It is in identification with the adults and the pleasure of becoming 'like them' that the child, from this point neurologically capable of sphincter control, wishes to go to the toilet, which is there for the use of everyone, big and small. He has always observed this; and if he has received answers to what the adults go to do alone in these comfort rooms, he too will want to behave like the adults, one fine day when he has passed 30 months. Thus, in two days sphincter control is acquired, and not to please anyone but himself.

Mothers who deny the child the freedom of his sphincter solely so that he doesn't soil himself, before he has the anatomical, neurological and sensory-motor possibility of controlling his sphincters and testing out the pleasure linked with their control, behave as if they are forbidding him from individuating away from her, from being at peace with their bodies and being interested in responding to and mastering their own physical states for their own pleasure.

Letting the child make his progress at his own pace is one of the keys to bring-ing up children, if one wishes to prevent future disturbances in his relationship with himself (that is to say narcissistic disturbances), and disturbances in relation to others. A mother who by her speech constrains the needs of her child, scolding him for urinating or defecating, also forces him to inhibit himself and prevents him from experiencing satisfaction at his own pace, although this is not what she aims to do. Her target is wee and poo, but this affects in a global way the child's physical and manual abilities, sometimes even his speaking ability, the ability to express himself. At this period of grabbing everything, the child needs to be taught how to handle all these things, by way of the speech of his mother or another familiar adult who shows him that he has hands, just like adult hands only smaller, but that can be skilful, if less strong. If he uses these hands intelligently, he will get the same results as the adults. If he does any old thing anyhow, he will not achieve his ends. This teaching of how to handle things through speech that accompanies the child's interest in manipulation constitutes a far more important education than that of sphincter cleanliness; this is the education of the symboli-sation of urethral and anal drives by the displacement of the part object onto all things. But for many mothers, only sphincter cleanliness and eating well are parts of their education. They will try, as abruptly as possible, to curb the child's interest in wee and poo while bypassing the transposition of the investment in the sphincter onto the hands, which before had been mouth-hands and now are anus-hands, and which by the handling and manipulation of various objects, including water and sand, have pleasure interwoven with intelligence. The ideas with which the child accompanies everything he does with his hands are firstly imaginary representations, and then symbolisations thanks to the speech of those around him, which the child takes pleasure in repeating, linked with his playful activities. His desire to do, undo, re-do, throw and collect – all this physical pleasure in manipulation originates in displaced anal drives, from the pleasure in peristaltic movements with regard to the solid or liquid part object onto all manipulable objects that are constantly available to the child.

We cannot suppress the interest in uro-anal pleasure that involves the desire for subject-to-subject communication, occasioned by the repetitive need linked with the pleasure of maternal toileting care, without the first part object (faeces) being replaced, for the better, by other things.

The vitality, intelligence and sensitivity of a human being are endangered by the forbidding of desire or pleasure linked with the satisfaction (however achieved) of desire without the libido having another outlet for appeasing its tensions.

Sphincter continence

In children who have gained good manual abilities with water, earth and all objects that support their fantasies and that derive from desire originating in anal drives, and who play physical games of motor agility and acrobatics on their own or in the company of other children, sphincter control happens spontaneously at around 22 months at the very earliest, but more usually around 25 to 27 months. It is usually a bit earlier in girls than in boys – between 19 and 20 months at the earliest – for other reasons, which are the complete independence of the excremental and genital apparatuses (continence can be requested of a girl a little earlier than of a boy). All these manual accomplishments form part of the pleasure of living for a child who loves his tutelary agent and who is able to anticipate his progress to please his mother or father. However, this anticipation should not be excessive. If sphincter control is acquired too early and by submission and dependence on the adult and not by means of a pleasure that he found for himself, the child risks losing it during his first trial in society.

The idea of human dignity comes very early. All adult actions and words that do not respect this feeling undermine the child's desire for autonomy, as if he were guilty of feeling pleasure in growing up and discovering the pleasure of mastering his physical needs and functioning in space, as allowed by his neurological development from day to day until the completion of his bodily schema at 30 months.

Sphincter continence – autonomy in the satisfaction of excretory needs – forms part of the exercising of human dignity, neither more nor less than autonomy in activity and rest, in feeding oneself and for pleasure with the techniques observed in older children and adults.

In order to master the means of autonomy of action that integrate the child into the family group as a human among others and respected by them, the child must not have been treated like a domestic animal, subjected to imperative verbal commands; the pleasure of autonomy and of daily discoveries (with the risk of sometimes experiencing displeasure and failure when body coordination has not yet been mastered) should not be stolen from the child because of the pleasure he gives to the adult in his dependency – a dependency from which he has to free himself; in addition, the child should not be made to feel guilty about his pleasure in autonomy by an adult who needs the child's dependency and his power over the child for his own narcissism, and who shows that he is anxious when faced with the child's wish to gain his freedom of existence.

All the conflict around the acquisition of autonomy and sphincter discipline, in the raising and early education of the child, comes from these contradictions of desire between the child and his nursing and educating mother; it also comes from the unconscious or conscious damage inflicted by mother on the feeling of human dignity of their boy or girl. The key here is the confusion that they inculcate in their child or that they do not undo if he confuses himself. The confusion is between his state as a child, his neurological impotence in controlling his sphincters and the shame that he can or should have about it. The spontaneous shame of the child in witnessing his own impotence, or the shame that is inculcated and cultivated (alas!) as an educational tool by the mother, spreads by contiguity to all the natural sensations of pleasure given by a bodily region that is also the genital region – the moral, erotic and aesthetic value of which should be preserved but taken away from parental control, which is intuitively experienced by the child as incestuous.

To go back to the narcissism attached to the body image and its functionality, the feeling of dignity is very tightly connected with this, as are all the conquests of the mastery of oneself and of space that progressively become possible for the child whose desire for this mastery long pre-dates his physical capabilities, which depend upon his neurological development that finishes at 28 to 30 months.

All children are proud to perform excretory functions like adults, in the same place and same way, alone and not with the help of the mother. Premature sphincter cleanliness requires the help of mother or someone else. When it happens at the right time, the child quickly manages on his own, and this is what is humanising for him.

One indication that it is not too early to start to ask a child to show voluntary sphincter continence is his ability and the pleasure he shows in going up and down a stepladder or stairs, and also the pleasure he may show in remaining squatting for quite some time while playing. These are proofs that the neurological system of the spinal cord is sufficiently developed to give co-ordinating and sensory-motor signals needed for experiencing pleasure.

Putting the child on the potty too early carries the risk of inducing serious psychomotor delays or even the foundations of an obsessional neurosis. In general, it is important that the acts demanded by parents of their children are pleasantly feasible for them. It is also important that father and mother give their children only prohibitions that are progressively modified according to their growth and neuro-muscular coordination.

It is important that children receive encouragement when they run small risks and congratulations when they succeed at something or attempt something but fail because of a small accident. Failures are educative, if one accepts and reflects upon them. When faced with difficulty in the absence of his parents, the child must be able to say to himself, 'ah yes, mum and dad did tell me this was a bit difficult'; so that when vexingly, he fails, he can console himself for his present impotence as would his mother if she were there, while having confidence for the future. He knows that every day, he is developing. This is an extraordinary moment in the child's discovery of the world and development of his motor skills, especially when he notices that everybody is happy about this development.

Errors of judgement and failures in actions must not entail feelings of guilt or of hopeless shame. These depressive feelings, like the contrary ones of disregard for reality and the casting of responsibility onto others, impede learning about things and investment in the bodily schema; both are the fruit of an anxious and guilt-making early education of a child of less than 20 months or in the months before primary castration (two and a half to three years).

Anal castration and its sublimations

A very young child is well able to understand a prohibition given to him on a temporary basis and that later, he will be told, 'You can do that now you are big, you couldn't before but now you can'; or a good neighbourly social agreement such as, 'people aren't allowed to do that and nor are you, and I wouldn't be allowed either if I were playing this game.' This prohibition follows on from the laws of social life; it is not related to the child's person or his clumsiness but to a place and rules valid for all, or at least for all of his age – rules applicable in this place by an agency above his parents and that are not aimed at him personally. When something is forbidden to a child who trusts his parents, he accepts this restraint because he knows that it will help him avoid too great a risk. It may not be pleasant, but it is not vexing as it is not felt to be tyrannical. When something is forbidden to all and in a lasting way, the child knows that it is in the general interest, which goes beyond the particular interest of each person, including that of the parents. It is important to fight the gregarious instinct, so easily exploitable in human beings – tribal mammals – and to educate the civic and social sense and the acceptance of rules, while allowing criticism of them.

After the anal phase, the child will have been able to accept the prohibition of taking without asking, and then without putting back after use, what belongs to others or even what belongs to the family group. If his human dignity is respected in speech and actions, he will integrate perfectly the forbidding of all behaviours detrimental to others, the forbidding of knowingly harming himself or another.

This prohibition of theft, of grabbing, of aggression towards people or objects belonging to others must be verbalised to him. The child understands and accepts perfectly well these restrictions to his drives when he sees the adults themselves submitting to the rules, especially if the adults do not use physical force against him in treating him like an animal or an object in their possession.

Until now, his bodily self is necessarily the object of his parents. How do these children manage when they really hurt themselves? Mother putting a bit of antiseptic and laying a hand on the painful part is enough to make them no longer feel anything at all – although the cut or the burn may take several days to heal. *Afterwards, the prohibition of hurting his own body or putting it dangerously at risk must be verbalised to him*: this is invigorating for the child, as it confers trust in him as a subject and a person. Some children, for better or for worse, see themselves as an object of their mother or father, of the person serving the tutelary role. It is important to awaken them to their personal responsibility. This is a very important moment, between child-rearing and education. The child's body itself is in reality not an object that particularly belongs to his mother or his father or some other tutelary person; it is a libidinal object in which the child experiences oral (imaginary and sensory) and anal (motor) pleasures – narcissistic pleasures – and the castrations applied to these constitute the humanisation of the child. *But for this to happen, both mother and father have to have accepted being anally castrated by their child.* What does this mean? That she doesn't always need her child for her own oral and anal pleasure, or need the enjoyment of his presence, or to act according to him, that she doesn't need always to fiddle with him, handle him, dress and undress him, adorn him, wash him, put him to bed etc. because he pleases her.

On the contrary, the child is called upon to take care of himself in all the ways he can, from day to day, to discover that he can do this on his own and that he wishes to do it himself. It is necessary that she is interested in him, that she is not indifferent to his progress, of course. If, after having said, 'You can do this yourself,' she leaves him on his own, he will feel abandoned and won't know what to do. Autonomously, he knows what to do to under the gaze of his mother and from what she says to him, which delivers him freedom as if this is part of the relationship between them; and then it is he who mothers himself, with her authorisation and, necessarily at the start, with her verbal help. He needs her to remain connected through her speech with his joys and successes when he comes to share them with her; and that she sympathises by consoling him, at least in speech, and sometimes with small maternal gestures – comforting caresses – during an experience that proves to be painful for him although rich in learning. She can, while consoling him, verbalise the facts without judgement, without scolding because he has failed and without always blaming another if he says that someone else has caused his failure. Does this come from the relationship between him and another? This is to be understood, if possible.

All this means for the child that he is considered to be a being who is constantly becoming, projected into the future in the imagination of his father and mother, becoming a big girl or boy, and soon a man or woman; that he is recognised by tutelary adults as a subject motivated by desire whose freedom and fantasies are respected. *The child talks about almost everything he does.* This is not in order to be heard by the adult: he cannot do otherwise. He talks about what he does because this is how he humanises his acts; but if one uses what he says against him or to spy on what he does and thinks, one destroys the freedom that was being constructed. When he is raised as I have suggested, he feels that he is esteemed as a living representative of the real genital desire of the adults. He feels himself to be their son or daughter in their eyes when they discuss him, and this prepares him to identify with the adult of his sex, which soon will be possible for him, thanks to his neurological growth, when he has fully assumed his motor and humanised being (around 30 months). Until then, the father and mother are seen as a two-headed tutelary ego-ideal (perhaps what the Kleinian school calls the combined parent).

Pathogenic effects upon the child of the parents' oral and anal erotisation: its retroactive effect, which is mutilating, upon weaning

A mother for whom the child's body is an oral and anal libidinal object upon which she exercises her discretionary powers for her own pleasure, that she cuddles and plays with like a doll, that she devours with her eyes and with caresses, that she doesn't allow to play with anything except what amuses her – this mother shows that she has remained stuck in her development at the anal and especially genital prohibitions, and her child plays for her the role of a pet. He is her dolly or even her poo-poo, like she calls him while hugging and kissing him with relish. The child therefore cannot continue to develop without becoming phobic or obsessional, and it is because symptoms of these two infantile neuroses impede his adaptation outside of the family that he is taken to a psychoanalyst (luckily, if this does happen).

Obsessionality is a means of stopping libidinal development relating to an anal ethos where the prohibition affects all part objects of pleasure. The child starts to relate to everything around him as if it were poo, prohibited by Mummy; even more prohibited, if she calls him her poo, as this proves that only he can be the valued poo. He is thereby invested with an erotogenic power over his mother, a power that inhibits him more and more, as it is pathogenic for the child to be an erotic object, and especially an archaic erotic object, for a mother whose image of development is not that of a woman with a genital attitude towards her husband and vice versa. The life drives of this child rekindle a dynamic endlessly stuck like a record needle in a groove: 'take' – eat this sweet, 'don't touch' – poo or wee; and in terms of emotional relations, 'kiss' – if the child is yummy or 'cute,' and 'spank-spank' if he is 'naughty' ('a little shit' to her) or has soiled himself. What further complicates this 'don't touch' attitude towards anything mother considers dirty is that these words are also spoken about the child's penis, so that in some cases he becomes so obsessional that he cannot urinate without help but needs his mother to get his willy out of his pants to let him do this, or he has to urinate seated like a girl. With little girls, they can't wipe themselves because they're not supposed to touch and it disgusts them (boys also).

These phobic-obsessive attitudes are developed by a mother who is not castrated and who frustrates instead of giving symboligenic castration. A mother (or educating woman) who teaches a child in this way is anxious about her own repressed genitality, trapped in regression to a fixation point that fetishises her child under the pretext of maternal love; she expresses a paedophilic eroticism. She strives to delay the child's use of his intelligence for fear that he will be interested in his physical functioning and his sexual organ. She makes him feel guilty about curiosity (the epistemological drive), which is the basis of the human mind. When he asks questions about his sexual organ or his excrements, she doesn't respond or only with: 'Be quiet, it's dirty, it's not nice to ask such questions, we don't talk about such things.' For him, every time he tries something new, there is immediately this pre-superego in play; even if he just thinks about an action, something says to him: 'Watch out, crocodile! Don't go there, hands off.' Because of the over-valuation of oral drives (eating requires fragmentation), everything becomes cut up into pieces, himself included; everything conceals danger. The frustrated human pre-ego is forbidden to individuate, is alienated into the role of a domestic animal trained to the desire of his master, the tutelary adult, and in this way perverted; the subject's desires are therefore projected into the pre-superego in imagining a voracious, devouring oral erogenous zone, frustrating of pleasure and mutilating – chopping off fingers that might stray towards something that mummy has said not to touch.

At the start, no child has a fragmented body image. He has an oral functioning that fragments objects of the external world – so that he can swallow them – and an anal functioning that fragments things inside him in order to put them out – this is how he does a poo. The repeated experience of these intake and output needs is accompanied by the fragmentation of the oral and anal part object, but this bodily experience is not experienced as a relationship of subjects. For him to have relationships with subjects, he needs speech about activities rather than the trading of part objects of the body and of bodily contact. For the child, the mother is still only a total object, as I have said, an object that is represented to him sometimes as two-headed – daddy-mummy or mummy-daddy – with which the child identifies without knowing yet that he is only of one sex, like only one of these two adults. He is therefore not fragmented. It is the mother who in some upbringings induces the imaginary inflation of dental or anal fragmentation of a part object, because she makes her child into her part object. She takes into consideration only her child's needs and leaves him playing the role of a functioning body, but not becoming a subject who takes initiatives; and outside of his real and supposed needs and the care of his body, she doesn't speak to him. This is how a subject comes avidly to want to give pleasure to his mother by creating his value through his own frag-mentation. If he has value, it is because he is a tiny piece, either of food or of poo, and mother becomes in the child's imagination a fragmenting mouth by which he needs constantly to be kissed (mimicking eating) or watched (consumed by her eyes) or heard or carried. He is her 'little bear,' she is her 'kitten,' he is her 'sweetie-pie'... whether girl or boy, they have nicknames but are never addressed by their given name; the child-object bears the characteristics of these nicknames, which are in reality soubriquets that express the mother's tenderness towards an object to which in reality she denies the quality of a human subject. The child suf-fers from desire that has been really perverted and that makes the little boy or little girl into an erotic object of possession for the mother.

If both parents behave in the same way, the time spent by the child as a liv-ing being is practically forbidden in their space. He has to live in frozen time. He has to behave like a larva, a statue, a walking phallus without head or legs – because Daddy and Mummy are for the child really cutting mouths or watching eyes (according to anal magical thinking, which is not experienced in sensory and spatial reality but in an imagination preserved from the oral stage). A child may be 'ruined' – engulfed in the call of the mother's or father's desire (less often, I must say, the father's, as he is ordinarily more often not at home). This is what happens when the couple are trapped by the absorbing or rejecting fascination that a child can exercise over them, whether he be beautiful or ill favoured by nature. Each tries to fill his existential lack by protecting the child, by exhibiting him, by having fun with him, overwhelming him and over-gratifying him, so that there is no risk of him looking elsewhere for the answer to the lack inherent in desire. Without him, the couple would fall apart. He is for each of them the decoy for the phallus.

However, the child subject is always there, present from conception though we may not know where or recognise him; and as there is a subject, there is a desire to be vitally linked with the id, and to the ensemble of the instincts that derive from the genetic heritage, represented by the present body. This – the belief in the exist-ence of the subject and his desires – is the basis of a psychoanalytic treatment, we could say the first article of faith, conscious or otherwise, of all psychotherapists, without which they could not do this job. The subject is present, we can't always know where, but as there is a body, there is a subject. If he cannot express him-self through his body, this necessitates the work of psychoanalysis, which will be to retrace the history of this poor soul in order to help the subject re-find the path he has taken to communicate to us his own desire, by means of his bodily schema and a body image that has not evolved but that has remained narcissisti-cally resuscitable.

However, sometimes this desire can neither show itself nor be imagined by the child. It may happen that a child is, in his person, completely the part object of the tutelary adult – like a teddy bear or a doll. And yet, somewhere there exists a subject with his own veiled desire that waits in passive drives until it is found by someone; or a subject, masked by a cautious indifference because of an invasive phobic state, who is motivated by active drives and who wishes to communicate by these with someone who accepts being totally passive and available in his presence. It is this availability to meet the most archaic drives of a human being that characterises the a priori attitude of the psychoanalyst, especially a child psychoanalyst. Sometimes there is liminal proof of the subject's desire, some phonemes that he dares to emit, that are neither cries nor laughter, therefore not in any known code, nor are they close in sound to those of the mother tongue, but they may be, as are the cries that imitate the noises of the natural world, signs that have some meaning for him, to be elaborated and interwoven in a symbolic way with the sensations of his visceral life in his moments of solitude. He also hears car noises, sirens, the hammer blows of workmen and builders, and these are interwoven for him with perceptions of his body in its states of need-tension or desiring fantasies, becoming indecipherable signifiers. These signifiers in sounds and actions become compulsive symptoms, and it is essential to know and to tell him that they have a human meaning that we cannot grasp. These signifiers are only valid for him, and I believe that even he does not know why he has chosen these sounds and then, by force of their repetition, given them value as signifiers. Do these signifiers not become magically conjuring, attaching a perception of the external world to snatches of fantasy, and providing him with an ephemeral but necessary link with reality? The symbolic function, which no longer links these subjects with the speaking world, links them nonetheless with the cosmic world, with nature and the objects around them. These children are very isolated, described as bizarre, speech-delayed; in reality, they are pre-psychotic and get worse if left on their own. They have failed in their learning during the motor, anal phase and its ethos – between 12 and 30 months. It is in this period that families constantly come up against the greatest learning difficulties. At the start, the child is inhibited in his desire, or is turned loose to satisfy himself – depending on whether the parents are demanding or inattentive; it is therefore their behaviour towards the child that is decisive, but secondarily, it is he who has lost contact with them and, on their own, they can do nothing to help him. After several clumsy experiments, after encountering failures in trying to be 'like the bigger ones' around him, the child may find a reconciliation with himself thanks to what is said to him in a generous way by his parents who, helped by a psychoanalyst, have understood what has brought their child to this state of isolation. Sometimes the parents, even with help, are not enough. Contact has been definitively cut and the child needs individual therapy, which takes a long time and is only possible if the child is anxious, which is not always the case. This 'Martian' – as described by the parents – is sometimes satisfied with his imaginary life.

The structure of a child said to be psychotic

The three body images in their constant linkage with one another bring cohesion to the narcissism of the human being; but they can become scrambled: instead of them preserving the human and ethical values the child should have acquired after weaning or in the course of anal castration, the child can invert or ignore these values. He obeys an ethos of archaic fantasies altogether inappropriate not only to his bodily schema[16] but out of step with the body image that corresponds to most children of his age. For example, he has a double squint or tries to touch or take with the back of his hand, or only with his mouth, or yet still, when he wants to walk, instead of opening his legs so that he can put one foot in front of the other, his feet cross over and he cannot walk and must be carried. I have given examples of this in other of my writings, and everyone in the clinical world knows of some cases. The child wants to grow up; his parents want this too – they express this – but at each daily renewed manifestation of his libidinal drives, their speech aims to prohibit, to put brakes on or, worse, to devalue his desire. At the very least, their acts and speech come to block his initiatives, whatever these are – putting his hands in his mouth or to his sexual organ, which is at least something for a child who did nothing until then.

This results in the child subject being integrated and structured within a narcissistic image that no longer promotes the realisation of the potentials of his bodily schema (which would allow him to acquire motor autonomy) because this would ruin his relationship with the tutelary agent. It is important to understand that the change of child-raising attitude (if for instance the parents, worried by the psychomotor delay in their child, do some psychoanalytic work) doesn't stop the child from staying in his delayed state. Finding liberty in his movements has become dangerous for him, even if he is now allowed them, because the baby human and especially the small child has introjected the image of the adults who look after him as an intuitive unconscious structure, especially if he is precocious and intelligent, as if these adults were the incarnation of his future self, a speaking-being, master of himself, autonomous and motivated. Before primary castration, the process of integrating the other as a knowledgeable self is learned from all those who are bigger and stronger, of both sexes. After primary castration (if this is done well), this integration benefits from the images of others, older siblings and adults, of the same sex as the child; and from the other sex, if on the contrary castration has de-narcissised him in his sex, instead of narcissising him. Or, still further, the child lives as if he wants to know nothing about his sex, and he can therefore regress to just urethra-anal functioning (encopresis) as an expression relating to his perineum. We have seen the problem at the point of primary castration. With time, what follows are dangerous experiences for the child and for others; before desire can be totally repressed, inverted or neutralised with regard to its genital future – which is in question regarding the facts of life and the principle of 'go forth and multiply' (as far as possible) – it accumulates through being opposed. The aggressive, active and passive life drives are reinforced. Unconscious acts emerge – without reflection, unpredictable, impulsive – so as to escape the deadly status of

16 See the case of Pierre, p. 162.

object, the child, reprimanded in his actions, at first too passive and then volatile, becomes a disaster of a child said to be a 'budding delinquent' – a biter, violent, predatory, destructive,[17] a terror in public gardens and shops. The parents'
reaction – as much coercive as anxious – constantly on the alert, confirms to him
day after day that he is an object, a thing belonging to his parents, so that he has
increasingly to stay this way; lacking the love and cuddles that his behaviour
makes it impossible to provide and also because all kindness and tenderness
exasperates his unconscious sadism, he seems to engineer situations that provoke reactions in adults so as not to find himself again in a relational desert, up
against only his active and passive drives. The tutelary agents, the educators,
mother and father, can be thought of as unconsciously mutilating and frustrating
of this child, unwitting abusers. In some cases, these parents, and others who
were more tolerant at the start, cannot repair the damage of a castration that has
not been given in time and with love. The child's pre-ego is no longer tameable
by a human being who loves him and whom he loves, a sanely human educator,
who allows the use of licit symbolisation of prohibited drives.

Such children, so raised, forbidden all desire, and introjecting the prohibition
of desire, often fall into psychosomatic accidents and become ill, prey to other
creatures, microbes, who are ready to take over the body of he who no longer
assumes it, or certain bodily organs that lack vitality. If their bodies resist, they
become dangerously ill-tempered children. Their nights are full of nightmares
and insomnia, because in their imaginations what is prohibited emerges in a
confabulation that satisfies transgressive desires that the introjected parents forbid or disqualify. In his vigilant sleep, the child is in a constant, merciless war
with his desire and the ethical contradictions of his body image, that remain or
return non-castrated.

I will not try to list all the cases here where an experience deeply distorting
of narcissism develops in the last neuro-muscular developmental period of the
spinal cord, that is to say between two and four years. I must specify that it is
always in the unconscious failures of education, during conflicts between the
child's libido and that of the educating adults, with the best conscious will on
both sides, that these serious future sexual and psychosocial disturbances originate, through perverse fixations or psychotising processes. In many upbringings, there are moments of failure. Fortunately, they mostly show themselves
in health problems (psychosomatic) that provide a diversion and allow, thanks
to a period of regression, a re-start. But when the body does not pay its debt
to the law of symboligenic castration, the failures are embedded in psychosocial habits and it is these that later are found in those who have the courage to
undergo psychoanalysis, made very difficult in adolescents and adults who are
physically healthy but who suffer from maladaptations that allow them neither
love nor creativity.

17 Even a firestarter.

The temperamental, the pre-psychotic

When the narcissism of the child's body image is split off from the bodily schema of his physical age, the child's oral libidinal desire to take in – to know, to understand – and his anal desire to do – to act, to experiment – awaken in the mother such an eroticised or repressed emotional response (in the unconscious – it comes to the same thing) that her irrepressible anxiety causes a more or less controlled expressive reaction – 'watch out!' – in which the child always perceives the unsaid. If she reacts to her anxiety with superego-ish guilt – which dates back to her own childhood – this guilt is expressed by contemptuous looks, hostile attitudes or words of blame and a withdrawal of love that she believes to be educative. The child loses even the possibility of a recourse to the fantasy of archaic pleasure – that of being consoled by her in his ordeal, of a reconciliation with himself through identification by introjection of a loving mother of a still helpless baby that she knew how to reassure. He believes that she no longer loves him, and is right not to (as he judges himself through her eyes); and if that is so, then she must only desire him, and if that too is not the case, then it must be that she needs him. She still feeds him, but then dogs get fed too. There is no way out.

He is therefore subject to the introjection of freakish feelings without representation, or sometimes with his given name as the only representation associated with him; his name vocalised aggressively, sometimes with his surname, the family name of his father (or mother, if she is single), that his mother links with him when she is not pleased for him to be *her* baby and hers alone. 'You really are a (so-and-so – surname)'; his or her given name with the added surname, severely spoken, are for the child who hears them accusatory, rejecting, the sign of his most depressive feeling. The effects of the death instinct resurge in the unconscious and invest this or that functional or erogenous zone of the body, in part or completely, and provoke for example anorexia, vomiting, encopresis, enuresis and insomnia. One hears mothers and fathers who believe this is aimed at them, as if these are oppositional twists and turns by the child they wish to train.[18,19] The more he shows the symptoms, the more they want to train him out of them, and this gives a dramatic and libidinally perverse situation between humans who can

18 Translator's note: Dolto's footnote, below, is effectively untranslatable, as there is no equivalent common expression in English to '*il m'a fait*' – literally, 'he did that to me.' Dolto's footnote gives examples of everyday verbal formulations used by French parents that express the idea that the child has done something with an intention of in some way persecuting, worrying or inconveniencing them. The closest English translation I can suggest would be that after complaining about the child's act, the mother might add something like, 'he does that to wind me up' or 'she does make my life difficult.' Dolto's footnote follows next.

19 Who does not recognise this discourse in every mother: 'He's got diarrhoea – he does that to wind me up, he/she got whooping cough – he/she makes my life difficult.' (*il m'a fait la diarrhée, il (ou elle) m'a fait la coqueluche,*' while fathers tend to say: 'he/she is pushing me, provoking me. I won't take this from your son/your daughter. He/she is taking the mickey out of me.' Mothers suffer and fathers feel provoked.

do nothing but destroy each other. The child loses even the sensitivity of his distinct sphincter sensations, the sensations of transit; he is totally given over to the death drives because his basal, most fundamental image has been affected – that which is linked with the mother, who as I have said is both life and death. If the mother no longer holds any characteristic of life for the mind and the heart, then for the body that cannot live without mind or heart, she becomes as death, or even a hoped-for death; and the death-mother will be the reference of anti-existence and of existence at the same time. Without taking into account the fact that the signifier 'dead' in French – dead, dying, death, biting[20] – inscribes itself in the body image, these children who have reached the limit of being alive and who are extremely intelligent subjects cannot swallow or chew any longer; their anorexia, which is a generalised lack of the desire to love, of the desire to desire, of the desire to exchange, is very particular and psychotic. At the same time, it is not unusual that their gullet no longer knows how to drink. When you want to help them to drink, it all spills out – they have lost their bearings in their relationship with the oral swallowing zone (erogenous and functional). Life – it is death . . . although without human witnesses, the child can still have solitary meals and may sometimes eat from the ground because this way of muscular and skeletal functioning is for him linked with that of small domestic animals who are exempt from the prohibition that he has introjected in his body.

These bizarre behaviours of children in great difficulty, called pre-psychotic, are not capricious. However, many children have fleeting whims of this kind that leave no mark; every psychotic child thus enters into a chronic state that could have been passed through in a few hours, a few days or a few minutes by a child who comes out of it, and who was expressing something that could not be otherwise expressed through transitory bizarre attitudes of the body. But the psychotic child cannot leave this state. He is trapped in impulses that manifest themselves only once in those who have developed healthily, be they unusual impulses triggered by a fantasy or a real event or aggressive impulses against the tutelary agent. In the child who becomes psychotic, it is very unusual that things stay this way. In general, the death drives of the desiring subject are localised in certain erogenous zones and the only way he can combat the anxieties of his relationship with the parents of today is to take refuge in memories of the parents of yesterday, in an archaic self. It could be said that this is again an autistic process, a de-phasing of the subject in its relation to the rest of his current relational lifestyle and of his existential image; this results in the return to some components of the child's body image that cannot remain constantly focused within his current bodily schema and match the manifestations of the subject's desires.

The body image, the passive and active language of the incarnated drives of his desire, causes the subject to preserve the narcissistic conviction of a

---

20 Translator's note: the French verb 'to bite' when used with the first-, second- and third-person singular is a homophone of 'to die' – 'mord' and 'mort.'

bodily schema earlier than the current one, in which his drives were differently expressed, for instance those he had before fifteen, ten, nine or seven months. The death drives reign over the rest of the current bodily schema like a prohibition of consciousness – the earlier respiratory, circulatory and digestive images can alone continue to exist as non-prohibited. The child feels possessed by enemies occupying his body, which he doesn't know how to control. He wants to express what is happening within him but comes up against an absence of words and even of facial expressions, as these desires are reflected back to him by tutelary adults in ways that do not express a humanised life, so that in return, the life of the adult is a corollary of what is inexpressible in his own life. And, as there are always three parts to the body image, the subject detaches one of the three components, either the erogenous, the functional or, more seriously for health or anxiety, the basal image. What follows is an illness of the autonomous nervous system or the growth of inexplicable anxiety, which causes him to have an accident; if the basal image is affected, he falls ill for a long time. The detached image escapes from the subject in the present, who regresses to an earlier body image and to archaic nar-cissistic behaviour, passive or aggressive, in order to retrieve his narcissism and not be mutilated – which happens when the basal image is damaged. This archaic behaviour is shown in fragmenting rages that escape consciousness, but which are less dangerous for the child's future development than states of almost catatonic stupor[21] caused by regression to passivity.

In certain cases, a child who has previously known a satisfying vitality may preserve, despite his nightmares, good sleep; and as some fantasmatic vitality dating from the oral phase remains and reappears in dreams – the guardians of sleep and of unconscious fantasies – we can see the life drives prohibited from the current bodily schema try to retrieve their focus through projection onto the bod-ily schema of another body, because of his inability to retrieve a current or even a past bodily schema.[22] This body may not even be that of another human – this is how the child fantasises and confabulates scenes of enjoyment, pleasure and dan-ger. To a witness of these games, he may appear delusional. He is not as yet, but he confabulates strange beings – powerful and threatening – especially towards sundown, as real objects lose their contours and external life some of its rhythms and human sounds. The child may feel himself to be the subjugated participant in an imaginary life of which he no longer is the architect. Some children seem to come 'unstuck' from reality, and their fantasies can be taken for hallucinations (and sometimes are); but in fact every time I am sent a child in this state, or am tel-ephoned during a dramatic pseudo-hallucinatory crisis in one of them, it confirms that if one talks very gently and calmly to them, while giving them some foodstuff

---

21 See the case of the flower-dolls in *Au jeu du desir*, op. cit., the case of Pierre, p. 162 and of Leon, below, p. 189.

22 This process remains in artists and novelists and serve as 'primary matter' (underlying themes?) in their work, which is one of sublimation.

that they liked when they were very little – a cup of milk or cocoa, or a yoghurt – and when you speak to them about the images that come to them and by which they feel invaded, one can release them from their trap. They relax because they are understood without causing fear, and one can tell them that there is no crocodile or snake, robot, lion, wolf, extra-terrestrial or Martian; it is they who imagine it, and the person who is there with them absolutely can reassure these authors of black humour or of science fiction or Douanier Rousseaus-to-be, dropped in the middle of the jungle. There is nothing harmful, bad or worrying if others speak, represent or mime what they imagine. A child who has fallen into this state will not come out of it if he is met by people who become anxious to the point of taking him to a professional, putting him under observation and separating themselves from him or abruptly placing him in a psychiatric hospital – and also if he is ridiculed. His body, in solidarity with a bodily schema attacked by an archaic erogenous image, suffers a fragmenting process, and the fragmented bits become the object of these imaginary agents that are his only companions. The said imaginary agents have real effects: they can cause illness in organs (there are always infectious germs ready to attack the human body when a part of the functional image causes the bodily schema to be affected by reactional inhibitions). This can also be organised into hallucinatory sensory and visceral processes, brought on by the trial of solitude if the anxiety of the child's entourage causes them to leave him alone.

Let us remember that it is when the child shows his desire and receives a non-response from the mother that there is a disjunction of the erogenous or of the functional image (though this disturbance does not go as far as attacking the basal image) and that fantasy appears – fantasy of a lion, a man in black, a big bad wolf, a witch or the devil – which in the eyes of the child are the allies of the tutelary agent. The child may also be contaminated by other children with such fantasies, and if the mother not only allows them credibility but in addition uses them as means of pressure – to frighten and enhance her power over the child – then we can say that this upbringing sets up in the future man or woman mental fragility and difficulties, including feelings of impotence: there is a risk that the libido will slip out of reality during hallucinations or psychotic crises.

These manifestations are caused by the subject's resistance in the oral libidinal period to accepting primary castration given in a manner felt to be sadistic, or to a clumsy Oedipal castration felt to devalue his genital desire; and in the treatment of adolescents – young adults to be – it is very important that they re-find the memory of these manifestations. It is in speaking about that distant period that the present hallucinatory period comes to gain meaning and to make space for his desire to experience and speak of himself in the transference. What was translated into a pseudo-hallucinatory fable is a way of expressing the desire of the individual today, who seeks by way of the breaks in his body image and in his transference onto the psychoanalyst to retrieve old or archaic experiences. The adolescent or adult's genital drives are expressed in part in a fantasmatic syntax and according to an anal-phallic/oral-phallic and an anal-passive/oral-passive ethos. This is what leads to psychotic episodes. The processes are the same in the relationship between the conscious and unconscious mind in human beings who live 'normally' (shall we say) and those who live terribly unhappily and in a neurotic or psychotic manner. For those who may fall into and be trapped in psychotic states, the difference lies in a non-homogenous libidinal economy; and in neurotic cases, it lies in enclaves that play a chronic role in inhibiting certain types of drive, cause the re-emergence of archaic body images linked with early intersubjective relationships[23] and, thanks to transference, become concretely expressed in the working process of a treatment. This is why the detailed analysis of situations in which the child was structured in the course of his development is very important for the adult psychoanalyst.

When the fantasy cannot, during waking hours, lead to any clear imagining expressed in games or verbally, then in sleep it takes the form of dreams – nightmares; or on the contrary gratifying dreams that for example give the satisfaction of killing the tutelary beings in dangerously anthropomorphised objects or wicked animals. All of this is favoured by the over-investment of the autonomous functional image that is implied by sleep. The functional image that I call autonomous is concerned with organ life and what is suffered in the body, in opposition to the animal life that corresponds with the skeletal-muscular activity, to the activity of the body animated in the bodily schema and that is controllable by will, be it external or that of the subject. What is reproduced in the dream is the possibility that the autonomous functional body image, which originated in the pre-weaning oral phase, could prevail; while in somnambulism, what is in play is the animal functional image of the anal phase before the prohibition of causing harm (or before the knowledge of this prohibition).

Once again, it is thanks to the universality of such processes that psychoanalysis is possible, because there is a regression of the drives in the confabulations verbalised or mimed, in games and free association within the transference in psychotherapy sessions and in the thoughts reported to the psychoanalyst. The expression of the child who uses his libido in the transferential relationship allows the return of the repressed, without the regression being enacted in the body or expressed in social reality. The presence of the therapist and his acceptance of fantasies without judgement but with a curiosity about their origins in lived experience, from the most recent to the early childhood of the patient, reconnects these words and images with the affects relived in the transference. These affects of a past era, while having been traumatic and anxiogenic, are expressed in ideational, emotional and relational elements relived in the here-and-now in relation to the psychoanalyst. Unconsciously remembered, often distorted, they bring time past and other spaces into the session, and feelings and expressions dating from that era and the child's relationships with others at that time. The fruits of a castration that has not been given can be given late, in the discrimination between the

---

23 See *Le Cas Dominique* (a 1971 publication of Dolto, not in this book): 'it is prehistoric.'

imaginary and reality made by the patient in analysis in hearing his words. The events that accompanied the neglected castration are relived with the psychoanalyst who, by listening, allows them to be verbalised without any judgement other than that which regards their inappropriateness to the reality of the supposed relation of the psychoanalyst to him or her (the patient).

I am going to clarify all that I have said by giving the illustration of a case. The reader will understand much better what I meant in all these pages where, I admit, the setting out of work with body images can appear very complicated.

The case of Leon

Leon was brought to the clinic by his mother on the advice of his school and the doctor, who after a several consultations could not find any neurological reason for his strange habits. Leon had a very particular way of moving around, seeming unable to carry himself as a big 8-year-old boy – he was soft, his subcutaneous tissues thickened and a little swollen, like that of a younger child.

I saw him enter the consulting room and from the door, follow along the walls, pressing against them and then in order to sit down, reach out a hand for the support of a table before collapsing into a chair. Then, he slumped onto the table – his arms, elbows and thorax pressed against it, as if when seated, he could not support his trunk vertically in his seat. He always walked this way, holding onto furniture and walls, or to an adult or a school-friend when on the road, a bit like a baby who is starting to stand upright and who cannot yet cross a space without auxiliary support. The school had advised his mother to bring him to the Centre where I worked as he could not follow lessons or play with others. Other than this, he had no problems with his temper. Within his peer group, he had no enemies; they would even help him to get about, and nobody was annoyed by him. At home, he was loved. He was an almost totally passive child.

His IQ was tested and found to be 63. He had an expressionless face, round, expressionless eyes that moved little, and a mouth that always hung a little open. He lived seated, slumped. His mother said that from earliest childhood he had had a tuneful voice and could sing any song he heard on the radio, but without enunciating the lyrics. He spoke with a curious tempo, chanting words and separating the syllables to a very slow rhythm, in a monotone. In response to my questions about this way of speaking (that his mother had not noticed was bizarre), she confirmed that this was how he had always spoken since earliest childhood. His sister, who was two and a half years younger, had been a saucy chatterbox since her early childhood and the two children got along very well, despite being so different.

She said her husband (whom I had not met), spoke with a very strong accent, being of Polish origin. She herself spoke at a completely normal rhythm in a pleasantly modulated voice. I was astonished that Leon could modulate songs with his larynx, while not being able to modulate phonemes. I said that Leon seemed to me a musical child. She responded that he had indeed been noticed by a teacher who, hearing him singing and knowing about his academic failings, had suggested he would teach him the piano. He tried this for several months. A letter from this teacher, included in his file, related that the child showed himself to be very talented and that contrary to his habitual style of motor functioning, when seated at the piano, supported by a seat back, his hands and fingers are very agile. Leon had the gifts of a virtuoso, according to this man, which is why he was interested in him. He had advised the parents to seek this consultation. Leon's tiredness obliged the teacher to support his arms by the elbows, or his shoulders by the armpits. Muscular effort by the shoulders was as difficult for the boy as the effort of walking. On the other hand, he could easily manage the use of the piano pedals, fitted with an extension that brought them to the level of his feet. When Leon played the piano, his teacher would hold him beneath the armpits while the child's fingers showed remarkable agility.

It was this piano teacher who alerted the parents and advised them to take Leon to a specialist in motor functioning. A children's hospital had taken him in for observation and a thorough examination over several days; and the diagnostic conclusion was that there was nothing neurologically wrong with him. The doctor had spoken to the parents about nutritional supplements, general apathy and mental and education delay in their child. I learned later that the doctor had alluded to 'psychotherapy' without the mother taking note of this. Acting on the views of the specialist and the confirmation of learning disability given by the IQ test, the school advised the mother to place Leon in a medically specialised boarding school. His mother had been very upset by this as he was well attached to his parents and sister, loved the piano and took lessons almost daily; the teacher lived in the same building as the family and she saw that he would miss all this in boarding school. This was why on the recommendation of the piano teacher she came to the Centre and willingly accepted the idea of psychotherapy, a resource that the recent opening of this Centre in Paris made possible. The child also agreed to come regularly to see me, knowing that this could help him to avoid going to boarding school and allow him to stay at home and perhaps even at his own school.

Leon had been coming to the Centre for consultations for around five or six months before I saw him. From the beginning, he had been taken on for psychomotor remediation and had just completed around 20 sessions. The occupational therapist was discouraged as, far from improving, the child seemed more absent than before, as much with her as with the mother and his entourage. Leon's willingness was not in question, nor that of his mother. They never missed a session, despite mother's work and difficulties in getting around (we are right in the middle of Paris and this was during the war). And so, the Centre's director thought that psychoanalytic psychotherapy could be tried, as occupational therapy had failed.

We have here a picture of a child whose speech, motor and thinking rhythms were slowed down but who sang in tune and whose finger and laryngeal rhythms were normal. Where does this come from – this neuro-muscular weakness, this need for physical support for his back by leaning against a wall or a seat back? What is the meaning of this lack of tonicity of non-biological origin? Why could this 8-year-old child not read or write while showing such manual dexterity exclusively at a piano keyboard? Why was he terrible at maths when he could learn music theory and play music by reading a graphic transcription of sounds and rhythms?

I asked the piano teacher for his current impressions about this last (as his first letter dated back more than ten months, from the time of the general hospital consultations for Leon's motor functioning), and he wrote me a letter saying that Leon could read music perfectly with his eyes but could not name the notes he was reading. The evidence was that he could read and assimilate music theory but that what he read was transmitted immediately to his fingers. This very slow child could very easily decode a piece of music he had never seen and play it at tempo. The letter confirmed that Leon was exceptionally talented for a child of eight years and that he could even be called a virtuoso, if he wasn't so weakened. The teacher added that as he lived in the same building, he knew the parents well – their workshop was on the ground floor – and they were good and honest people who were interested in their child. Leon had spoken to him about me and said that he trusted me.

This was indeed a complex case. When the school pronounced him unable to read, I thought this could not be true as while not being able to say the notes, he could read them very quickly. It had to be the same with letters – that his eyes could read them very well without him being able to pronounce the phonemes as he read them.

Leon was sweet-tempered, and in the eyes of his mother, this was another counter-indication against putting him in a special school that, as she well knew, had many very temperamental children. At school and in everyday life, other children never attacked him. His schoolteacher and his sister said they sometimes helped him, but in a special boarding school, what would happen with the difficult children?

By putting questions to his mother about the beginnings of Leon's motor functioning, I learned that he sat up in his cot very early, that very early he had wanted to suck his thumb but that she had stopped him by pinning shut his sleeves with safety pins, and also that as soon as he could sit, she would put him in a high chair. He would remain there quietly for hours and whole half-days, at the height of the work-table of parents who were sewing in a family-run clothing workshop. He would smile, watching them work. Later on, it was on his potty that she sat him: it was both his potty and a low armchair – an armchair in which he was held by a wide belt; and it was his little sister who took his place in the high chair. When he needed to do his business, they unbelted him and removed a wooden board to reveal a cut-out seat – very convenient for him as he was so late in walking. 'He never left our side, never disturbed us.' Thus, Leon had lived seated, tied, with nothing to do with his hands, watching his father, mother and their colleagues working, for three years. But when Leon started going to nursery part time at the age of 3 and a half and the parents tried to put his sister on a little cut-out armchair similar to that of her brother, she refused this – arching her back and screaming so much that her mother had to give up this system of containment of her and leave her on a rug on the floor, as the little girl also refused to stay in the high chair. It was only now that the mother freed poor Leon from his usual seat. Leon had never crawled, and when he was freed from the seat on which he had been tied, he remained seated, leaning against a wall. Sometimes he would go towards his sister by bottom-shuffling, and when he stood up, it was by holding onto furniture. He started to walk, in the manner I observed, at the same time as his sister, when she was 14 months and he more than 3 and a half years old. His mother thought, as did her colleagues in the workshop, that being with other children at school would be good for him, and she tried out this experiment at Easter 1939, when Leon was 5 years old. The events of war interrupted this experience. Everybody was evacuated from Paris and the mother herself fell back to the maternal grandmother's home in Brittany.

In the course of his occupational therapy, Leon had always and at every session drawn the same thing, in black lines: a square house with a sort of trapezoidal roof, windows without cross frames – empty – a smokeless chimney and a door. Between the house and the top of the page, there was a sort of very flattened 'n,' which was the 'sky.' The bottom of the house coincided with the bottom of the sheet of paper and therefore was not underscored by a line. These stereotyped drawings were in the file containing the observations of Leon handed to me. Mother said he had never done any other drawings while at home; his sister drew but not Leon. He never used colour, although there were always coloured pencils available to him at the Centre.

We began the treatment. The first sessions were very poor in speech and activity. I saw mother before the boy, then in his presence, and then the boy on his own. He brought the same drawing to every session, made while he waited or when I spoke to his mother. He answered the questions I asked him about the drawing with very little speech – slow, chanted as I have described, without any facial expression: the-roof-the-sky-the-door . . . From his manner, I could not tell whether he was interested in his psychotherapy, although his mother said he always remembered when it was his session day. After some sessions, his piano teacher's letter confirmed to me his interest in the therapy and his transference onto me. In the course of the sessions, I learned from mother that she was Breton, and that the father was a naturalised Polish Jew. She had not known, when she married him, what 'Jewish' meant and had never learned anything about it from what her husband said, because he was not religious. It all happened between 1934 and 1935 when she was 19 years old. She had met him one Sunday while out walking with a friend from her village, who like her had been sent to Paris. She was a maid-of-all-work, with board and lodging with her employers. Her husband was 15 years older than her and was the first man she got to know, as she was shy. They were married at church in Paris according to her tradition, and her mother came from Brittany for this. She herself was not a practising Christian although she said she was a believer and had some special devotion to Mary. Her mother and childhood friends would not have understood if she didn't get married in church; her husband was not religious and was happy to please her. The children were baptised together one summer in Brittany, when Leon was 5 years old, which was the first time she returned to her mother's after having left her home region (this was the summer of the evacuation). Father had agreed to the baptism in a letter but they had never spoken of it again. Of her religion, she still retained some hymns in Latin or Breton dialect that she liked to sing in the workshop, the tunes of which Leon knew well although he never pronounced the words. The couple got on well together; both worked in the same little family clothing workshop that had welcomed her husband on his immigration from Poland seven or eight years earlier. She was the sole surviving child in a family of five children of which some died very young and the others a little older, but she had only vague memories of them. She had not passed the school certificate and said she had not been capable of it. She had done an apprenticeship in needlework with some nuns in Brittany. Her parents were poor, which was why she came to Paris, at first as a maid, and then after meeting her husband, she gained employment through him at the workshop where he worked. A friend of hers from Brittany had taken her as a lodger for a while, then she married and lived together with her husband and then Leon was born. It was a very close family; mother never had severely to scold or correct the children, and father was very gentle with them. Father was very industrious with his hands and set them up in a small dwelling in the suburbs with an adjoining kitchen garden in which he grew vegetables; but despite the interest he had in Leon and that Leon had in his father, the child was too weak and easily tired to help his father in the garden. He would sit and watch him.

Mother worried about the educational future of Leon; she wasn't able to help him, having herself not studied much and being able to read only slowly, she said (privately, I thought the chanting speech of Leon might imitate the way his mother read). Father, not having been educated in French, could not help his son either, and he was the only emigrant from a family that had remained in Poland. Mother had seen photographs of a sister of his who had written him a very nice letter upon his marriage. Leon's sister, almost 6 years old, was already at primary school and learning very well. In contrast with Leon, she could not sing but was lively and nimble and was already helping her mother around the house and her father in the garden. I also learned that in September 1939, father, as a naturalised French citizen, had been mobilised; all primary schools had just been closed and mother left for her parents' home in Brittany. There, Leon did go to school, as he had been going a little to a primary school in Paris that was right next door to his parents' workshop.

In Brittany, his school attendance was quite irregular; being 6 years old, he should have been going, but the school was not close at all and his way of walking made him tired, even when accompanied by his mother. There was no canteen and the children had to return home for lunch and then set off for school again. Mother felt that this missed first year at school was a handicap for Leon in what followed. After the defeat of 1940, father, whose unit had fallen back, was demobilised in the south of France and returned to Paris, where mother rejoined him and they both returned to their work, despite the disappearance of the boss of their workshop and some other workers (mostly Jews who had left Paris and, unlike Leon's father, not returned). Under the Germans, Leon's father should have worn a yellow star but refused. This was when he explained again to his wife that he was a French citizen and had been mobilised, and that because of this believed he would have nothing to fear; but that he was also Jewish – about which she had no understanding. She had thought that what Germans held against the Jews was that they were usually rich, but why take against her husband, who wasn't? Anyway, her husband had to hide; he stayed at home to work while she continued to go to the workshop in the same locality where some French, non-Jewish friends who were kind to her gathered. The work was very different to what they had been doing before the war: mending rather than making new things, because of the lack of cloth. She brought clothes to her hidden husband and when they were done, returned them to the workshop. Having total trust in me, she told me that her husband had dug a hole in the garden, camouflaged it with branches, and slept there at night as the Germans had already come to arrest Jews in the neighbourhood and always came at night or in the early hours.

During the day, her husband worked from home; she left in the morning with the children, who went to the school next door to her workshop. They returned four and a half hours later, and it was there, in the same building as the workshop, that the piano teacher lived. Having heard Leon singing, he started to give him almost daily lessons in exchange for no payment but that the workshop sometimes did things for him and she sometimes gave him some black-market flour and butter brought from the suburbs by one or other of her colleagues. Mother also recounted to me a 'ritual' of hers, which involved her children coming into her bed on a Sunday morning, as there wasn't time on other days; and while father was preparing breakfast, she would go on all fours with just her head above the sheets, with the two children underneath her and they would play, yapping, at being a mummy dog and her puppies. This game and been inaugurated in Brittany where her own widowed mother lived alone with a bitch and her puppies. Playing together, she and her children had invested in this game that had become a weekly moment of happiness for the family. Father would laugh watching them entertaining themselves in this way, and she saw no harm in it. She spoke to her husband like a little girl might to a big person of neutral sex. She described herself as a little unsocialised when she met her husband – shy with boys and quiet with girls, knowing only her friend from her home village who had like her been sent out to work – this was up until she got married, when her husband became everything to her. She got along very well with her friends at the workshop and they had become a second family for her.

In terms of sexual relations, she was indifferent and what she loved was to be cuddled, close to the husband who was so kind to her. Her pregnancies went well, she had breastfed the children completely for almost a year, which was the way in Brittany; and she took them with her everywhere until they were too heavy to be carried by her, and then it would be in a pushchair.

During the first two sessions, Leon appeared to me dazed and mute, or almost, in front of his drawing. If I asked him questions about the drawing, or about what his mother had said about him in front of him, he did not answer. It was only in the fourth session that I understood what had happened. I could have understood by the third, but didn't until the fourth and then more clearly in the fifth: in fact, Leon was responding eight days later, when he came to a session, to questions I had put to him the week before. When I understood this and congratulated him for not answering without thinking properly about it, telling him that this was a sign of intelligence, his eyes – until then a little bulging and expressionless – shone with joy. I then asked him to make a plasticine model. He appeared not to have heard (this was the fourth session). When he arrived at the fifth, still with the same drawing and behaviour (holding onto walls and slumping onto the table), he quickly took the modelling clay and made some pieces out of it – four sausages of exactly the same size that he put on the table, lined up next to each other. And then he stopped. I congratulated him and said that he certainly had in his heart something he wanted to say to me about this model – maybe that there are four of them in his home, four of the same, of the same family – or perhaps he had another idea. The following week, he arrived still slowly and clinging to the walls and with the same drawing. In complete silence, he took the model and his idea of four sausages of the same size and did exactly the same as in the previous session, and then having contemplated the work and still sprawled on the table and resting on his forearms and part of his hands, continued to make another two sausages of the same length but slimmer. He then tried to assemble the six cylindrical pieces without my understanding what he was trying to do. I made the same statement – that he was surely trying to make something and to say something by what he was making; I didn't understand it but I wanted to understand and maybe would see a little more the next time. The following week he presented in the same slow manner, but this time hardly touching the wall in the small space he had to cross before reaching the table – and managed to cross this space without putting his hand on the table to support him as he sat down, as he had done on every previous occasion.

His drawing was different – a boat, also geometrical and empty as had been the house, but the spread-out 'n' that had been the sky above the house was now below the boat (doubtless representing water). Leon said not a word and immediately took to making models. Using the same elements as previously and quickly creating cylindrical sausages and adding a quite neatly made plate, he constructed a seat with a plate for a back and said to me: 'It's a chair,' chanting the syllables. I asked if the chair was happy with its fate of being a chair and if he had made it for someone. There was no response either to the first or the second question. The following week he came with a drawing of the same boat as the previous time, but this time the sheet was not big enough to contain the boat. The front and the back as well as the top of the triangle of sails were outside the frame of the page. The boat's hull came to the bottom limit of the page like the houses of the first drawings. He found a few elements of the chair in the plasticine box and began again, slowly and carefully to make the object.

> 'It's a chair,' he said after a silence in which he looked alternately at the object and at me, and added, 'It's happy to be a chair' (the answer to my question of the previous week).
> I said, 'Is it waiting for someone?'
> 'Yes.'
> 'So, someone might come and sit on it?'
> At this point in time, he started to make a little man. An ovoid, smooth body with a ball-head joined to it, two curved sausages for the legs. Then a triangular plate, pointed at the top, for a hat like the triangle of the boat's sails, was joined to the head-ball. And on the front of this, he stuck two little balls as eyes and in the space between them scored a hole with a pencil for the nose-mouth. No ears, no hair, no neck, nor arms. He put the man figure lying down on the floor in front of the chair.
> 'What's this?'
> No response.
> 'A man? You?'
> 'Yes.'
> 'Do you want to sit on the chair?'
> No response.
> 'Does the chair want you to sit on it?'
> Without saying anything, he put the man on the seat, bending his legs to make them touch the floor in from of the chair's legs; then he pressed the back of the man very hard against the back of the chair.
> 'Is the man happy?'
> 'Yes.'
> In silence, both of us contemplated the object he had made for a long time.
> Me: 'What is he thinking, this little man?'
> No answer.
> 'Is he a friend of the chair?'
> No answer.
> 'Is the chair happy?'
> 'Oh, yes,' said Leon with conviction and added, 'It is happier than the little man.'
> I looked questioningly at him.
> 'And yes, when he leaves, she will keep his back and the little man will no longer have a back,' and he smiled a sarcastic little smile.
> I asked: 'But will he have kept his head, his bottom and his legs?'
> No answer but a facial expression that looked to me like that of a child on his potty, straining to pass a motion and bloating out his tummy. That was the end of the session.

The following week, mother asked to speak to me alone. They had come early one weekday morning to arrest her husband; luckily, he had been hiding in the hole in the garden and they had not found him. They hadn't looked there. They had woken her up and also the children, and questioned her. She said what she had to say: that her husband had gone to the free zone and that she had no news of him. They had questioned the children and they had not replied, they were barely awake. They had undressed Leon; she didn't know why. And they had told her that she had the right to a divorce. They then asked the children what had happened to their father and they had said they didn't know. Since then, Leon had been distraught. He had wet his bed, he had vomited after the police had gone, and he had had diarrhoea all day afterwards. I asked, 'Had this diarrhoea already begun before the police visit?' (I was thinking of his mimicking of defaecation and my perplexity about what this might mean).

'But yes,' she said, 'He started having diarrhoea the day after his last session.'

And what had most surprised her was that it was not during the day but when he was in bed. On the other hand, he had not vomited until after the visit of the Germans, and also for the three days since then he had urinated in bed. She was keen to tell me that he had been clean very early, because she had been very attentive, and that she had always changed her babies as soon as they were wet to avoid a murderous cold reaching their abdomens (her brothers and sisters having died at an early age). I asked if she knew why the German soldiers had made her son undress; 'no.' I explained that it would have been to see if Leon had been circumcised. She knew neither the word not what it meant. Had she not noticed if her husband was circumcised? No, she said, but she didn't know how men were made (she meant the penis). She remembered that when they had first had sexual intercourse, her husband had told her she could look and that she had to know that he was Jewish. She had answered him by saying that she didn't know what this was, but that it changed nothing for her, as she loved him. And up until the obligatory wearing of the yellow star, which he should have accepted because he was Jewish, she had known no better and was still ignorant of the rite of circumcision.

'Ah, that's why they undressed him! It was to have a look. Because they asked me if the children were Jewish and I answered that my husband was French, that I was French and the children too.'

In her reasoning, her husband, like lots of Jews, believed himself to be a citizen under the protection of France, having been naturalised and even mobilised under her flag. She added that faced with the risk of arrest, her husband had gone to try and see if he could get to the free zone and if he managed to find accommodation there, she was to join him with the children.

Mother left and Leon arrived, seeming very tired. He went directly from the door to the chair without once pressing against the wall and without slumping either onto the chair or the table. He sat normally, looking at me – not drawing, not making models. I spoke to him about what his mother had told me. Leon told me that his father had left 'for good' and that he would go and find him with his mother and sister, once he had found a house there where there was no war. I spoke to him about the last models he had made and about how the chair-back had wanted to keep the back of the boy. He told me what his mother had already told me at our first sessions, usually alone, as Leon, being so slow with the drawing he was making, left her alone with me for a while.

> 'When I was small, and my sister too, Mummy wanted us to stay on the potty and would tie us to it.'
> 'Did you like it?'
> He did not know if he had liked it, but his sister hadn't. She had cried so hard that her mother hadn't done it to her; and when little sister was not tied, mother no longer did that to him. Did he remember how old he was when that happened?
> 'It was before I was 4 or 5 years old, in Brittany, according to what they told me or at least what I understood of what they told me. I understood mostly that grandma didn't want the little one crying and that's why Mummy stopped doing it,' – and then stopped it for him, although he didn't cry. It was certainly the same year that they had begun the ritual of the bitch with her puppies. I spoke to him about his new bedwetting.
> 'Mummy said it was because the soldiers came to look for Daddy and they frightened me.'
> 'And is that true? Were you frightened?'
> He didn't know.
> 'What did the soldiers want?'
> 'They wanted to see my willy,' he said, looking a little embarrassed.

So I explained circumcision to him and that this was how one knew if a man or boy was Jewish or not. If one is Jewish, you are circumcised; it is like baptism, only it can be seen. One removed the little bit of skin at the end of the willy in little boys – and I gave the real name of both the penis and the foreskin. I said that in his father's family, that of his father's father, the day of circumcision was when the boy was given his first name, that this was a day of celebration, like that of baptism in his mother's family in Brittany. When he had been baptised at church, his father had not been there because he was away being a soldier, but he had written and given his consent for him and his sister to be baptised Christians. On that day, his foreskin had not been cut, they had had water poured on their heads and they were given their first names. I took the opportunity, as I was talking about the willy and foreskin, to mention the erection of the penis, and saw that Leon was paying close attention. I noticed that at this session, when speaking about the departure of his father and of his undressing by the Germans, his verbal rhythm had become almost normal, with at times little frozen silences, with an indifferent air – a little like a stammerer who stops himself while looking for the word that will allow him to continue his sentence. After talking about the penis and circumcision, I was silent for a while and then said, 'Do you know the difference between girls and boys?'

> He said: 'Mummies have boobies, girls don't have them and fathers neither.'
> 'And you – do you have them?'
> 'Yes, I have them a little bit, I have more than my sister but less than my mum.'
> 'And haven't you noticed that your sister can't do a wee like you do? That she is not made like you down there?'
> He answered: 'No, they have hair that hides it, except Daddies who have in on their tummies and also their faces, and they don't have blond hair like girls.'
> Their hair colour? His sister was blonde, like her mother, and he was chestnut, like his brown-haired father (and whom Leon said had the same hair colour as he when he was little). He would become brunette when he grew up. I told him in precise language about the reality of sexual differences – about the absence of penises in girls and women and asked him what he knew about or could say about that. He replied that he thought it was good that it didn't grow on his sister but with his mother – he believed she had one. She hadn't said anything about it to him.
> Had he asked her?
> 'No, I didn't ask her, but cows have four with milk to be milked. Goats have the same – I think two of them. With dogs, it's like for mummies. They haven't got hair there.' And he indicated the spot of his belly-button in the middle of his abdomen. 'They have lots of babies, and need lots of nipples on the belly to feed them, but they get drowned afterwards.'

I am quoting the text exactly as I had written it, while he was speaking – at a normal rhythm. We were witnessing a loosening of speech, like a loosening of excrements, could we say, about the fantasies of confused and disparate body images. All this began with a seat, a piece of furniture and a back that had become a thing. The models revealed vague ideas and anxieties about being grabbed, of castration, confusion about sex, hair, breasts, navels and moral judgments. It was good that his sister hadn't got a willy or breasts, and good that he was like his mother – incredible that mother had no penis – but nipples were as good as.

The treatment was coming to an end. I was aware and hopeful that the family had soon to leave for the free zone to be with father, if he had succeeded in crossing the demarcation line. For the subsequent sessions, mother deliberately came alone before Leon to speak to me about the questions I had advised her son to ask her. After our meeting, I had told Leon to tell his mother all that we had talked about. She had been quite embarrassed – she didn't know how to address questions like those. So, we had a session together, all three of us; he and she would talk together and she would look at me for help in responding to him. Parentage, that of Leon, erections, conception, pregnancy, birth, that of Leon, breastfeeding, that of Leon, the birth of his little sister, the sexual forms of girls and adult women, the social futures of his sister and himself, the prohibition of incest in humans – all of this was addressed by the linkage of words and ideas. At the moment when incest was in question, mother intervened by talking about the bitch at his grandmother's house in Brittany. Leon cut her off, saying, 'Yes, she had puppies with her son.' This allowed me to say that what happened with animals was not allowed to happen for humans. Leon then told me that his piano teacher was not married, that he had told him that he was married to his music and that that was much better. Mother smiled, amused. I answered saying that he was anyway a man and that there were musicians who were married to women while being married just as much to their music, and who had children – not with their music but with women.

Leon replied: 'But if you are married, you have to get divorced, the Germans said that, and it is very expensive.'

His mother stared at him, astonished.[24] I told him that when people loved each other like his mother and father did, they didn't get divorced; that the Germans had only said this because they believed that people like his father, who were Jewish, were bad; and I added that it was because the Germans were stupid that they thought this. His mother would not get divorced and soon they would join their father in the free zone. I quickly drew a map of France to be able to explain to him what I meant by the occupied zone, the free zone and the line of demarcation – words commonly used by us and all around us at that time.

At the end of the session, mother asked me if she could also bring her daughter, who like her brother also wanted to know things, as she didn't know how to answer them having herself never been taught any of these things. She just didn't know what to say. Leon was in complete agreement that his sister should come too. The following session, which was in fact the last, was spent with both children and mother. The little girl knew about the absence of a penis in girls and also about motherhood, but she did not know about the penetration necessary for fertilisation. She made an immediate link with her grandmother's bitch and the packs of dogs in the street, about which she and her friends would talk: 'They climb on each other, they are stuck together – it's not nice . . .' I mentioned the prohibition of incest for humans, which left her contemplative. Then I saw her exchange sideways glances with her mother, who said: 'There you are – she's got you! You who are always saying you are going to marry your father!'

> I said: 'We always say that when we are little, it's just a joke; but when we grow up we learn the truth. Your mother didn't marry your grandpa – her father – and your dad didn't marry either his mother or his sister.' (They had seen their father's sister in a photo.)

24 It was a wedding in Brittany and the journeys of the couple and a witness, a friend from the workshop, would have been too expensive. This is why they got married in Paris and paid for her mother's journey from Brittany.

She laughed and said: 'Well, without this rule we wouldn't have Mummy!'
'Exactly,' I said. 'And the children you will have with your husband, who is
now a boy whom you don't know, will have your mother as a grandma and
your father as a grandpa. And if your brother marries, you will be the aunt
of his children, and he will be the uncle of yours.'
Leon joined the conversation, saying, 'I won't get married, ever . . . or
maybe . . . well, if I do, it will be with my piano teacher . . . or maybe I will
be . . .' He could not continue as his little sister had burst out laughing:
'That can't happen – a man marrying another man! A man always marries a
woman . . .'
'Yes,' said Leon. 'Well then I will do like he did and marry my music.'
I said, 'Yes, maybe . . .'
His sister said angrily: 'That's not fair! Music is not a lady. I want to be an
aunt, so you've got to marry because if you don't, I won't get to be an aunt!
Music doesn't make children!' The children bickered on, mother smiling
and amused, and so the family said their adieus to me and left.

I received a letter from mother telling us that she had too much to do, she was
too busy to bring Leon here, she was packing. She was going to leave for the free
zone where her husband had found work and accommodation for them. Leon was
doing very well – her friends at the workshop considered him transformed. The
letter continued, detailing this for me: at school, he had begun to read well, to
write and to count and he came home with good marks every night. He enjoyed
hopping and had even begun to play ball games and to run. The letter continued:
mother had been very scared one day when she came home to find her children
not there; she had found them hidden in the hole in the garden, playing a trick
on her. She continued, saying that she couldn't wait to see her husband and then
thanked me: mothers should be told, she said, that it was incredible that the doctors hadn't found out earlier what it was that made her son not like other children;
and she added that she no longer played at being a bitch with puppies (following
my recommendation). She missed this a little, but she had understood what I was
saying and that it was for the good of the children. Her husband and children were
everything to her and she would do anything to make them happy and well.

I have recounted the case of Leon in full and in detail for it to be understood how
child psychoanalysis allows us to grasp the organising unconscious functioning,
the symbolic of the body at work from the oral and anal stages of the libido before
conscious reflection, and how the narcissism of the man- or woman-to-be invests
his sexual future, which therefore depends on the manner in which the child is
mothered and brought up, well before knowing the particularities of sexual differences. Here, we can very easily see how desire is damaged according to the
constitution of the body image and its effects on the functioning of Leon's bodily
schema, the damage of this loving upbringing of a child tied to his seat. The body
image of the subject whose desire was forbidden to act upon the motor functioning of the bodily schema itself prohibited healthy neurological potentialities that

nonetheless remained intact. Motor skills, the agility of distal parts of the body – hands, fingers, larynx, eyes and feet – were possible but not the cohesion of the images between these, and therefore the linking tonicity of the bodily schema. In addition, we can observe how in representing a chair, Leon made the back and the seat absent – illustrating the absence of the seat and back in his own bodily schema. We can understand that this child, who never had toys to hand and who, belted to his seat, could only watch the adults living, while developing an apparent ideational, verbal and corporal delay, but who preserved and even developed, unbeknownst to the adults, a potential agility with his fingers in watching the sewing work of all those nimble hands in the clothing workshop and had introjected what he saw. In this case, we saw how the same upbringing was submitted to and integrated, with damage, by the boy but not by the girl, who was 30 months younger. She too could not resolve her Oedipus complex but at least she had set it up. By 'setting up the Oedipus,' I mean that she had fantasised the incestuous marriage to her father, while Leon had not even set up his Oedipus, because of his canine identification, which made him a puppy and like his sister the puppy of a canine mother – without doubt imaginarily incestuous with regard to his beloved father, the husband and father of the children, but not sexually desired.

And what I have not mentioned is that added to all of this was the truncation of the paternal surname – mother told me about this in I don't remember which session and it was noted in the file: 'such-and-such' known as 'so-and-so.' They had used 'Karpo' for 'Karpocztski' or something even more complicated, mother being unable to pronounce the surname of her husband. Leon had heard this altered name, different from the one he knew, and had always been called this when he was at school in Brittany, but not at nursery school in Paris, where they called the children by their first names. In the workshop and in everyday life, his parents, school friends and he himself spoke only the first two syllables of his paternal surname, the whole being judged too complicated for French mouths. It is likely that this mutilation of his paternal surname and the revelation he had had at school added their symbolically mutilating impact to Leon's relative imaginary confusion about sexual difference, with regard to which he had not received a humanising castration. That must have overdetermined a symbolic undermining that led to the identification of the human subject, whose hair colour was the only bodily characteristic similar to that of his father, with a feminine or asexual half-individual mammal.

The game of bitch and puppies, which had continued every Sunday for at least three years, had been kept up ever since that important summer of their baptisms, from the time that the sister came to live with Leon and his mother in the absence of father. That was the year they were separated from their father, who was mobilised for more than a year, up until the end of 1940. The game with mother had perpetuated the canine identification of that time, when grandmother's bitch had had puppies that were said to be those of her son. This is what gave an imaginary authorisation of incest within the family relationship of Leon and his mother when they were together in the absence of the father, but without Leon ever speaking of it. He had displaced this fantasy onto the chair, slowly constructed from assembled phallic-shaped elements, and which took possession of the plasticine man (who prudently had hesitated to give himself up to it), took a sadistic pleasure in stripping him of his back and his pelvis. It was through associations referring to Papa who was not to know (the marching song known to all children from primary school age onwards: 'I've lost the doh of my clarinet – oh, if Papa knew this . . .') that I understood that this must have something Oedipal about it, but was never made explicit either by him or by me.

We can see how in the psychoanalysis of children, expression by model-making, drawing and the words that the child connects with these have for the session the value of a dream that can be decoded; the work of the unconscious, given the opportunity of being psychoanalysed and with the psychoanalyst putting his unconscious free associations in the service of the treatment reveals its problematic. At the age of 1, Leon, in his boyish narcissism and as the subject of desire that had not yet been prohibited by weaning, could manifest his active drives in the dexterity of his fingers and the vocalisations of his larynx in the fast tempo of a song without words, which defended his future integrity as a man. Leon's sexuality in its path from the oral to the genital stage, had been blocked almost completely after weaning at the moment of the blossoming of anal libido, because of the restraint imposed on his hands, arms and then his whole body. He was impeded in all articulations – labial, dental and that of the phallic laryngo-tracheal air column. His anal sexuality did not invest the phallic drives active in his body in the skeleto-muscular bodily schema. This prevalence of passive drives inhibited the tonicity of the scapular-humeral and the sacral-iliac joints, the hips and the knees, giving an absence of vertical structure that at first sight you could think was the result of a sort of biological myopathy. His strange way of speaking allowed him not to identify with the accent of his father or the way of speaking of women – his mother and his sister; unconsciously, this is how he resisted feminine identification. But everything had to be frozen, in his active cognitive linkage, in his vocal, lingual and buccal articulation and in the links to be made between his optical perceptions and his speech, in pronouncing the phonemes of letters or of musical notes that he could read. According to his schoolteacher, he could neither read nor write, but it is probable that with some patience, one could have allowed him to recognise letters and read with his eyes without pronouncing the phonemes, as his piano teacher noticed he could with musical notes, whose graphic representation, decoded by his eyes, passed directly through the intermediary of his fingers to their execution on the piano. In short, his fundamental narcissism remained marked by a passive oral ethos or near enough; but Leon as a subject retained a masculine desire in his relationship with the world, things and space. His interpersonal relationships had become set in a concrete pattern that the stereotyped drawing of the house illustrated. The impact of occupational therapy was to increase his obsessionality into an invasive inhibition. His bodily schema was invalidated by a body image where, to have value in the eyes of his mother, he had to accept to be her erotic part object, oral or anal, that is to say fragmented, the fragments being kept together by an external seat, like a grabbing mouth. In order to keep some cohesion between the fragments and to keep his bodily schema whole, he was obliged constantly to find relay points upon which to lean – things or people – physical supports – exterior to his body, which was about to undo itself like a puzzle.

Through this clinical case, one can understand how the seat, which to start with in the embryo is a caudal region, becomes successively a region emitting urine in utero, then a uro-excremental and genital region, then a region of a muscular tone specific to verticality for the bodily schema of the pelvic girdle, with its two out-buddings that are the lower limbs that are at first non-functional. Then, this region of the pelvis develops a uro-genital focus and an image of needs, and a third focus – that of sex in the form of a third member in the boy (the penis) which at first has no other substantial sensation than that of the urinary function. However, the penis is erectile during urinary miction in boys until around 28 or 30 months. Then in a few days, because of the development of the organ named *verumontanum*, the penis when in communication with the bladder is flaccid, while when in commu-nication with the seminal vesicles becomes erect during this period of their non-functional development. Genital desire, as much as urinary need, is accompanied by an erectile penile image in the boy until 28 or 30 months. In the girl, the visible signal of sexual sensation, the penis, is absent, but the urinary function is present. The clitoris and the vulva are erectile organs – one phallic and the other orbicular at the entrance of the vagina; they are invisibly sensitive in the encounter of the girl with other people who elicit in her an emotional or physical attraction. The excretory urinary function could be confused with the anal function; and in lan-guage, mothers talk about 'front bottoms' and 'back bottoms,' 'small business' or 'big business.' Except through the sense of smell, which discriminates very well the emission of urine from that of faeces, children are allowed in language to make no difference between poo-ing, weeing and sexual matters. The seat can become the object of obsession, becoming like a static thing if the sitting posture is imposed for too long in babies, who must progressively experiment in space for their bodily schema to become dynamic and motor, their agility becoming pos-sible because of their neuro-muscular development. They need to displace objects and furniture by pushing and pulling, to grab and change the places of portable things, to throw them away and recover them; they need to show that they are masters of these part objects in the space outside their bodies. This mastery of external objects linked with adults is a displacement of the mastery of digestive part objects in the internal space – food, faeces, urine. When the development of the spinal cord allows it, children of both sexes have to sit, crawl, move their bodies around on their bottoms and then on all fours, and the development of the *cauda equine* gives sensory-motor feedback thanks to the completion of fine nerve endings in the feet and perineum; they have the pleasure of moving around on all fours and then on two feet while pushing a chair or leaning upon a fixed support, before being able to let go and walk, then run, climb and do acrobatics just for fun.

For Leon, a passive child with swollen tissues, his identification with four-legged dogs, animals, did not authorise verticality. This identification related to the close merger, to the heat of mother in the nest with little sister, all concomitant with an image of incestuous and fertile sexuality between the son dog with the mother bitch. This motherhood of the bitch – giving birth to puppies and suckling them, as he had been able to observe his mother breastfeeding his sister – these consciously registered scopic images in his memory were therefore not totally without human references, but human symbolisation had been scrambled at every stage. The oral and anal stages of the pelvis made him into a part object that could be additive (taking in food) or subtractive (putting out excrements) linking both of these with the functions of addition or subtraction symbolised in arithmetic. What should have allowed reading and arithmetic was invalidated by the fragmentation of the body image and its effect on the bodily schema. The uro-genital stage was confused with a static ventral and caudal basal image (men's genital hair supposed to be at their umbilicus and called the belly). Bellies were what others had – mummies and daddies – but not him.

The linkage of scapular girdle–pelvic girdle by the vertebral column causes the cohesive linkage and imaginable tonicity of the bodily schema. However, in this child there were only fragmentations that impeded the cohesion usually acquired through the experiences of moving around and of free play of a body that constructs by way of trial and error the possibility of speaking this body and building up a representation of the bodily schema: a preconscious and conscious abstraction of the real and current powers of the animate body, as ego (me) or object (you), among others in time and space.[25] For Leon, the oral stage was linked with the supposedly penile teats and with the milk-producing belly of the bitch ('but afterwards, the puppies get drowned'). The mother herself was confusing human subjects with a phallic animal entity – the bitch who had a dog-son who was the father of her own puppies; the mother was playing in identification with the dogs and the children slotted in with her fantasy.

For Leon, his father was reduced to the truncated signifier of the first syllables of his surname and to the foreign accent that vaguely justified this reduction, connected with the nudity forced upon the boy by the Germans and the fact that according to the law, Jews should be divorced – as was said to mother by the police officer who came to arrest his father. What this man said triggered a loss of sphincter control, perhaps inducing Leon-the-puppy to drown himself in his nocturnal wee. No, the man did not scare him but he had said that the temporary companionship of Leon's female-mother with his male-father-Jew-more-than-man

25 Translator's note: This is a highly complex sentence in which certain theoretical constructs are implied but not spelled out. It seems to imply that the abstract concepts (or pre-concepts) of 'me' and 'you' – ego and object – are constructed upon the physical capacities of the developing body. These capacities along with the bodily schema are in turn developed through the trial and error of free play and movement linked with speech. Leon's lack of motor experiences, because of the strapping of him to the seat, did not allow the development of his bodily schema; his body image remained fragmented and, consequently, his ability to construct very basic concepts was also impaired.

had to end. His father, preparing Sunday breakfast, could pass as a breeder of children who are incestuous puppies. It has to be said that Leon did not know his maternal grandfather, the grandmother from Brittany having been widowed for a long time. Despite the birth of his sister, the masculine and paternal imago was not brought into a genital coupling – probably because his mother was frigid. For Leon, the masculine paternal imago seemed to be held by the music teacher – the only person who allowed him to invest the dynamic motor functioning of his fingers upon the piano keys (immense teeth of a sonorous piano-thing, through which Leon's virtuosity could be manifested) and the speed of his eyes in deciphering the musical score – a sheet where the notes and rhythm are printed on two staves of five parallel lines, perhaps associated with the five fingers of the hand in the bodily schema – fingers invested by him and perhaps fragmented from his body image, but nonetheless efficient in expressing his exceptional taste and talent on the piano. It is his beloved teacher who recognised him as a musician, who looked after him and who respected his parents; he at last allowed the subject to express himself by compensating for the child's weakness with the help of his own body, by supporting the child's body whose shoulders and arms were not able on their own to support the weight of the forearms, wrists and hands. The complete recovery of this boy of 8 happened through transference onto me, a 'me' associated in a triangular situation (me–him–mother), and then with the letter from his piano teacher in another threesome (me–him–teacher). Lastly, with me, him, his sister and his mother, it was a situation of four in which we talked about the father and the danger for him in moving around – the reason he was not able to meet me. But he was very interested in his children and in particular in his son, and to the coming and going to treatment that his mother took time off work to facilitate.

The recovery of Leon says more than many theories about the weakened bodily schema of a neurologically healthy organism and about the way in which the unconscious body image can be the origin of the symbolic dysregulation of the body's functioning: his boyish desire, progressively becoming more phallic at the genital stage, could not be invested without endangering the ethos developed in his early childhood intersubjective relationships.

We saw that for Leon, the body image:

1 Had no clear human reference.
2 Was fragmented at both the passive oral and anal stages – neither oral castration (although he had been weaned) nor anal castration were followed by a symbolisation of drives whose expression in bodily contact was thenceforth prohibited.
3 The body image was genitally ambiguous, not to say absent. It is certain that the psychoanalytic work did far more than any placement in IMP[26] and specialised knowledge in re-education.

---

26 Translator's note: IMP stands for *Internat Medico-Psychologique* – meaning a residential setting for children with emotional and behavioural difficulties.

What was psychoanalytic in the story we have related (as opposed to a psycho-therapeutic re-education of psychomotor functioning) is that the transference allowed Leon himself to speak the words and signify in language what allowed him as a subject to re-find his desire. The psychoanalyst knew nothing about the passive masochistic pleasure, both fascinating and dreaded, taken by Leon and that had sustained him in living. The turning point of his treatment was my notic-ing the sadistic satisfaction in his smile and the quickness of his reaction in speak-ing about the pleasure experienced by a thing (the chair) in snatching something away to the detriment of a living being.

It is always like this, whatever the case that comes our way, even if we have some inkling of the generalities of the body image at a certain point in the evolu-tion of the child. The essence of my work is to shed light on the unconscious pro-cesses in children, in their relationship with this and that mother and father, and to try by clinical example to make psychoanalysts listen to others. Anyway, we know nothing about the lived experience of each case, beyond common processes. Only he, the child, this other, can know. Thanks to this work, perhaps what we gain is a sensitivity in listening, in the widest sense of the word.

Whatever knowledge we gain through the testimony of others, nothing can replace the observation by all our senses of what comes from this other human being. Leon, whose presentation was that of stupefaction, debility and even psy-chosis, proved what we know – that behind even such an aspect as this, there is a desiring subject. He tried to communicate with the subject present in us psycho-analysts, who are another desiring member of the human species. How do these meet? How do these two halves of a shell, these two interlocutors, meet each other? How, symbolically, do the adult psychoanalyst and the child patient, both of whom have demands and desires on their part, manage to do this?

The psychoanalyst, an ex-analysand, is only informed by his own experience of analysis, of his history and the relational difficulties that belong to his own his-tory, those he could have re-found and relived with his analyst. This is why what we, who have become psychoanalysts, witness of the treatment of children is precious in helping other children in the course of development. The language by which the desire of a developing infant is expressed, and the language of a young child affected by disturbances who recovers his order by the expression of past relational difficulties that he relives with his psychoanalyst in the treatment – this is what serves as our working medium and that allows the extension of psychoa-nalysis to the treatment of psychotics.

I don't know what would have become of Leon in IMP, a place of education and socialisation where the educational staff are extremely devoted and often even informed by psychoanalysis, in other words tolerant of the children's modes of expression that don't conform to what an ordinary school would expect of them. We had already seen the failure and even the worsening of Leon's state over 20 sessions of psychomotor therapy. I think this case proves to us just how necessary it is for every child who presents a low IQ (Leon had a tested IQ of 63, where he had been a precocious baby), or where some mental debility is apparent, whose behaviour seems impaired (without any organic lesion being detected), or who shows aberrant verbal and motor language, to undergo a psychoanalytic investigation before any re-education, rather than after its failure. Before a decision about re-education of the child is made, what is needed is a psychoanalytic investigation that takes the time needed to listen to the parents, who have after all brought the child to a psychoanalyst with a request for help: a decision as to whether the child suffers, if he needs specialised re-education, with or without psychoanalysis in parallel, and above all if he would benefit from a separation from his parents, and a preparation for this, and the same for cases where it is the parents or other children who would benefit from the separation. The whole family – grandparents as well as parents – are stakeholders in the history of this unhappy child. This doesn't mean that they should feel guilty. Leon's mother was guilty of nothing in what happened, while at the same time what happened was because of her; but also because of Leon's complicity and particular sensitivity. His younger sister could not bear the constraint upon her motor functioning that her well-meaning mother wanted to impose on her. The responsibility of the entry into a developmental disorder is not only incumbent upon the parents; sometimes the connivance of desire between the child and the parents can warp the future of the child and even the future of the parents' relationship with their child. It is precisely what psychoanalysis allows us to study. Leon was trapped, 'perverted' is the right word, by his love for his mother, probably because he was a boy; his sister did not fall into the same trap. But Leon had an exceptional sensitivity, a reflective and intuitive intelligence, some precocious libidinal potentialities rich in passive drives – and God knows that he exploited these passive drives. There will be no end to the search for reasons for this trapping of Leon in a static fragmentation anxiety. The important thing was how to help him find a way out of this shell that obstructed his communication. This is what the analysand-psychoanalyst training and the analytic study of the transference relationship can help us discover.

From there, once again what would have become of Leon in a medico-pedagogic institution is difficult to predict, but this would have been an artificial separation, intolerable for him and for his family. Leon would have been supported in an IMP, all children with difficulties are, and every or nearly every one of them triggers the interest and affection of adults devoted to marginal children; but for each of these children, who in their own way is a badly steered 'drunken ship,'[27] there is an adult who tries to help them navigate. But what motivation could Leon have had to get out of the prison in which he was? What would have become of his musical education? Attacked by volatile children, Leon's fine sensibility and slow reactions would have driven him to shut down more and more and maybe even to masochistically enjoy these attacks.

27 'Bateau ivre' is a reference to a poem by Arthur Rimbaud referring to a ship that has lost all bearings, drifts and eventually sinks.

The educative spirit that presides over the work of IMPs is expressed through methods that attempt to use in children what is left of their not-yet awakened abilities, or maybe not-yet repressed. A tolerant pseudo-familial emotional social milieu – quasi-familial – exerts upon them an enlightened guidance in a climate aimed at making them feel safe. Some children, neglected by parents who are not available to them, find an educative attention that they are ready to trust immediately. The personalised friendship and calm authority of the specialised staff returns some trust in adults to children who had lost this, and gives them support and models for their physical growth and psychosocial development. For children caught up in academic failure and inaptitude in emotional exchanges, speech and language therapy, psychomotor therapy and even supportive psychotherapy allow them a new apprenticeship of being in the world. The maladapted child is supposed to have been deprived of maternal and paternal love that would have given him the education he should have had. The idea of remediation in these residential and therapeutic settings is to 'repair' the effect of damage previously experienced. In an IMP, people act as if the child's relational link with the mother, the nanny, the first 'others' who looked after the child, did not have sufficient quality to ensure the good behavioural and language development of the child. This is the working hypothesis, and why not? Education in an IMP aims to create a new relational bond between the child and the adults, so that the child takes them to be his developmental support and models. The staff team elaborates for each child a pedagogic project that the child's keyworker tries to carry out. This personalised interest plays the auxiliary role to the remaining healthy developmental forces in the child – forces that the adult who has taken on the emotional relationship of parental substitute tries to use to best effect, to elicit the child's effort to adapt to the group to which he belongs.

But the child's own desire, that which had been developing from birth, elaborated in harmony with or in contradiction to the desires of those who looked after him, is forgotten. They cannot take that into account. The past is to be left behind, and here, the child is expected to have a fresh start. Desire and its past structure cannot be taken into account; these are not conditions in which one can take account of or examine the pathogenic role of the child's desire and motivations, or of his unconscious acceptance of failure and marginalisation, or for that matter his submission to being the object of medical and pedagogical concern.

The desire to communicate in a new way can be elicited from a child as a result of the attachment his educator forms with him. This means of motivation involves the eroticisation of the child's relationship with the adult, who can thereby mobilise new libidinal drives upon a foundation of transference of previous relationships. To limit the eroticisation, the educators engineer themselves into a parental and inevitably artificial role, and in doing so play out their own maternal or paternal transference onto the child. Both parties, child and adult, are more or less tricking themselves. At any rate, this transference cannot but be manipulated to the benefit of the child's development, which tends to favour his preferred educator; but the relationship itself cannot be demystified. The transference cannot be analysed because one cannot analyse and enjoy the relationship at the same time. A relationship is acted out in reality and is not only expressed in subtle gestures or spoken. *It is impossible that there be a psychoanalytic treatment* – an analysis of transferences and resistances – *at the same time as education or re-education*, whether it be in a family or IMP setting: in a place where psychoanalysts and analysands live and meet each other, there cannot be psychoanalysis. What I mean is that transference that could be analysed becomes too mixed up with real relationships with reciprocal libidinal benefits, as much for the adults as for the children. Psychoanalysis, whatever the age of the analysand, can only be engaged with by means of the manifest and persevering desire of the patient who suffers and who wants to work to escape from the bad life he finds intolerable. Children's symptoms are the means by which the subject can use his suffering and make it less painful to bear. This means that few children actually want to be analysed, and because they cannot foresee the future that will be denied to them by these symptoms, they may not be anxious about it as may be the adults who can predict a very difficult future for them. The child may come to want this talking therapy because of what his parents or teachers say, if they have confidence in this method and can make him hope for better, and if despite his symptoms, he suffers; and especially when they support his courage in the course of a treatment that may at times be painful, if it is efficient – painful for not only him but also his entourage.

For Leon, what made possible the visit to the Centre was the threat of separation that weighed upon him and his mother. The IMP was the only possibility for Leon's education proposed by his teacher and headteacher, who knew him well. Recourse to psychotherapy had been suggested by the doctor who had examined Leon's neurological state and chronaxies two years previously, who had not detected any organic anomalies and who had said to mother in conclusion: 'Psychotherapy could help your child. His motor debility, like his mental and academic debility, is not organic in origin.' However, mother had not at the time been ready to accept understand or accept this.

It was lucky for Leon that he had reached the point of being placed in an IMP and that both he and his mother were confronted with the pain of imminent and inevitable separation. This was needed to motivate them to turn to a medicopedagogic consultation about a pathological state of passivity that caused psychosocial incapacity. It could be said that Leon was presenting an extremely early hysteria linked with a potentially perverse libidinal state while still being innocent and unconscious of it, as were his parents.

Leon, who came to the Centre on the advice of his piano teacher, had at first been assigned to an occupational therapist, who tried to free up his movement. It was a complete failure. The OT, the doctor who assessed him on arrival and referred him to the OT, his family and everyone who knew him found him even more stupefied and slower than before the referral for remediation. This is what led, in the assessment letter I was given, to the words: 'evolving towards a schizoid state.'

Leon's conscious good will was beyond doubt, as was his mother's, who persevered despite her work, the difficulty in travelling with Leon and the scarceness of public transport. Maybe it was about the unsuitability of the working method. The remediation, with its pedagogic aims, did not take into account the superego prohibition of the unconscious desire of the subject, his body image probably forbade body movements, threatening him with fragmentation.

One could try psychoanalytic work that doesn't aim at breaking down resistances but gives them a chance to be expressed in language other than that of the body itself in his habits and functioning. My desire was to give back to this child his subjective freedom, which was masked by his state as a slow and badly articulated puppet.

With an a priori assumption due to my psychoanalytic training, I was expecting the existence of a fundamental narcissism in conformity with the ethos of his sex, that is to say in agreement with his own bodily schema by which the subject in reality becomes present and is in a relationship with others and with the world. There were no lesions, no organic dysfunction in Leon's body. His physical presentation was therefore linked with the body image he had constructed, and with some imaginary and unconscious motor and tonic incapacities. Leon did not suffer physically apart from 'fatigue in muscular efforts.' If the subject of his desire remained impermeable or even unconsciously resisted remediation and a positive relationship with someone who he hoped could improve his state – which would have allowed him to stay in his family and at his school – it is because the work of the occupational therapist did not address the subject in his history, the subject in the history of his desire. It only addressed Leon's body, a body that was the pathological result of his relational history. The origin of his disability was without a doubt psychogenic, but his disability was truly physical, embodied. His body was really disabled even if that could not be organically explained. I was thinking that as Leon had such hopes from the Centre there was an argument for trying a psychoanalytic psychotherapy.

I therefore planned to listen to what the mother–son dyad had to say, first mother's side of the story (and father's if possible) and then the son's, without aiming to modify anything of the present effect of their pathogenic libidinal fusion, pathogenic at least for Leon.

The psychoanalyst had to trust these two subjects, mother and child, misguided in a fusional magma that neutralised their sexuality, in any case that of Leon, with both of them preserving the pleasure of an archaic, incestuous, reciprocal and unconscious sexuality. It was necessary to listen attentively to what Leon was trying to express mutely in sessions while apparently half asleep. His presentation, his repetitive drawings, poor and stereotyped plasticine models had to be accepted as they were, while knowing quite well that they expressed a message to be decoded; but what? Only Leon could know what his slowness, his clumsiness and his hands were saying. Leon had to be able to give to his creation – representations of things through rudimentary models and drawings – an imaginary life and retrieve the meaning of his desire by lending words to these little bits of plasticine – lending them intentionality, feelings and pleasures. It was for the psychoanalyst to make Leon connect his words and what they expressed with what his mother had said of his history and with the memories that he had kept of it himself.

It is this decoding work by the proxy of transference objects that allowed the analysis of his projection onto the chair of his mother, as the robber of his motor cohesion, who fragmented him – a fantasmatic construction of the passive enjoyment of a loved oral object, available to a cannibalistic subject who was more or less consciously supposed to be in any interlocutor who was interested in him. This way of thinking about oral enjoyment is, for the growing child who faces fantasies of penile mutilation and later genital castration, a source of anxiety. In his history, these anxious fantasies come to the aid of the prohibition of incest, the acceptance of which supports the dynamic and symboligenic effect known as the 'Oedipal resolution.' Leon was 8 years old, but where was he in his development? I could not know. My desire was to understand Leon through his transference relationship with me. I also desired to make him speak rather than mime his resistances, which I respected, so as to allow the return of repressed drives.

My work as a psychoanalyst has been supported by my epistemophilic drive, which made me hope that Leon, if the subject within him could prevail over the ego, could retrieve ideational and psychomotor intelligence included in his human genetic capital, as son of Man and not only son of Woman and subjugated by her; maybe he would be able to retrieve the narcissistic ethos of a human being born healthy from the body of his mother, an ethos that validates the bodily schema of the boy's body itself (or a girl's in other cases), as he goes-on-becoming a man (or woman), that every stage of development calls into question. This calling into question relates bodily schema to the phallus and to the active and passive drives of desire, and castration anxiety at each stage causes a reorganisation of these for the survival of narcissism.[28]

We have seen in the narrative of the sessions *how the symbolisation of the body image can be accomplished through the mediation of made objects.* Transference onto the psychoanalyst helps the child express what he experiences through drawings and models – in this case, Leon's fragmentation anxieties and his enjoyment as a subject who has been entirely alienated as the object of desire of the other. The verbal expression given to these representations allows us to see the child's desire through the imaginary focus upon these objects of projection, created and executed by the child himself. These objects represent him to himself as a subject: they are endowed with intentionality and act like the people who for him have been models in his childhood – transferences made anew upon the person of the analyst. My analytic work was to question him about what in his behaviour raised questions for me, and about those aspects of our relationship in which I felt he was raising certain questions about me.

---

28 I remind you that my suggested definition of narcissism is of a continuum from foetal life until the present of the going-on-becoming in the creative potential of his sex.

What clearly emerges from the case of Leon and explains why any method other than psychoanalysis was doomed to fail is that transference onto someone who wishes to help him, however positive on his side, could only make of him in his relationship with the helping person an object of cannibalistic consumption. In his transference relationship, everybody was like the chair towards the man, mutilating the sketchy unifying cohesion of his body and prohibiting the phallic ethos through the threat of mutilation.

This is what he felt in the pedagogic attitude of the occupational therapist and that he also felt about me during the first sessions, despite the fact that I was only listening and of my acceptance of how he was. This is why he could not answer my questions – questions that interested him, as they resulted in eight days of cogitation! I was interested in what he felt and thought more than what he made for show. Everyone who wanted help, support and guidance for him was felt by Leon to be like the armchair – the armchair toilet of his infancy, which turned him into a somewhat paralysed voyeur, initiated into doing nothing that could be a pleasure for his hands, during which time he would watch everyone else – his parents and their workshop colleagues – show a lot of animation and taking pleasure in working with their hands. It may well have been worse for Leon not to submit to this undermining of his desire for motor pleasure, as this would have confirmed his belonging to the feminine sex (unlike his sister, he accepted his mother's whims and in this way preserved his potential virility). His little sister had refused the coercion of the armchair and kicked up a storm when faced with the seated restraint imposed by their mother. Behind the screen of a caricaturally great motor weakness, the griffins of sexual destiny and entry into flesh had, in defence of this first and last bastion of his human belonging, kept for him a masculine libido and a boy's narcissism that saved the intelligence and sensibility of the future man-in-becoming that was Leon. Behind the weak and badly articulated puppet was a subject whose eyes ran with speed over scored notes and transmitted their meaning to his fingers, which in turn ran at speed over the piano keys; a loving heart, a son and brother loyal to his family, a being with sublimated desires – in brief, a precocious child and a rare being – this was Leon . . . but caught in an early hysterical neurosis and the sexual perversion of a phallic part object of an innocently infantile and incestuous mother.

Leon is one story among many others. There are also a great number of children who present with early anomalies of adaptation when they reach the age where the parents have to give them to society for their instruction and psychosocial training – that is to say to compulsory schooling. Whatever the psychodynamic reasons, taking into account conditions of foetal and post-natal development and then upbringing, all children who do not correspond to the new physical, mental and personality demands laid down by institutions are excluded from attending mainstream school. For them, it will be schools intended to help and re-educate the maladjusted, the poorly socialised, the inarticulate, the physically challenging and the wrong-doers, as if they were not to be respected for what they are – by other children as well as by the teaching adults – which is beings of language, though misguided in a mode of receptivity and expressivity that makes them difficult to integrate. The suffering that is at the origin of this maladaptation of children in living with others of their age is not completely avoidable, as there are many among these who behind their pseudo-organic mask of various delays, incapacity and psychosis are precocious children who have not been recognised as such in the first weeks of their lives, and who were definitively discouraged from trying to communicate with an entourage that did not understand them and did not respond to the questions often posed by their body, as they could not yet speak.

Psychoanalysis brought not only the plague, as Freud said, but also a means of study of the development of the human, for so long immature and dependent on its parents, before the blossoming of its genitality. It especially allows the clarification of those fragile and inevitable moments where the psychic structure is organised in early infancy, the insoluble contradictions between physical needs and relational emotional desires – misunderstandings and contradictions that leave their traces in the future libidinal economies of the subjects, and especially of those precocious in their intelligence and sensibility. It is my wish that if there were sufficient numbers of psychoanalysts interested in the prevention of psychosocial problems by bringing up each child in a manner appropriate to them, we could elaborate rules of behaviour for adults – rules to be respected by all adults living in contact with children, be it in nurseries, hospitals or schools, so that the most gifted do not become, as is their destiny today, clients of institutions for psychotics and the learning disabled. Anyway, it is a pity, especially as it is avoidable.

From birth onwards, the anxieties of desire and of death festoon the axis that links the imaginary with sex, linking our attraction to someone with the fear of displeasing him. The narcissism of each of us is unconsciously obliged to make do with what is the fate of man, masculine and feminine. A human being cannot survive on his own. Harmony with the nursing mother, the male or female tutelary adult is a condition of survival for the baby. We individuate by way of this first vital language-based dependency and we need others in order to be able to bear the dramatic destiny of being both an imaginarily powerful and desiring individual as well as one who is in reality quite powerless. Contact with other humans with difficulties different from or similar to our own brings the possibility of recognising that we all have difficulties and can speak to each other. Psychoanalysis has brought proof that the child, however young, understands what is being said about his being in the world, and proof also that speech can liberate the human being if he succeeds in expressing by these means his suffering to him that listens attentively and without judgement.

We have also learned that the child, before being able to verbalise his affective states, expresses his joy and well-being in good health, and his relational difficulties in functional health problems. Paediatrics is constantly being confronted by functional disturbances in small children, and most of the time, these are of psychogenic origin. If we could allow the mother to talk about what has been happening, and if we say in words to the child what he wants to say but is translating into body language, we see most of these reactive symptoms disappear, without having to prohibit the functional manifestations of bodily disturbance by means of medication and chemicals. It is possible to help human babies to live their inevitable and difficult destiny by helping them to express themselves and by deciphering the meaning of what they enunciate without prematurely stopping them from trying to signify their desires in their own way. I think, for example, about the meaningful screaming of babies who suffer from the anxious ambiance around them and people who want them to be quiet; what these non-sleeping, vomiting babies need is that we understand the meaning of the suffering that they are showing in this way. The work of child psychoanalysts in hospital consultations is all about this. In general, we corner these children by intimidating and medicating them into prematurely stopping signifying their desire in their own way. The impediments to this regulatory activity come from what the adults cannot bear of the expression of their children's suffering. And then they sometimes become anxious themselves, for their own reasons, and their anxiety secondarily contaminates the child, who had been trying to rid himself of his own anxiety by expressing it.

Whatever the cause, these little ones, inhabited as they are by anxiogenic desire for the parents they love, feel that these desires have to be falsified to the point at which they travesty, counteract and pervert them – and all this very early – to suit their parents. Parents are not educators by profession. They serve as initiators and first models. The huge work of prevention and early treatment of the failures of children's psycho-affective health and behaviour falls to the ensemble of the adults within a society and in particular those who dedicate themselves to the education and care of humans – those who mix with the children and are not, as parents are, narcissistically implicated in their imaginary relations with the child. They have to know that an immediate cure of the functional disturbances of the child's *body* will aggravate the *repression* of the feelings and emotions, as long as speech does not come to their rescue by enunciating what their bodies are trying to express.[29]

29 In paediatric departments, mothers and father have to be allowed, even obliged and helped to enter into the cubicle in which the child is isolated, and to touch him, hold him, change him, feed him, speak about him to the nursing assistants and about them to him, as they replace his parents in their absence, and of the doctors who care for them in this temporary place in order to return him cured to his parents. For babies and sick young children, the repetitive sensory contact with mother and father several times a day is indispensable to the preservation of at least the basal body image, and also of functional images. This preservation guarantees a quick retrieval of overall psychosocial health without psychic consequences in the affective or psychosomatic range, after the return home and to health. Two pretexts are put forward for prohibiting or advising against contact with parents: 1. the avoidance of the child's crying at their departure; 2. the avoidance of distress caused to the nursing staff; whereas the emotional reaction of the child is the guarantee of the cohesion of the pre-ego subject in his suffering body. The parents' anxiety is also that of the child and what the nursing assistants say about it allows it to be symbolised and, later on, allows an understanding of what the child says of memories of the period in hospital that was such a trial to him and his parents.

Pathology of the body image in the latency phase (after an Oedipal phase resolved in a timely way)

We have seen that with the Oedipus complex, secondary narcissism is established in the child, that is to say an emotional attitude (active and passive) vis-à-vis oneself as presented to the world by its body, with its given sex, to which pro-creative acts with family members are definitively prohibited. I would say that by the age of 8 at the latest, the latency stage has been established in most children; at the same time that the organic intensity of genital glands quietens, the emotional intensity of the parent–child relationship also becomes muted. This said, we shouldn't forget that from birth every child is unconsciously informed of his sex, because his intuitive and elective desire is attractive to representatives of the other sex. This desire is felt by the child in a confused way in intimate feelings. And this desire is global, although in growing up it will become increasingly focused on the genital region. For the observer, it plays an undeniable role in all emotional choices with regard to the father and mother, as representatives of not only the sex that is attractive to him but also the safety and loving warmth that the subject vitally needs to replenish his being.

When they reach what is called the age of reason, children know that the love of their mother and father for them is not of the same kind as love linked with physical desire between adults of which they have some intuition. Children know that their more or less fantasised desire to access the genital act with their mother or father will not happen, but they need to be told this and it must be signified through the emotional or passionate actions and non-actions of the adults towards them. Unfortunately, when the parents have not had castration from their own parents, children are faced with ambiguous sensual behaviours under the pretext of parental love. When two parents love and have esteem for each other and live their desires and love in a quietly conflictual way, that is to say friendly most of the time, in contact with society where they have friends of their age, the latency stage is easier to live for the children. But this is not obvious when parents don't get along or don't have a social life that their children can observe. The father's body, whatever happens, has some emotionally affecting value to the child – as much for the daughter as for the son; but how he presents, how he is and how he acts, is not always very admirable. It is not always easy for them in the face of society to be the daughter or son of this man, their father, or this woman, their mother.

For example, it is difficult for children to feel safe and to use their libido in a creative way in society if their parents get divorced and are in a legal conflict – a conflict that has to be resolved by the placement of the child with one or other parent. The emotional distance necessary with regard to the two parents becomes impossible because of either their conflict or placement decided in favour of one or the other. These children of divorce are often taken to a psychoanalyst for clinical disturbances. As a symptom of their suffering, one finds alterations in the communication of the subject with his bodily schema, where again the disturbance found is due to the weakening of the sublimation of oral and anal drives, a sublimation set in motion by castrations in earlier, pre-Oedipal childhood. The difficulties caused by the fact that the Oedipal castration can no longer be sustained by the parental model coincide with the family conflict, and this double disturbance devitalises the libido that was engaged in previous sublimations.[30] These sublimations, which give value to the child within the family and society in accordance with his sexuation, were constructed at the time when the parent who gives the castration was incontestably credible. But for the child in the process of growth and structuration, the parents' separation has changed both the value of the model and the credibility of the adult as one who is esteemed.

And then in addition to the modesty that first appeared at the period of sexual difference and even more at Oedipal castration, there is a *symbolic* modesty in play in showing or not showing oneself to be happy while feeling the parents are not, or feeling obliged to succeed just in order to console father or mother for their marital failure. And so, the child regresses or remains trapped in a prolonged, pre-Oedipal binary relationship.

The case of Marc

I remember a child, let's call him Marc, whose parents, while not being divorced, lived a marital drama of mutual incomprehension since the death of their eldest son, a very brilliant boy who had died in an accident three years previous. Marc, the second son, who in early childhood showed as much promise as the first and had never presented any difficulties up until then, was for the last two years being excluded from everywhere. Because of his displays of temper at home and intolerably provocative behaviour towards his father, both parents – who were teachers – took the advice of psychologists and placed him at a boarding school. When I met him, he had just been excluded from the lycée for repeatedly falsifying his report cards and again, for provocative behaviour towards teachers and teaching assistants. With him, I looked over the falsified report cards his parents had brought me and in speaking to him about these, discovered to my astonishment the meaning of the falsifications.

From the boy and his parents, I learned that when he was a day-boy, he was always losing his report book and never gave them to his parents to sign; and after several months of this conduct, he was finally expelled. At present, as Marc was a boarder, it was difficult for him to lose his report card. So, what was he erasing? In the table of honours for the first months, which was written on the card, he was falsifying his place and his marks, which had been excellent during the first weeks after his arrival at the lycée, replacing them with bad marks and bad places. This report card, crossed out and falsified, had fallen into the hands of the headmaster of the provincial lycée in which Marc had been placed for a little more than a term.

---

30 These halts and reversals in development of which the child feels himself to be the victim are for him not unlike a game of snakes and ladders.

The headmaster, having seen the card and heard continuous complaints about the boy's behaviour, had decided to exclude him for a week to set an example.

> Marc was 12 years old, well developed, nervously tense. Guilty? No, annoyed and defensive. 'I am not mad. I don't know why they have brought me to you.'
> I asked if his headmaster had asked him for the reasons why he falsified his report card.
> 'No, he never spoke to me about it.'
> 'But why did you falsify it?'
> 'Oh, so that my parents wouldn't know' (that he was a good pupil).

And why must the parents not know? This is where it became complicated. He emerged from his embarrassment to explain that if his parents knew that he was a good pupil, he could no longer be one. For a start, it wasn't fair. He never really tried but good marks seemed to fall his way. And he wasn't there to console his parents for the loss of their eldest son – he was the wonderful pupil, always first in class. And he, Marc, even with good marks, could never be as good a pupil as had been his older brother. And here, Marc cried. Also, if you worked well in class you might die. Friends of his parents had said this: after his brother's death, from the age of 9 to 12 years, Marc had been stewing on a little comment made by friends of his parents: 'He was too intelligent, too perfect. This child was one of those not meant to live.' He gave too much satisfaction; he was too good. 'It's always the good ones who die.' We know phrases like these, said in moments of grief, as the speech of intended consolation between adults around the deceased: 'Poor thing, it's better that he died . . . it's the best ones that go . . .' etc. Marc took these words as prophesies of his own death should he have success comparable to that of his brother's at school. Because he was exceptionally intelligent, he could not do other than well and this terrified him. And then, he knew that he had been a disappointment at birth to his brother who wanted a little sister – and having said this, he cried again.

My work with this child was not very psychoanalytic. He had come to stay with his parents in the Paris region for the week in which he was excluded from school, which was just before a two-week break, after which he was supposed to return as a boarder. At the second or third session we had, with his permission and in front of him, I spoke on the phone to the headmaster of his lycée. He was astounded to learn from me that the report card had been falsified by the substitution of bad marks for good ones. He had never thought to find out the motivation for the crossed-out card, but then he had never seen such a thing! In the end, it was this headmaster who succeeded in treating the boy – not a psychoanalytic cure but an educational and humane one. He spoke to Marc and they decided together than when he returned to school, he would first of all go and speak to the headmaster. What I found out from the headmaster who phoned me once or twice during the second two terms, was that he had made a pact with Marc: there would be two report cards – one on which there would be his marks and commendations in their original state, and this would be kept by the headmaster and Marc's parents would not know about it. Then there would be a second report card, concocted between the child and the headmaster that was be seen by the parents, with completely ordinary marks and class places, and as this is signed by the headmaster, the parents would feel that the child was tolerated, was getting through his school year and nothing more. In this way, they would neither become anxious nor would they gain too much satisfaction. It was unbearable for Marc to give them that as he said, 'I am not here to please them.' As the counterpart to the headmaster's involvement in the secret report card, Marc was to commit himself to no longer disturbing classes and provoking the teachers.

It was a clever pact. Marc was relieved of a magical guilt about his brother, who prohibited him from succeeding in class – as well as the deceased – and also from his fear of dying in his turn from being, like the elder, a model son. He no longer had to provoke his teachers in place of his parents, and he made a promise to the headmaster. But more importantly, the source of his behaviour had dried up. The source? Marc had been driven mad because in the home of his depressed parents, he felt that they expected to be comforted by their son instead of by each other, as would be a true couple. The headmaster had quite understood that this child had submitted to a mechanism of self-punishment, and decided to help him. The situation was a difficult one for the educator and this was also why he telephoned me. He would have liked to telephone the parents behind the son's back, and tell them the secret that he was finding difficult to keep; but he had made a promise to Marc. I told him: 'You have to see this through to the end, otherwise it will all fail.' And he had held firm, pleased to be helping the son of a teacher, being one himself, to get out of a bad situation. At the end of the school year, Marc had done very well, while letting his parents believe (and believe they did), by way of his letters, that week after week he was on the verge of exclusion but was just about managing, etc.

When Marc returned to see me with his father, on the advice of his headmaster, we had a session between the three of us in which the truth came to light between the two men, in which they were able to speak truthfully and to be understood; but Marc made his father promise not to say anything about it to his mother, who would not, he said, accept his lie. I think that this was so that a secret pact should exist between these three men – the headmaster, who was a little older than his father (and who doubtless had the place of a grandfather here), father and Marc himself. Afterwards, I learned from the father that he himself started a psychoanalysis.

This is a story in which after an unproblematic Oedipus, the drama of losing a brother brought a boy like Marc to make himself misjudged by society and to destroy the image he had given, as severe anxiety, both of death and of castration, would follow should he satisfy his parents.[31] The boy's Oedipus complex had been resolved well before the death of his brother, but the fatal accident had weakened the libidinal balance of the rest of the family. If the boy had been willing to engage in a psychoanalysis, which wasn't the case, we would certainly have found rivalry between the brothers since early childhood, a rivalry that the second had completely repressed by being in admiration of his brother, a doubtlessly mutual rivalry between boys only two years apart and both very gifted. This rivalry would certainly have been re-experienced otherwise at the time of Oedipal fantasies, and then again in the rivalry towards his father shown by Marc in the form of continuous provocation. Mother was, like father, a teacher, and depressed since the death of her eldest son. All this would have been made explicit with the awakening of what had been repressed but not fully symbolised in Marc's early infancy, including his guilt about not having been born a girl. In life, these repressed libidinal energies play their role in other ways. Why? Because the resolution of the Oedipus complex and entry into the latency phase of the child characteristically involves the introjection of the ego-ideal and of the pre-Oedipal superego into the ego itself. The narcissism of Marc's ego, a primary narcissism mutated into secondary narcissism, was exacerbated by the introjection of an ego-ideal that developed around a prestigious brother and a father to be satisfied. The maternal aspect of the ego-ideal – that of an esteemed teacher – also played a part, and this image kept of the real mother, who became a source of anxiety because she was depressed, was superimposed over the ego of the boy, accentuating a sort of feminisation of the passive drives that happened after the death of the brother. Mother was no longer strict with him and made no demands, she was too depressed. On the contrary, she would beg for peace at home, that people be kind to her, that the father did not get angry etc. All this had a depressive effect upon Marc, who reacted with aggressive active drives: this mother should have been repaired but it was not his job to do it, it was her husband's. In his mind, she had to forgive him for having remained alive, a second child who did not satisfy her as well as the firstborn, as she too would have preferred a daughter as the second. Marc would have had to be a substitute for his brother. It was impossible – and at what risk? If he was a substitute for father and soothed his mother, this would be perverse for a child who had accepted the prohibition of intimate cuddles and sensual love with his mother, which precisely characterises the child who has gone through Oedipal castration and entered the latency phase.

All this would have been clarified during a psychoanalysis, but all these unconscious libidinal forces were unconsciously acting to forbid him from being impressive and successful in his social milieu, wherever he was. If a solution had not been found to his race to self-destruction, self-dereliction and social rejection, this child would probably have fallen into a depression similar to his mother's, or even worse, he would have lost himself in it. His mental state was worrying

---

31 I am talking about the ego-ideal that he had constructed as the second child.

enough for the provincial psychiatrist who saw him that he advised father to take Marc to a psychoanalyst, as he feared that his anger and behaviour issues would evolve towards a more serious mental state – he did not say what – involving school failure followed by delinquency. In reality, it was for Marc as a traumatised post-Oedipal subject to save his own skin.

With Marc, we can see the fragility of a post-Oedipal structure that had been successful and healthy at the age of 9: the child, shaken at this point in time, began an anxiety neurosis and depressive state at the age of 12 against which he was desperately fighting. While in his Oedipal and post-Oedipal state, Marc did not know how to distance himself from his parents, as he had become a single child and their only hope after the difficult mourning of an exemplary firstborn son.

Of post-Oedipal fragility

If psychoanalytic theory proposes that after a well-resolved Oedipus complex, the individual's libido is solidly structured for the future (and this is true), we should add that this solidity still requires the help of the entourage, and above all does not survive a cascade of traumatic emotional incidents. Clinical psychoanalysis allows us to grasp the unconscious dynamic in play during the latency phase after a normal Oedipal resolution – that is to say when the prohibition of incest is clearly assimilated and the child has integrated into his age group in society.

Evidence from consultations shows us that children of both sexes remain fragile and pervertable (while this may not necessarily be visible), because their successes or failures elicit de-narcissising effects on their parents, or on the contrary narcissising ones, in particular on the parent of the same sex, in reference to whom they will arrive at an adult stature. So, while they might have seemed completely healthy in their family and social lives up until the age of genital awareness and after the Oedipus complex, while there were no incidents in reality, this is where puberty brings anxiety to some adolescents and young adults, causing exhaustion that disorganises the psyche – inhibiting, destructive and psychosomatic effects. In the case of Marc, all the advice pointed to 'putting this young and depressed man in the process of becoming temperamental in a special school'[32] where the fresh air would do him good. Why not? Well, it wasn't a lack of fresh air that he suffered – unless one means the lack of a harmonious atmosphere between his parents.

All these young people who are ready for adolescent and adult sexuality suffer at the moment where this should appear from a real impotence that unknown to them must be called sexual, which is characteristic of the latency phase and will not consciously preoccupy the subject until adolescence is reached. But this

32 Translator's note: Dolto refers to *lycée climatique* – special schools typically in the mountains or by the sea, on the model of sanatoria built for recuperation from tuberculosis and other organic illnesses.

potential genital impotence strikes not only the subject in his desire to meet others and to be confirmed in his ascent outside of the family; this impotence also strikes at the sublimation of already castrated pre-genital desires. This is what is seen in those who have difficulties in concentrating, academic difficulties.

There may also be mortifying states of anxiety that provoke depression and the acting out of despair, for example at a so-called betrayal by friends. This hasn't got to be in consciously sexualised friendships; it may be in intensely sentimental relationships either heterosexual or homosexual, but vague, as these are at this age.

When parents get divorced, the child of whichever sex in the stages of latency or puberty will feel betrayed again. If many children of divorce have recourse to psychotherapies of various kinds, this is most often (as long as they are authentic psychotherapies) for the support of pre-genital castrations, which tend to give way to anxiety about the parents' separation, and of the choice between one or the other that the child believes he has to make, as he listens in turn to the partisans of one or other partner in the couple. It is very hard for him to continue to esteem both of them, and so a very strong friendship marked by narcissistic exclusivity serves as a refuge; and if that friend betrays him, it is a drama.

The fragility of adolescence

There are also adolescents who seem to have been through their Oedipus but have not at all understood the prohibition of homosexual or heterosexual incest because they had not earlier coherently experienced their power of expression as a boy or girl, and perhaps because they had neither homosexual nor heterosexual erotic temptations regarding their brothers or sisters, or their mother, before the age of 7 or 8. This consciousness of eroticism may appear suddenly with developing sexual maturity, and pre-adolescents may feel disturbed – girls with regard to their father or uncle and boys to their mother, aunt or sister – because they don't know how to speak about what they are experiencing. Impulses are experienced without words, without images; the body is moved and they don't know what to do or who to speak to. This may elicit perverse and often compulsive behaviours, often masturbatory, about which they feel guilty and by which they in fact avoid the work of reaching their goal, which is to speak to and be with the one they love in their fantasy and in the secrecy of their masturbation. How are these impulses going to play out if not towards human beings and in particular those that fill the imagination of the adolescent? They will elicit in the emotionally solitary adolescent the illicit and compulsive conquest of things, of stuff – in place of a conquest of friends, girls or boys, for activities of shared pleasure. They elicit passion for animals they pet and who pet them in return, which shows esteem, in place of knowing how to write love messages to or how to get petted by those who preoccupy their minds. These boys and girls often repress their active desires, feel socially guilty and enter into passive, impotent withdrawal, which is sometimes translated into a state of chronic fatigue that is in fact and unknown to them hysterical fatigue. They cannot do any sport; as soon as they are faced with competition or social obligation, they oblige their parents to call upon doctors – everything exhausts them. They show dark emotionality, pounding hearts, eclipses of tonicity. Are they ill? It is the climate of emotional loneliness in which they live that depresses them.

The failures to gratify their desires have ambiguous effects on these children. They feel themselves to be odd; they don't know how to speak about this; they feel alone in their experience of overwhelming sexual feelings upon seeing or meeting the beloved object or the object of desire that they don't even love. They would like to behave as they see everyone else behaving, and this gives them every sign of an anxiety-linked illness. Compensating processes sometimes make them wish to become not exactly murderers but delinquents – passive delinquents, exhibitionists looking to shock, fearful, conglomerating into a group of misfits that can act if subjugated by a leader. Sometimes, the excitation they get in preparing a coup – e.g. the transgression of rules as Marc did in ceaselessly provoking his teachers and the rule enforcers at his lycée, or the transgression of the laws of civil society, very tempting for inhibited boys and girls – is what allows them to enter into contact with others of the same age, something they would not dare to do if it was not about being in league against the defenders of laws in an attempt to sidestep them. Girls usually favour shoplifting as a way of experiencing the thrill of the fear of being caught. I have had several women and young girls who call this kleptomania; but this is not kleptomania but hysterical stealing to experience sensations verging on orgasmic in tricking the security guards and transgressing the law in department stores, and also the pleasure in being caught and pleading their case – that they are ill, they didn't do it on purpose, making up any old story to take in the security guards. There is a game of cat and mouse with plainclothes police officers that provide moments of relief in the empty and anxious lives of these boys and girls. And then, in some cases. there may be a wish to have their parents harshly judged because of their child, or to cause them trouble because they did not care enough for them, their children. In this, one finds a return to the twists and turns of the child in the face of his suffering in no longer being the exclusive object of desire and love of his parents.

In young people of both sexes, homosexuality may appear – but it is a homosexuality of behaviour claimed to be a deeply rooted homosexuality, with passive arrogance in boys and active cynicism in girls. In this showy display of homosexual behaviour there is an abandonment of competition in this case concerning sexuality; but this giving up of competition can be seen in every area – educational and professional as well. There is also a group of young people with a 'meh' attitude – unclear about their sexuality, incapable of taking responsibility for their desire and their independence in order to assume a romantic relationship. In fact, the sexualities on display, homosexual or heterosexual, are decoys – reactional. They are cries of demand from children of extended childhoods, who are ignorant of themselves and of others. The show themselves to be other than that which society admires and values, so that society will notice them and take account of them. Alcohol and drugs, when these young people start to use them, play a part in their dereliction, their giving up of competition and become, we could say, a slow and progressive mode of suicide.

All of this could indeed end in real suicide, the equivalent of the primal scene of their conception in which the adolescent refuses to recognise that he played a part in the initial act of his life. These young people cannot admit that they were born from their own desire, that this was reassumed day by day and made them survive until now. We often hear, 'I never asked to be born' spoken in a tone of persecution and grievance; sometimes, 'nobody loves me,' which in reality translates as 'I have no one to love' or even, 'I can't stand myself.' The loneliness of the heart causes despair, but instead of recognising this and talking about it, the adolescent turns it into a magnified grievance; dare I say he phallicises it into 'I love my defeated self.' And it is in a fit of self-love, I believe, an impulsive acting out of the desire for something else, something new, for escape, that they commit suicide – in the ultimate hope for an erotic sensation of nirvana. Fortunately, some of them fail in this, and it is by the psychoanalytic study of these that we can trace the processes that lead them to this point. The subject stayed awake during the coma and is more lucid afterwards than before the suicide attempt of the ego. And perhaps he feels less guilty of living having been through the experience of near-death: because this has been refused him, it could mean that he has to play the game of life.

Most children that psychoanalysts have to see after latency and at the start of puberty are those who lack creative means that would have helped them to discover the desires that underwent castration in the early stages of their development. In the clinical cases that I have studied, these castrations failed in that they never led to the symbolisation of drives, which were simply repressed with regard to their object, without being used for the conquest of legitimate objects offered to the child – objects involving pleasure and socialisation linked with the sharing of pleasure with others. They are also sometimes children who have suffered a mutilation of their body image at the mirror stage or at the age of primary castration. These would be children said to be psychotic and maladjusted.

But what really corresponds with neurotic, post-Oedipal disturbances are those subjects seen clinging to the mirror in the eyes of those who look at them, those who succeed not for themselves but in order to be seen and without being able to project this success into an adult future. These young people are clinging to an image of their face, their body, their look, the surface of their visible appearance. They inflate what can be seen to hide their internal distress. At the slightest doubt of their eventual success in an enterprise whose goal is the realisation of their desire, an imaginary wall rises up like an obstacle between them and the world. It is the anxiety of the void, the absurdity imbued in the meaninglessness of the project, followed by a lack of dynamism in defending and taking responsibility for it. They withdraw to the mirror to find themselves, in order not to lose themselves completely. It is much less serious if they withdraw alone to the radio, to music to calm and carry their anguish – less serious especially if this music brings them to rhythmic movement in dance or skating as there is in this a whole-body pleasure that tires them out and that allows them to show themselves not to care while in the midst of others. They can feel the joy of being at ease in their bodily schemas. Also, running and fast acrobatic gymnastics during which they cannot even think, which may stupefy them but also sustain a false elation in exhausting the body, are nonetheless better than passivity and drugs: they allow physical survival with bodily ease relieving bodily tensions in the moment, although at the cost of satisfying the tensions of the heart.

There is also fragility in the face of first love – first romantic love or first romantic love linked with future projects, because desire is now involved. Up until now, these young people have only known friendship. This time, it is a love-desire; at last they get close to the object of this love-desire – and that person rejects them. The young man or girl does not seem to consider that the experience may be due to the inaccuracy of their imagination in idealising the beloved, who is then discovered in reality to be quite different. Instead, they experience an immediate and unbearable devaluation. There is an immediate resonance for them, a resonance decipherable in the dreams they recount, of neglect they experienced in their childhood, neglect of them by their consciously loved parent. All of a sudden, the unconscious association of these two trials makes them feel guilty, as if it were in itself incestuous to have loved someone who did not respond to their hopes. We may see young people attempt suicide and not fail, or others who cannot speak about their depression enter into psychotic states with serious organic effects. What is absolutely necessary here is for someone who is not a parent or in a parental position towards the child – not necessarily a psychoanalyst, sometimes grandmothers do this very well – to listen to the despairing love story of this boy or girl – listen and sympathise without consoling, criticising or judging, but discreetly supporting the narcissism of the forsaken one.

It may also be that the love object of the adolescent or young adult is put on such a high pedestal and idealised to the point where it becomes unthinkable for him or her to enter into communication with such a sublime entity; and the subject loses all ability to do anything. He becomes like a setting dog, searching for his love and spending his life waiting for the gaze that will never come and for good reason, as the other whom he dares not inform of his love has no inkling that he or she is desired, as he or she lives in a completely different sphere from this frozen lover. This erotomania of young people is seen in the creation of groups of fans of a star, hero or heroine of their dreams. For some, this is not that dangerous – it just fills their leisure time and allows them to meet other fans – but others experience true distress in not being noticed, loved and supported in life by those they love.

There are therefore two ways of being de-narcissified for a subject who has attained the secondary narcissism characteristic of a healthy post-Oedipal stage, both of which have serious, rapid, de-creative and mortifying effects. A negative response to his desire may destroy all his body images and leave him with nothing with which to continue to live – neither his right nor any means of even trying to seduce. Or if his desire went completely unnoticed by his desired other, the lover interprets this as if his desire was forbidden by pseudo-magic, and this awakens in the adolescent the pangs of the Oedipal period – the terror of being surplus, the penetrating jealousy of those they see being welcomed while they themselves are not; and rather than a feeling of abandonment leading to slow or fast suicide, this may provoke a vengeful act aimed at the more successful rival. In particular, this can be seen in subjects whose history shows that they did not experience the period of castrations as narcissising and promoting of their development, but as painful trials, realities to be suffered in the face of their dreams, at a time when their brothers and sisters seemed to be the preferred objects of their parents.

Badly given and badly received castrations, delivered without respect or compassion to children who experience them as slaps in the face may (after a more or less bearable latency period and beginning of adolescence), cause the young person to be seized by guilt upon his first failure in love outside the family, be it clearly heterosexual or homosexual love or only vaguely tinted by sexuality. This guilt is completely imaginary and has nothing to do with any logic or with the responsibility of an unfortunate act that would have jeopardised their possible happiness. There is a psychological test that tells a story where a little boy or girl (according to the sex of the child being tested) has an altercation with his father or mother whom he had disobeyed, while another child is on very good terms with his/her parents. In the test, which is a spoken one, the two children are supposed to use the same way to school and go over a bridge that by accident collapses. One of the two children is killed in the accident – which one? A very young child or a child in the latency phase or start of puberty whose Oedipal resolution has not been symboligenic will, in both cases, immediately say that the one who has been killed is the one who disobeyed. On the contrary, a child who has had a good experience of his latency phase, or a self-confident adolescent who can bear to be excluded by their chosen ones – these will immediately say, 'But how can one know?' In those who give the accidental death to the disobeying child, there is a projection upon things of this world of magical thinking regarding the parents' omnipotence, of the superego. It is obviously a failed castration because a parent should be experienced by their children not as omnipotent but as feeling responsible for the child and able to bear to make him suffer in order to help him; who empathise because they have been through that themselves and know how to explain that to the child. The non-castrated child has not been helped to understand this through conversations with his parents about real incidents, stories heard or current affairs – all things that parents concerned with education and development should talk about to their child. For example, the child has not been initiated in the knowledge that disobeying can sometimes be necessary to gain autonomy, to get him out of a blocked situation, on condition that the one who disobeys has thought through what he is doing, measured the risks and decided to face them, including the risk of displeasing his parents and being told off by them. It is true that experienced people, which is how adults seem to be to the child, know how to foretell dangers that children cannot. Unfortunately, many parents foretell also dangers that do not exist and through abusive prohibitions or absurd prophesies inhibit the desire had by every child to become autonomous – the duty and the desire to think for themselves and to take risks when he has taken a decision.

I return to this leitmotif: it would be the role of school to support the critical faculty in children towards what adults say and the often absurd regulations to which they are subjected and that the child believes himself to be guilty of transgressing, while in fact they have a duty to do so.

Awakening the critical faculties of children regarding the holders of power is also very important and, if parents cannot do it, it is for school to do it. The holders of power are in the eyes of the law those in charge of enforcing it. But those who want to use power to manipulate and identify with their role are bad masters; we can help children tolerate them for a time, but we also need to support the exercise of their critical faculties when they face these authoritarian behaviours that are not sensible and are authority for its own sake, that is to say they are deprived of socially useful human meaning.

Anorexia

Adolescent girls at the start of a responsible life in society, who after Oedipal castration and the following latency phase have pathologies of body images, very often present problems that appear clinically as anorexia, sometimes minor but that can become very serious. One has to understand this symptom in relation to the body image. It does not go back to the Oedipal period but well before that, between the ages of 3 and 6. All that the Oedipal period did was to reshuffle what happened when these little girls were younger, at the period of primary castration, which is to say when they accessed the knowledge of their sexual belonging and their narcissistically gratifying pride in becoming women like their mother. This is a period that is dialecticised also according to the value of the name-of-the-father, a value of which mother makes the child aware; as it is around a man, a valued phallic representative, that all sexuation in little girls is organised. Little girls who, at the period of primary castration around the age of 3, accepted the delaying of their sexual life until puberty, but who were convinced of their personal value as the daughter of this man or woman – these girls rarely (and I have never seen one) develop anorexia. When they reach puberty, they know how to keep the phallicism necessary for their archaic drives, that is for industrious activity, activity in the service of play, in social life; they succeed academically and socially. With modesty, without shame about themselves, they are happy to show themselves to advantage and to attract the gaze of others when their bodies develop and they become young women. They compete with other girls without feeling guilty.

One must also understand that among these girls who reach puberty after a successful Oedipus and a socially successful latency period, there are some who at adolescence dress up as boys. This is not always a sign of a developing homosexuality; it is sometimes a sign of an overflow of feminine wealth, sometimes of a resistance to allowing the expression of passive desires of seduction, and it may also be a prudent tactic – as it is difficult for a girl who attracts the gaze and desire of boys and the rivalry of other girls to continue to acquire weapons for social life. She may be tempted to give up academic competition, and in the present day, we know how important it is for a woman who wishes to be autonomous in every situation to be able to earn her own living, especially when she is responsible for children or may even have to raise a child on her own, when her salary becomes really needed. The passive drives dominant in girls at puberty can hinder career success, and 'tomboys' are often far more heterosexual in their desire than supposedly very feminine girls whose feminine charms are recognised and vaunted by all and who are sometimes neither girls nor boys but passive in the extreme, and who expect to be the chosen object of a phallic being, whatever it is, who will give them all that they don't try to obtain for themselves – possibilities of life in society – as legal or illegal parasites. While they seek a man to look after them – a legitimate spouse or regular lover – what this is for them is a phallic social respondent from whom they can benefit as a baby benefits from the maternal breast and the tutelary adult upon whom they were dependent. When they become women and, unfortunately, mothers, they are incapable of raising their children. They can be good in pregnancy, during breastfeeding, but their children will be raised by them in their own sexuated narcissism. They are not able to give castrations to the children or to elicit in them the symbolisation of drives of which the raw expression is prohibited. They raise children who eat well and appear well but who do not become girls and boys who are autonomous desiring beings.

Anorexia nervosa and bulimia are far more common syndromes in girls than in boys at puberty or in adolescence and are also symptoms with libidinal roots in the period of primary castration that was very poorly supported by the upbringing given by their mother. In boys, bulimia is sometimes seen as a syndrome of the Oedipal phase, while anorexia is seen more during the latency period; at adolescence, it is again bulimia. In girls, anorexia occurs at the start of puberty or afterwards. This arises from what the girl's genital drive takes from an economic organisation somewhat similar to that of her oral drives: it is likely that at the time of weaning, the oral drive relating to the desire for the breast (I am not talking about the need for milk, I am talking about the desire for the breast as a part object of the mother) may have been repressed without the symbolisation of the pleasurable subject-to-subject relationship between baby and mother, which should replace and exceed the pleasures of touch and taste of the breast for the mouth of the baby girl. In girls who become anorexic, interest in the relationship with mother and with sexual desire in the widest sense is completely repressed without becoming transformed into interhuman relations with the mother and women.

At puberty, phallic interest, represented in men by the penis is in girls represented by the breasts, which grow during puberty; the development of breasts and the onset of menstruation signify consciously or unconsciously for the young girl her possible fecundity. Most commonly, the parental couple in this case lives in an infantile mode in an either pleasant or unpleasant atmosphere, and the unconscious idea of pregnancy is unbearable for these girls. Their conscious shame is about getting fat; they live a conflictual magma in which adult sexuality is lost, marked by a negative sign, a horror of having a bosom, breasts, a horror of being fat. This needs to be analysed, and it is to do with disturbance in the real relationship between daughter and mother, between the girl and food, between daughter and father, her imaginary femininity and inexperience of boys, between the girl and her mirror. To get fat[33] – an expression that has unconscious links with pregnancy – is dangerous for the aesthetic of the young girl who wants to seduce: it will supposedly stop her from being pleasing. But it is mostly she herself in the mirror, in her own eyes, that she wants to please by effacing all the feminine roundness of her body, even the most discreet. Her desire for the father is therefore disguised either in a complicated and conflictual affection, or on the contrary in a manifest flight from his view and refusal to answer when he speaks to her. Her problem is rooted in a conflict between love and desire with regard to her father and in a conflict of feminine rivalry with her mother in which the child remains as her kitten; mother of course worries about her but never really considers her to be a girl in the process of becoming a woman. The narcissism of the girl is caught up in a complicit game of bluff. She experiences unconscious and completely autonomous conflicts that date from when she was 3 to 6 years old and that have only very little to do with the current behaviour of the parents towards her – behaviour within a secondary reality linked with their justified anxiety about her dilapidated health.

Pregnancy and body image

The nausea of pregnancy also comes from a conflict that dates back to the body image of a very young age, that of weaning and of the start of the Oedipus complex.

Appendicitis in both boys and girls is a psychosomatic disorder relating to the period where they imagined conception to happen according to some digestive technique. Although these fantasies are far in the past, there was a time when they were operational and left possibilities of later infection in this part of the bodily schema, because the body image of a pregnant woman was seen as full of magic poo. Boys and even girls imagined that behind giving birth lay a peculiar anal power in the mother. The incestuous baby that every pre-Oedipal child unconsciously wishes to carry, like mother, as a pledge of the love and of the desire they have for their father (and I am not talking only about girls but also boys) – this unconscious, incestuous baby must absolutely be aborted before the Oedipus complex can be dissolved. This is how the appendix becomes the seat of an inflammation and must be removed, in order to save the subject from an archaic trap in which the fantasy of a desire that could not be clearly articulated by the child long ago would become real in the dysfunction of the bodily schema. It is therefore the body, in the appendix, that signifies and repeats an unspoken thought – a

33 Translator's note: in French, *la grossesse* means pregnancy while *grosse* is fat and *grossir* is to get fat.

thought that currently has no meaning for a child who is 7–8 or 14–15 years old. The reader may be very surprised by what I have just said, but if they are often with children, they would be surprised by how many of them fantasise and trumpet to everyone that they are going to have a baby and who assume and show that it is in their tummy. There is clearly nothing to do but laugh and say to them: 'Ah. You believe that?' They said it. And for these children there will be no appendicitis later; it is those who repress this desire and don't speak of it for whom the body will have to signify it before they leave childhood behind. This is the difference: speech expresses a desire and avoids it having to be expressed by the body, if not now then later. This is why children's fantasies, when expressed, should provoke neither repetition, denegation nor any show of feeling; the child has to be left to speak – that is all, and enough. His discourse is liberating of what is in the process of being healthily repressed, after which it will be symbolised in a cultural way rather than in the body. The boy's feminine drives will be sublimated in other ways than in bearing a fruit of flesh, and the emissive genital drives of the girl otherwise than in the desire to herself have a child for her father.

Hysteria and psychosomatics

The developments given all throughout this work to the notion of a body image both related to the bodily schema and distinct from it brings me to clarify the relationship between the real body and the unconscious, libidinal, dynamogenic image made of it by the subject, and the differences with regard to narcissism between hysterical and psychosomatic symptoms.

We have given the name of *hysteria* to behaviours that unconsciously aim to manipulate the other, while we call functional impairments to the body that are not due to organic causes *psychosomatic* – there is no infection, not even lesions, at least at the beginning, no neurological problems, and yet the individual suffers from a health disturbance. His body is ill but the origin of the physiological dysregulation is an unconscious psychological disorder.

In any case, be it hysteria or psychosomatic illness, the invalid really suffers and is hampered in psychosocial activities. In those problems called hysterical, it is said that the individual is most often a woman: I doubt this.[34]

The hysterical individual is in overall good health but with expressive disturbances that come on suddenly; he unconsciously indulges in manipulating the

---

34 I think that hysteria is spoken of mostly in relation to women because of the fact that society values the phallocratic and haughty behaviours into which male hysteria is often transformed, which is narcissising for the subject and may be effective in his dealings with others. What makes us track hysteria better in a woman is that when she fails to obtain her goal and her narcissistic suffering is over-excited by this, she sometimes perseveres with the same behaviour, unconscious of its source, and that the hysteria, by this fact, appears without any link with social success. All this to say that what we call hysteria in women are the methods admired in men as accessories to their social success.

other, by what I would call low means. In the hysterical woman, frustrated libido is translated into spectacular scenes in which she is paralysed and which confer guilt on her partner, who is not satisfying her sexually; but she herself suffers something in the order of an unconscious orgasm at each of these scenes: she has a libidinal economy that in each crisis leads to an unconscious nervous discharge followed by a feeling of well-being, like in an orgasm.

It is the inter-individual life – the life of relationships – that the hysterical individual hinders, either in the smooth functioning of a partnership or in relations at work; while the psychosomatic does not hinder the functioning of his emotional relationships with others – for him, it is the doctor who becomes the object of manipulation, confused by if not really worried about his chronically ill state.

Hysterical paralysis impedes or causes suffering to an individual, who is unconscious that he has caused it; his unconscious goal was to manipulate another who was frustrating him, but in the end, he becomes a prisoner of what is said by his body, which he believes to be attacked by an external agent, for example microbial or an accident due to clumsiness, and which stops him from moving. He feels himself to be the victim of a cause foreign to him when in fact, unbeknownst to him, it is he who self-victimises for an unconscious aim, which is to act upon his entourage or to stop himself from acting. Psychosomatic illness is about the effects of an unconscious (to be decoded) battle between agencies of the mind, fighting inside the individual; while in hysteria the imaginary fight is between the individual and another, from whom he unconsciously desires or dreads a satisfaction in a reality that he otherwise cannot control.

Freud cites a case of the hysterical paralysis of the arms of a young woman who was secretly in love with the friend of her brother who would come to visit while the brother had broken his leg, but who stopped coming to the house when the brother recovered. Without knowing it, she wanted to see this young man again and without being able to admit or say this, she paralysed her own arms in imitation of her brother. Her arms were as if in an imaginary cast with the unconscious magical logic: 'If a member is paralysed, the young man will return.' Freud enabled the girl to speak under hypnosis about the meaning of her paralysed, apparently broken arms. In the hypnotic trance, the desiring subject was completely lucid about her ego – the hypnotised girl knew that her immobile arms were a call for a visit from the young man. The ego, adapted to the language of the environment, had no access to the signifier of desire because of the resistances that developed in it and prevented the subject from going beyond the taboos of her upbringing. In trance, the girl could speak of her hope of a visit from the young man. She could not have had this understanding of herself awake, if Freud had not told her what she revealed under hypnosis. And it was in the face of the narcissistic emotional damage brought by this revelation that Freud realised that it was useless and even harmful to cause a sudden rapprochement of the unconscious to conscious mind by work under hypnosis that is revealed afterwards to the patient – it could only cause trauma.

Freud showed that it was worth much more to work with the conscious subject and his resistances to reach the truth about his unconscious desires, as once these have been expressed and the period of their organisation analysed, the resistances have no reason to remain. More precisely, during the work between analyst and analysand, the transference of the emotional relationship with the people of his childhood is established upon the analyst, and once the resistances in this are exhausted, the desire can be spoken and put back in relation to the time that it first appeared.

Instead of an often traumatic, unusable and wild revelation of repressed desires, Freud inaugurated the treatment of psychosocial problems by the mediation of transference made by the patient in the course of meetings contractually spaced in time, always in the same place and requiring payment. The relationship between these two participants becomes the opportunity for re-living past experiences, or of new ones for the patient, who finds himself confronted by a margin of difference between the psychoanalyst and himself in their appreciation of the imaginary and real aspects of the material brought to each session. From this comes a maturation of the patient and of his expressive language, and from that, the elucidation without guilt of his desires about which he can speak here, without acting them out. The work leads him to grasp the relative value held by his various desires, whether to speak of them or silence them, according to the ethos that he critiques day by day on the couch. This ethos is readjusted according to the evolution of his consciousness, which emanated from an archaic preconception, and of his conscious judgement, both of which are developed through the link with the psychoanalyst – a link that is 'dis-intimised,' and becomes ordinary and disenchanted. The analyst, the guide to the patient's subjective work, never intervenes in the reality that gives rise to actions to be made, decisions to be taken according to those of the patient's desires that have to be negotiated with the social world, and this non-intervention allows him to assume them as best he can. Treatment ends with reciprocal discharge between analysand and analyst, the former being no longer motivated to continue a repetition of his life story that no longer interests him, with the latter preferably in agreement.

A case of hysteria in a young boy, Alex

I had the chance to know a boy of 13 who had broken his right arm several times and who could not move his elbow when the cast was removed. His arm remained frozen although radiography showed no obstacles to the flexion and extension of the forearm. In the course of the two weeks of rehabilitation that followed, the boy broke the same arm; there was a new plaster cast followed by its removal. Again, the mobilisation of the right arm seemed impossible. There was then a third fracture of the same arm, a third cast and of course, once again, no mobilisation possible after the cast's removal.

To confirm that the elbow had complete freedom of movement (x-rays having shown no anomaly in the articulation, and the surgery had been done in a children's hospital), the boy was given a general anaesthetic: under anaesthesia, the arm was shown to perfectly free in passive movement. Functional recovery should therefore not have posed any problems in this case. But when he had woken up from the anaesthesia, we would have had to break the boy's elbow if we had tried to make it bend. He himself tried and could not do it, although he felt no pain in this invalid upper limb. At this point, the consultant head of the service in which I was a junior doctor, knowing that I was a psychoanalyst, asked if I could take charge of the boy and make him accept that nothing in reality was preventing the recuperation of mobility in his arm.

I and the boy both accepted to work together and so Alex came every other day to the surgical department. We would sit together for a good half hour on two sides of a table; he would draw and we would talk. I had not myself treated him for his fracture, and was not present when he was anaesthetised for at any of the attempts at physiotherapy. I was therefore in a classical way able to play the role of a psychotherapist. After very few sessions, the unconscious desire that forced Alex to mobilise his arm appeared clearly. He lived on a rough estate – a deprived area near the hospital. He had a sister four years older than him who might have seduced him when he was 8 years old and she was 12 – therefore five years earlier. At least this is what he said – true or false? He liked this sister and he also had a brother four years younger than him whom he liked. He talked to me about his real desire for his sister. Real desire? He confessed with some embarrassment to having played at believing he was the husband and she, his wife during a tender, pseudo-maternal scene involving his older sister, himself and his younger brother. But this is not what was important, he said. During another session, he told me that what was important for him was a dream that troubled him but that he could not tell me. He was drawing knife attacks mechanically while talking and his drawings were associated with the unsaid of this repetitive dream. From session to session, he associated from this dream and according to the various characteristics of his narrative, he would also mime it while telling it.

One day, while he was miming a scene, a variation of the dream in which his 'big sister' was represented (this is how he always named her in his dream, while in normal conversation he always said 'my sister'), he started to move his right arm, to his own astonishment, as if his hand was armed with an imaginary knife aimed at me, who represented his older sister in the dream. We managed to talk about what he had just acted and at the same time, to compare this with the drawing that mechanically he had been doing while talking. This could signify that his right arm, armed with a knife, was inclined to deal a mortal blow to his sister, or maybe to his mother when he was small, as he was talking about a big sister and to another woman like me. To have his right arm paralysed would obviously stop him from causing a misfortune. This impediment came from his humanised conscience – unconscious conscience maybe – of the prohibition of incest, and of the prohibition of murder. The prohibition of murder, as we have seen, comes from anal castration and the prohibition of incest from Oedipal castration. This was translated for him into guilt – the guilt of an incestuous transgression that his

sister had tried to force on him; at the same time that the guilt of the potential murder of his sister – murder that could be the symbolic displacement of his archaic
incestuous desire, as in the body image of a small boy, the magnificence of penile
erection and the desire that accompanies it for the chosen maternal object makes
the child dream of killing his love object.

It was a response to his sister – at that time 17 years old and he, 13 – who
wanted him to share with her the big parental bed where she had been sleeping for
some months while their mother was in hospital. She was pressing him to accept
this, saying that they would put a bolster between them, but he refused. This was
the current conflict. Alex preferred to sleep on the floor or in the other room (there
were only two in the accommodation) where his father slept, when he was there,
and also his little brother. Yet he and his sister had shared the same mattress in
their early childhood and before their mother's hospitalisation. In response to a
sister who was suggesting a semblance of bodily contact that would be pleasurable for her, he wished to respond with bodily contact that would kill: and it is this
that he was unconsciously defending against.

His hysterical paralysis was an imaginary self-mutilation – painless, inconvenient, but far less serious than the truly self-mutilating fractures. It was just
an unconscious act – he fell, and it was always the same arm that was broken,
repaired and then broken again. The hysteria disappeared under general anaesthetic but as soon as he regained consciousness returned to freeze into total impotence his murdering arm, which became immobile. Alex was nearly 13, growing
and going through puberty, which awakened in him the memory of a seduction,
which he said happened long ago – a seduction in which his sister had, he said,
made him masturbate her, after which she did the same to him. This memory,
if it was not a fantasy, was told with very little affect and was undoubtedly at
the root of an unconscious desire. It was, perhaps, a screen memory of a fantasmatic desire when he was a little boy – a heterosexual desire, as yet little to rival
father's, but still a male desire expressed by the desire to penetrate the body of
his sister or mother before the Oedipal phase. He replaced penile penetration
with the penetration of a knife. Although his arm was paralysed, his hand could
draw graphic representations. One could see a hand armed with a butcher's knife
but never the person targeted by the knife on the same drawing. It was around
these drawings, and the dream that he could not recount, that all the analytic
work revolved.

What was his father like, and his grandfather? A difficult migration had brought
this family from the east to their insecure situation near Paris. Although the child's
arm did not need rehabilitation, the physiotherapist, who got on well with Alex,
offered to restart the work with him after psychotherapy had relieved the psychogenic motivations behind the strange loss of motor functioning. And Alex like to
chat with this male physiotherapist. The fact is that he told him what he had told
me, and the physiotherapist found himself playing the role of an excellent educator for the pre-pubescent boy, whose father, either absent or very preoccupied,
neglected to play for his children. For reasons unknown to me, the mother was in

a hospital, also unknown to me, for many months, and it was the older teenage sister who kept house – if one could call the hut divided into two rooms a house.

We could say that what is hysterical is always a cry for help addressed visibly to an other, aimed at obtaining a more or less clearly erotic libidinal satisfaction that is desired and repressed at the same time. This ambivalence of desire provokes in the subject a regression of drives that is unconscious, although they were probably conscious to begin with. This regression expresses drives by linking them with an archaic mode of satisfaction.

In Alex, the drive for genital penetration was transformed into the drive of a penetrating limb that Alex did not want to act out. This was the meaning and function of the hysterical symptom, the displacement of the penis onto the arm and the knife and the arm's subsequent paralysis.

Psychosomatic problems arise from a pain aroused by intimate suffering – suffering due to a disappointing relationship with a chosen being, which is translated into an imaginary wound, with a return to an archaic body image and to a time when the subject was in a relationship with someone other than that currently in question. The current psychosomatic problem is a sometimes amplified repetition of a past dysfunction, real or imagined, of the patient's own body. The body becomes a substitute for the companion present at the initial trial who is linked with the trial currently being endured – a companion whom the subject thinks understands him and will not leave him to suffer alone with his current illness. Therefore, it is not the same narcissism that seems to be disturbed in psychosomatic illness and hysteria. *In hysteria, it seems to me that it is secondary narcissism that is in danger; in psychosomatic illness it is primary narcissism.* In hysteria, what one might call the erotic ethos is organised around genitality; in psychosomatics, it is organised around dependency in feeding and doing, of autonomy in relation to the loved one in childhood – a loved one in a chosen relationship who could accompany him through the trials of oral and anal castration.

There is therefore something more archaic in psychosomatic illness than in hysteria. Let's look at a case – that of a mother – which seems to me typical of psychosomatic disturbance. During the funeral of her son, who died as an adult, at the moment that soil was being shovelled onto the coffin, she felt a blow – like a punch in her stomach. The medical examination that followed shortly afterwards found that she had stomach cancer and she died soon after, a month to the day of her son's death. It is highly likely that she had suffered from this cancer for quite some time without knowing it; this is what the doctors said to the husband, but she had felt its bite on that day, at the moment when her son was being put in his grave. It was as if the death of this eldest son, the first she had nursed, had awakened in her an impossible weaning. Perhaps she had unconsciously remained attached – flesh to flesh – to this firstborn son, even beyond the weaning period. At the point of her son's death, the definitive detaching of her body tore from her the visceral substance of her own stomach. The death of the 'me' that had transformed the woman into a mother upon the birth of her firstborn son (and women know very well that there is a firstborn for each sex and for fathers too): becoming a mother for the first time involves a mutation – a mutation of the ego, of the narcissism of the woman, but not of the desiring subject. The subject's growth is out of step in time and space; it knows neither birth nor death but only the verb *to be* for *to love*.

As subjects, we only know others by way of ego relationships – our ego with theirs and vice versa. And this is where psychosomatic problems lie, linked with the relationship between the symbolic and reality, of time interwoven with space, which constitutes living flesh, mediated by linkage between the body image and the bodily schema.

The subject has no words to speak about the suffering that breaks the continuum of a vital relationship. The body seems mutilated in a place specific to the history of the broken love bond, and the suffering that could not be expressed remained, albeit partly anaesthetised, and was signified by the curbing of part of the body's functioning.

On this subject, it is well known that someone with a heart problem should avoid strong emotions because these touch the heart – the heart of the body image, of emotions; this heart has an impact on the bodily schema and the visceral functioning of the heart. The 'feeling heart' and the 'flesh heart' – as one child I was treating taught me to say – are distinct, can be differentiated, but sometimes in pathology they interfere with each other.

It is well known that dramatic discussions within the family could awaken a stomach ulcer in someone who has the potential to have chronic ulcers. The analysis of a subject with a stomach ulcer confirms the archaic nature of this psychosomatic disorder. His libido stayed marked by the love of his mother mixed up with his desire for her. The dream representations during the analysis followed a cannibalistic ethos, the analysand re-living the time when his mother breastfed him. This ethos of maternal love, of being eaten up with kisses, plays its role down in the stomach, in relation to the people who share with us our meals and whose angry outbursts have emotional repercussions on others.

The case of Tony: psychosomatic father, hypochondriac (or hysterical) child?

I knew a man, let's call him the father of Tony, who was the last born in a family of five boys. For years, he had a stomach ulcer and suffered gastritis from the age of 14. He was the only one of the five brothers to have a regular social and genital life – he was married and Tony was his only child. His four brothers were delinquents who spent most of their time in prison.

Their father, the paternal grandfather of Tony, was a child under the care of social services (as was Tony's grandmother), and died in an accident at work when Tony's father was a small child. He did not remember him. As to the mother, she was alcoholic (or became alcoholic after becoming a widow?) and died of delirium tremens when Tony's father was 10 years old. Tony's father said that she breastfed all her children. He had tears in his eyes when talking about her, who was so good, but who lived in a disorganised fashion and had been rejected by society because of her alcoholism. Furthermore, at her death Tony's dad, who was 10 years old, and two of his closest brothers were put in the care of social services.

This mother, rejected by everyone, induced in her sons when they were babies and loved her an intimate conflict of frenzied love and then shame for her vis-à-vis society. They grew up in material deprivation. The four other sons constructed their libidinal structure keeping the beloved mother of when they were small as the only ego-ideal! This identification was their only support, as their father's work killed him at a time when there was no social security, no benefits and no compensation for workers accidentally killed. Growing up with her, they had no other family, having become, like her, individuals maladjusted to laws and objects of rejection for society. They all began their juvenile delinquency at the age of 14, and it is at the same age that Tony's father paid through his gastritis for a sort of delinquency of his digestive tract. He kept the same fixation to a mother that had been such a good nurse and so sweet and tenderly loving in his memory. His brothers started by stealing, then drinking, then it was prison and armed assault. In their recidivism, two of them became murderers. Tony's father was a psychosomatic delinquent: it was his stomach that he would attack or that would attack him, or more precisely he self-devoured, in the absence of the maternal breast that he had suckled last and that because of this, he said nourished him for longer than the others.

One can see here, distributed in a family, the distinction we were talking about between hysterical and psychosomatic disorders. Three of the brothers – those who were more than 4 years old when their father died – were hysterical; they were active, hysterical delinquents. The fourth was a passive hysteric. The fifth, Tony's father, was psychosomatic.

The reason I knew this man and his history is not, as one may believe, a psychotherapeutic treatment for his ulcer. I met him in my hospital outpatient clinic when asked to assess Tony, then a 10-year-old boy. *For several months, Tony had been missing school under the pretext of acute pains in his knees.* The observation in hospital and all investigations did not allow us to understand the cause of this pain. Was he putting it on? What was his cognitive level? People said that his pain really stopped him from sleeping and interfered with his walking. During a prolonged period of observation in hospital, Tony did not appear either temperamental or educationally behind. His IQ was 105 – in short, he was a puzzling case. This child was neither delinquent, temperamental nor delayed; he suffered. He was hypochondriac – knees?[35] I or we? What about us – my father and I? It sounds like a pun, but it is pain. But it is truly this that was coming out in sessions when I was listening to him. He stated the problem of his paternal family through

35 Translator's note: Dolto uses here a pun that cannot work in English. Knees in French is *genoux*, and she follows this with the homophone *je, nous*? – or I, we. Her point is that the signifier knees sounds the same in French as if you say 'I, we.' Perhaps if the patient had been English, he would have suffered from enuresis? I wee . . .

a call for help that had taken the linguistic form of this symptom, translated as a pain in the knees.

Originally, there was what a neighbourhood doctor said, having been called one day when he did indeed suffer from a slightly inflamed knee for which the doctor ordered rest and no school for a week and diagnosed growing pains. This happened a few months before Tony celebrated his tenth birthday, the age at which his father lost his mother and was placed in care. It is probable that at his son's birthday all these old memories returned to the father but he said nothing of them – nothing of his childhood or his family had been spoken of to his wife or his son. The wife, who was also a child of the state, had been abandoned much earlier than he had and had a good memory of a nurse in her childhood, who had unfortunately died shortly after retirement. Of her husband, she only knew that he had his mum until the age of 10 and that the poor woman etc. . . . and she knew only vaguely about the delinquency of a step-brother she had never seen because of 'papers and letters from a lawyer' that her husband once received. He told her then that he had to speak to a lawyer about his brother's misdemeanours – the brother who was closest to him. She was discreet and loved this husband, who like her was orphaned and marked by misfortune. The child knew nothing of his kinship origins, on either his father's or his mother's side. And it is this psychoanalytic treatment of a grandson that allowed me to understand the libidinal destiny in a family when narcissism is wounded during its development.

The ethos of desire in Tony's father was rooted in the oral stage, in the narcissistic problems of the phallic value of his mother and, for his brothers, around secondary problems linked with the contempt for and abandonment by a father defeated in a work accident. Thanks to the hypochondriacal problems of the child, I got to know the history of this family; and by the words through which the unsaid was at last being spoken, I could help the child recover his health. Traumas of the heart that are not expressed in words can be expressed by the body, which feels traumatised through the intermediary of the body image interwoven as the weft and warp of the fabric of our narcissism. In the case of this painful knee, it was about the heart of Tony's father and of his own – his heart linked with his dad's heart – in short not of the knee (*genoux*) but of I–we (*je–nous*).[36] These two hearts represent the emotional link that binds a human being to the one who makes him, to the one that he loves at the beginning of his life and makes him love himself – I mean the father or the one who holds that place. This is the same father, responsible for his child, girl or boy, who from the age of 3 detached the child from the binary relationship with his mother, to make of him a sexualised social being according to the law. This is why all the spoken and unspoken knowledge regarding a father is so traumatic, in the sense of structural elements in the unconscious life; this is also why this trauma is transmitted to the next generation. This is one of the most important discoveries of psychoanalysis: the heritage

36 See footnote 31.

of an unconscious debt that saps one of the descendants in the second or third generation.

As Tony's father had not known his dad at the time of his weaning, he could only develop and detach from his mother by way of what society told him about her. Also, society did not help his older siblings, who were father substitutes for him. For a small child, older siblings represent other 'big people' in contact with mummy – paternal substitutes in some way. These older siblings were unable to serve as references to the law as they themselves were traumatised by the decapitation of the family and by the distress in which the mother remained, with her five children. The trauma due to the abandonment of the children by one or other parent is different according to the developmental age, not physical but emotional and sexual, of each child in the same family. Following a trauma that hits all the children and the parent who looks after the children alone after the disappearance of their partner, if everybody managed to talk about their suffering to someone who can listen to them express themselves in their own voice – they can manage to overcome the trial and even work through it; and if able to express everything that a living being in this distress has to say about the event, they may even emerge stronger from the experience. Every trial is an experience of survival of the body, and it is as if the body had the psyche as a metaphor; but for the psyche to stay alive, language needs to be exchanged, to be expressive in the moment to a listener who accords the speaker the value of being the subject of his own history.

Every trial is an experience in reality that could be processed psychically if the body survives. But for this, work is needed – psychoanalytic work – and this can only be done with somebody who by way of their listening and training gives to the speaker a symboligenic castration, that is to say helps him to understand by symbolisation what he has lost and then to begin to own it. Thus, this brave father who had to abandon the position of head of family because of a fatal accident at work – each of his sons could have honoured him by standing fast in their difficulties if they had been helped by another person, as they were all intelligent children. But this would have required the rehabilitation of both the person of the father of which they had no experience other than the abandonment in which the mother found herself, and the suffering mother whose only solution had been to drink so as to leave the food to the boys, at a time when wine was very cheap.

From begetters to the begotten: imaginary suffering in reality: debt and heritage

Putting words to the suffering of an ordeal for whoever will listen and lend his attention to the subject who speaks and trusts in him – this calms anxiety; and then, living and surviving free of anxiety will allow him to find the solution on his own, having worked through the acute experience of the trial. This means that drives whose satisfaction is prohibited provoke libidinal hypertension and from this, anxiety – like any hypertension in the human being. A libidinal hypotension provokes withdrawal and sleep; libidinal hypertension provokes anxiety;

anxiety through hypertension causes illness, and the illness is felt as guilt in the first place; and then as this freezes the life forces of the individual, he feels secondarily guilty of not facing up – of lacking the dignity linked with assuming responsibility for one's desire, which is rooted in the human being from the start of life. This is why anxiety has to be expressed. If it cannot be expressed in words, it will be in behaviour or in bodily functioning – by the behaviour of the body in society or in temperamental behaviours, or by an autonomic or motor dysfunction of the body.

Everything is language in the human being. The body itself is language, by its health or its illness. Health is the language of those who feel well; illness is a language of suffering and sometimes of anxiety. Being ill is the sign of a battle against an enemy of this equilibrium of exchange that we have named health. Therefore, all energy is focused on resisting or curing the damage that an external agent has caused by either an accident, wound or illness, or secondarily by a defence reaction. I have tried in these last pages to decode the development of the body image linked with primary narcissism, and then with secondary narcissism after the resolution of the Oedipus complex. I have said that this is erogenous and functional, but also that it originates in a basal image, any threat to the integrity of which is felt to be mortal. The image connects the body to the most autonomous language – cardio-respiratory and digestive. The integrity of this body image – when linked with the cardio-respiratory and digestive systems – gives the human being a sense of security in sleep, without which the desiring subject cannot animate his flesh, and gross psycho-organic disturbances may follow.

If the basal image is affected, there is partial or total devitalisation, up to the point of a lesional reaction. If it is the functional image that is affected by a traumatic event that remains unspoken, there is a functional reaction in the neuro-muscular or immune systems. The deregulation of homeostasis and of tonus begins unconsciously and to a greater or lesser extent affects the ego and the order of psychic agencies, and from there on behaviour as a language. If it is the erogenous image in question, there can be a sapping or on the contrary an over-excitation of desire, in a way that overwhelms the subject's ability to express desire within his bodily schema. Tony's father's older brothers, for example, endured suffering at puberty or pre-puberty, when their mother was totally broken down from a social point of view, and they were not able to construct themselves around a work ethic. Their father had been despised in his value as a worker, as work cost him his life and society showed no respect for his place as the head of the family in helping his children to survive materially, and not only educationally. The older brothers had been given the example of an honest and orderly working life by their father, but his death destroyed the castration he had begun to give them, and with this, the brake on the impulses to damage and to murder, taking with it the symbolisation of oral and anal sexuality, which is the springboard of a libido usable in education and work. In addition, when left to their discretion, their tender and loving mother became the focus of the incestuous feelings reawakened in them. All this was unconscious, but the result was that work no longer had any value, and in addition, filial love for the mother was frustrated as the children were not yet able to work to earn money to help her and could do nothing apart from observe when those around them accused her of putting up with hunger and insufficient food while continuing to drink. The older children were struck to the core of their human dignity – the basal image of their narcissism – by the degradation they inherited from their father and mother at the Oedipal and social phase, and could only become serious delinquents, with two of them going as far as violent crime, their crimes escalating as they went through the prison system and associated with delinquents worse than themselves, and who did not keep as respected an image of their mothers as that of each of themselves.

The brother for whom Tony's father had been summoned by the lawyer was the one closest in age to him. He was apathetic, a passive hysteric, did not like girls and according to the lawyer had been exploited by a gang but had personally not committed any theft or violence. This brother had been Tony's father's companion in residential care when their mother died. He was the one their mother weaned while pregnant with Tony's father.

Tony's father made no negative judgement of his brothers. He was a victim of misfortune and talked with resignation of his brothers but expressed an ardent and unwavering love for his mother, and an idealised regard for a father of whom he had no memory and about whom he knew nothing other than that he had also been a child in social care and had died in an accident at work.

Symptoms, be they hypochondriac as in Tony (grandson of a victim of a work accident), hysterical as in his uncles or psychosomatic as in his father, can be understood as the language of the unconscious ego – connected with the body itself in the place of the bodily schema. These symptoms, which obstruct the freedom to live, are means of expression of the suffering of a human being who has been narcissistically wounded – given that narcissism is moored to an unconscious ethos that develops from castration to castration, symboligenic or not, and ensures continuity and cohesion of the psychic and sexual structure.

This continuity of the psychic and sexual structure – this is what is understood by the term 'narcissism,' which is linked with the interweaving of the unconscious body image and the preconscious and conscious bodily schema. Narcissism is the condition of the construction of the subject, who is neither temporal nor spatial, in contrast with what can be said of his body, and is similar in nature to the ego by which the subject objectifies himself in his behavioural motivations, which he justifies in reality with fantasies or verbal rationalisations that manifest themselves in his exchanges with the cosmos – in other words health, his relationships with animals and humans and his temperament.

Other bodies also are objects belonging to the interwoven reality of time and space. Each body represents a desiring subject, if it is a human, but is perceived by others in the form of an object offered to their desire. Philic or phobic reactions to the other are elicited, by which I mean one may desire to enter with him into a relationship of pleasurable exchange or may refuse a relationship that would be unpleasurable.

It is the subject of desire – as the witness and also the actor of his own history – that is incarnated in this body on the day of its conception, and who trustingly renews with each breath his contract as a living being. One could say that from second to second, a subject's narcissism renews the contract of the desiring subject with his body. This is what being alive is for a human being.

This contract that binds the human subject to his body is the enigma of each human being. Whenever one speaks, one speaks of oneself under the cover of the word 'me'[37] – distinct from 'you' and 'them' – but at the same time also in the name of 'I,' who can either disavow the 'me' or consciously own it (and maybe also unconsciously). In sleep, the subject is the witness of this other immobile, almost vegetative 'me,' while at the same time this subject performs the work of re-assuming the body that had become tired by his desires while awake: it is thus that the basal narcissism ensures daily the renewal of his contract in life, the renewal of the enigma. This sleepy 'I,' unable to say the grammatical 'I' of a sentence, who from somewhere unknown watches over and allows the body to replenish its strength – this 'I' is the witness to desire in all desiring subjects back to the dawn of time, engendered from mother to daughter, from father to son, since the world began.

The human child approaches this enigma around the age of 3. Innocently, he believes that the adult, the finished image of himself, will give him answers to all his questions; but the adult expects of his child an answer to the enigma of the meaning of *his* life, a response to the enigma of the failures of the 'me' in relation to the desire of the 'I.'

And it is this bad hand, this incomprehension in which each expects of the other a response that neither can give that creates the problematic of the parent–child relationship. They cannot easily accept their impotence – the child that of his parents and the parents that of their child – their inability to give the other the satisfaction that their imaginary desire sought in reality. In any case, for Tony, who had a pain in the knees (*genoux*), this lower limb joint created an enigma presented to doctors who with their knowledge of the body had no solution to the problem, but who enabled the contact with a psychoanalyst, which clarified the other enigma of the 'I–we' (*je–nous*) presented to the father by his child's body – an enigma also presented by the father to the child, who in his love for his family was on the threshold of assuming his desire for himself. This story also allowed the young analyst that I was at the time to see how the unspoken suffering of two families can express itself in a 10-year-old child, their heir: Tony, who was deprived of normal life and of sleep by a hypochondriacal stabbing pain, was shouting out a suffering that went back to his father and grandfather and maybe even further.

---

37 Translator's note: in French, the word for the 'ego' is '*le moi*' or literally, the 'me' – which has the advantage of designating a view of oneself as an object that can be described. In this sentence, it seems to make more sense to emphasise this narcissistic aspect of the ego by the use of 'me.'

Obviously, nothing had changed for the father, but in talking to me, he reactivated in himself, at his current age, the emotions and feelings of his childhood. But he was not alone. He could, in rethinking the meaning of his life, talk to his son about what he did not know but that had created a problem for him, and of what he knew and had made him sad.

Tony did not ask direct questions of his father; it was through the intermediary of his body that the questions were asked, when no answers were found in the body as an object of medical knowledge. The enigma of the changes of growth and of the destiny of human beings causes them at different times in their personal history to recover some interior events of the past, sometimes even events of the dead. These are events that happened between their grandparents and parents and also those that happened during the life of the subject but that could not be spoken of during his developmental life. Tony's body appeared to stop him from living, but it was not that; it was the unsaid that his body represented that caused the problem. Tony allowed his father to put words, at last, to his history, for a psychoanalyst who was listening – words of a son who became a father and begetter of children, and of a grandson. He could, with these words, talk of his wife and his son, while he had never spoken in this way to anyone: he spoke about his mother, of the family misfortune, of the courage of this woman, of his unhappy brothers about whom he never spoke to Tony – the uncles defeated by their libidinal strength that a father who disappeared too early could not initiate into any law other than that of bravely working – a law that became absurd and redundant because of his un-honoured death at work. And what can we say about the distress in which his disappearance left his wife and young children – the same distress that the father of Tony's father experienced when abandoned to the state, a distress that Tony's mother also knew when also abandoned to the state. But one has to go back even further in the history of these desiring beings; one has to go back to the distress of the maternal grandmother and of the paternal great-grandmother of Tony, who were denied value by society during their pregnancies; women who had been used as objects by irresponsible men and had not been supported in taking responsibility for their child. All this was summarised in Tony's body – in his two knees, each of his lower limbs representing the support of his life, his two parents for whom the enigma was 'I-we' (*je-nous*).

In conclusion of this work

For each and every one of us, the enigma of our lives in its relation through our bodies to the bodies of others and through language to other subjects, through the mediation of the most substantial things to the most subtle looks and sounds, remains.

The body image, interwoven every microsecond with the bodily schema – the substratum of our being in the world – links the subject to the body in its palpitating substance, the lieu of his appearance: this is a way of articulating the unconscious desire. The enigma remains, linked with the weight of the flesh, always plural, with its needs and desires and where everyone's ego (with those of others) is exhausted. And then, what is to be done with that subject in his quest for subtle union with another subject? Desire that would like to be in tune with the other through the subtle harmony of love. The enigma 'I–we' (*je–nous*) remains from generation to generation while me, you, the others die; and language is the enigma that, separated as we are from each other, unites us beyond . . . below . . . by what? In whom? Would this unknowable be the Subject of the verb 'to be'?

Index

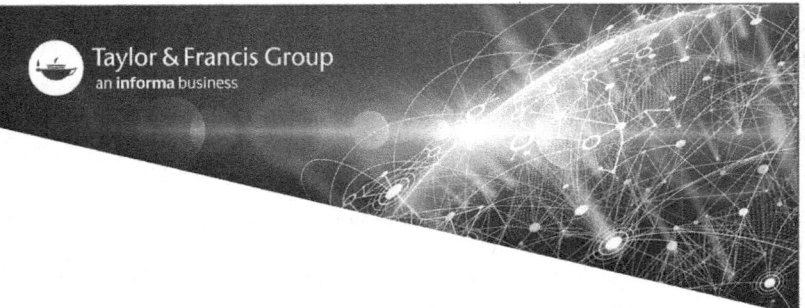
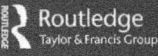
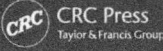